MW01528250

**LIBRARY**

College of Physicians and
Surgeons
of British Columbia

SPRINGER SURGERY ATLAS SERIES

Series Editors: J. S. P. Lumley · J. R. Siewert

W. E. G. Thomas · N. Senninger (Eds.)

# Short Stay Surgery

With 274 Color Figures,
in 415 separate Illustrations

Springer

William E.G. Thomas, MS, FRCS
Consultant Surgeon
Royal Hallamshire Hospital
Glossop Road
Sheffield, S11 9NN
UK
Phone: 0044 114 2713 142
0044 114 262 0852
email: wegthomas@btinternet.com

Univ.-Prof. Dr. med. Norbert J.G.M. Senninger
Direktor der Klinik und Poliklinik
für Allgemeine Chirurgie
Universitätsklinikum Münster
Waldeyerstrasse 1
48149 Münster
Germany
Phone: 0049 251 8356304
Fax: 0049 251 8356414
email: senning@uni-muenster.de

ISBN 978-3-540-41101-7
Springer-Verlag Berlin Heidelberg New York

Library of Congress Control Number: 2005938807

This work is subject to copyright. All rights are reserved, whether the whole or part of the material is concerned, specifically the rights of translation, reprinting, reuse of illustrations, recitation, broadcasting, reproduction on microfilm or in any other way, and storage in data banks. Duplication of this publication or parts thereof is permitted only under the provisions of the German Copyright Law of September 9, 1965, in its current version, and permission for use must always be obtained from Springer. Violations are liable to prosecution under the German Copyright Law.

Springer is a part of Springer Science+Business Media
springer.com
© Springer-Verlag Berlin Heidelberg 2008

The use of general descriptive names, registered names, trademarks, etc. in this publication does not imply, even in the absence of a specific statement, that such names are exempt from the relevant protective laws and regulations and therefore free for general use.

Product liability: the publishers cannot guarantee the accuracy of any information about dosage and application contained in this book. In every individual case the user must check such information by consulting the relevant literature.

Editor: Gabriele Schröder, Heidelberg, Germany
Desk Editor: Stephanie Benko, Heidelberg, Germany
Wissenschaftliche Zeichnungen: Dr. Michael von Solodkoff, Christiane von Solodkoff, Neckargemünd, Heidelberg, Germany
Production: Marina Litterer, Heidelberg, Germany
Cover: Frido-Steinen-Broo, EStudio, Calamar, Spain
Typesetting: K. Detzner, 67346 Speyer, Germany

Printed on acid-free paper 21/3151 ML 5 4 3 2 1 0

# Preface

Developments in medicine and surgery have resulted in innumerable benefits to our patients. Increased knowledge of pathophysiology, healing processes and early detection of disease have been accompanied by a rapid evolution of techniques making medicine and especially surgery safer, and therefore more capable of dealing with previously unthinkable tasks. However – as might be expected – such advances are also more expensive. This has put relentless pressure on the healthcare systems of the world, and there will be an increasing requirement for more and more surgery to be done on a short stay basis. Hospital beds are at a premium and in order to drive down costs, same-day admission and day-case surgery will become the order of the day. This in turn will require a major educational drive to inform both clinicians as well as patients as to the benefit of such short stay surgery, and we shall all have to adapt to this new way of working.

Short stay surgery will therefore play an increasingly important role in the provision of surgical care in the future. Adequate surgical techniques and postoperative management of pain and nutrition can now allow the conduct of procedures with a minimum of hospital stay, thereby cutting costs and increasing the quality of life for the patients. A perfectly functioning system of preoperative, perioperative and postoperative care and surveillance is of utmost importance to create a safe and secure environment for patients and to avoid harm or untoward incidents. Therefore clear guidelines and standards are the prerequisites of successful surgery, be it short stay, out-patient, fast track, day care or such a similar approach by any other name.

The editors therefore felt that it is timely to present the readers of this book with information on how to select and treat patients with short stay surgical procedures for a wide variety of clinical conditions. Such conditions significantly influence public health simply by virtue of the large numbers of patients involved and because they represent widespread need. It must be stressed that we are well aware that there are "many paths leading to Rome", and therefore it has been our intention to describe one safe way to reach the goal, not all possible ways. This applies especially to aspects of technique. Thus this book seeks to inform and educate surgeons about the enormous potential of short stay surgery and to provide the basis for such practice. It presents didactic advice on setting up a unit for the provision of such care and then provides information about the practical aspects of such surgery in each of the specialty areas. It presents clear descriptions of the actual operative procedures in order to stimulate clinicians to increase the percentage of their practice that is undertaken on a short stay basis. Many may feel that such a move towards short stay may be detrimental to quality care, but each of the procedures described has been tried and tested in a short stay environment and we commend them to the reader.

We are practising surgery in a changing world and we must be prepared to change with it or be left behind. There is no doubt that change for change's sake is unprofitable, but the move towards short stay surgery does indeed benefit the patient, minimise complications and utilise resources more efficiently and effectively. Therefore with discernment, clinicians will be able to dramatically increase their utilisation of short stay facilities, and we trust that this book will encourage many more to embrace this practice since this will undoubtedly result in the greatest benefit of all, the well-being of our patients.

**W.E.G. Thomas – Sheffield**
**N. Senninger – Münster**
**January 2008**

# Contents

# List of Contributors


**Mireille Berthoud**
Consultant Anaesthetist
Anaesthetic Department
C Floor OPD, Royal Hallamshire Hospital
Glossop Road
Sheffield, S11 9NN
UK

**Iain C. Cameron**
Consultant Surgeon
Royal Hallamshire Hospital
Glossop Road
Sheffield, S11 9NN
UK

**Mario Colombo-Benkmann**
Oberarzt der Klinik und Poliklinik
für Allgemeine Chirurgie
Universitätsklinikum Münster
Waldeyerstrasse 1
48149 Münster
Germany

**Andrew Kingsnorth**
Professor of Surgery
Level 07
Derriford Hospital
Plymouth, Devon, PL6 8DH
UK

**Christian F. Krieglstein**
Chefarzt der Chirurgischen Klinik
St. Elisabeth-Krankenhaus GmbH
Worthmannstrasse 1
50935 Köln
Germany

**Martin Langer**
Oberarzt der Klinik und Poliklinik
für Unfall-, Hand- und Wiederherstellungschirurgie
Universitätsklinikum Münster
Waldeyerstrasse 1
48149 Münster
Germany

**Siobhan Laws**
The Royal Hampshire County Hospital
Romsey Road
Winchester, Hampshire, SO22 5DG
UK

**Jutta Liebau**
Chefärztin der Klinik
für Plastische und Ästhetische Chirurgie
Kaiserswerther Diakonie,
Florence-Nightingale-Krankenhaus
Kreuzbergstrasse 79
40489 Düsseldorf
Germany

**Vaithianathan Natarajan**
Consultant Urologist
Department of Urology
Royal Hallamshire Hospital
Glossop Road
Sheffield, S11 9NN
UK

**Neil Oakley**
Consultant Urologist
Department of Urology
Royal Hallamshire Hospital
Glossop Road
Sheffield, S11 9NN
UK

**Friedrich W. Pelster**
Oberarzt der Klinik und Poliklinik
für Allgemeine Chirurgie
Universitätsklinikum Münster
Waldeyerstrasse 1
48149 Münster
Germany

**Dick Rainsbury**
Consultant Surgeon
The Royal Hampshire County Hospital
Romsey Road
Winchester, Hampshire, SO22 5DG
UK

**Franz Raulf**
Chefarzt der Abteilung Chirurgie II – Koloproktologie
Raphaelsklinik Münster GmbH
Loerstrasse 23
48143 Münster
Germany

**Emile Rijcken**
Assistenzarzt der Klinik und Poliklinik für Allgemeine Chirurgie
Universitätsklinikum Münster
Waldeyerstrasse 1
48149 Münster
Germany

**Matthias H. Seelig**
Oberarzt der Chirurgischen Klinik
St. Josef-Hospital
Ruhr-Universität Bochum
Gudrunstrasse 56
44791 Bochum
Germany

**Norbert Senninger**
Klinik und Poliklinik für Allgemeine Chirurgie
Universitätsklinikum Münster
Waldeyerstrasse 1
48149 Münster
Germany

**William E.G. Thomas**
Department of Surgery
Royal Hallamshire Hospital
Glossop Road
Sheffield, S11 9NN
UK

**Dirk Tübergen**
Facharzt für Chirurgie und Proktologie
Warendorfer Strasse 185
48145 Münster
Germany

**Shoo-yee Wong**
Smeestersstraat 3/5
3400 Landen
Belgium

# Part I General Principles

CHAPTER 1

# Organisational and Anaesthetic Aspects of Short Stay Surgery

Mireille Berthoud

## INTRODUCTION

The very first operations under general anaesthesia were performed on patients who could be described as day cases. James H. Nicoll, a surgeon working at the Glasgow Royal Hospital for Sick Children, reported to the British Medical Association 8988 operations he performed on children over a 10-year period. Between 1899 and 1901, 460 of these operations were for harelip and cleft palate. All of these patients were day cases. Ralph Waters, an American general practitioner-turned-anaesthetist, founded his Downtown Anesthesia Clinic in Iowa in 1912. This clinic was dedicated to dental and minor surgery under general anaesthesia, with patients returning home the same day. He went on to establish the first academic department of anaesthesia in the USA.

Following these early pioneers, little interest was shown in ambulatory surgery until 1953, when two dedicated ambulatory surgery units were developed in Durban and Johannesburg. These provided a safe anaesthetic environment for dental procedures. Then in the early 1960s, hospital-based short stay units were developed in Canada, the USA and South Africa. The first freestanding ambulatory surgical unit in the USA opened in 1970. By 1994, 60% of all surgical procedures in the USA were being done as day cases, with 10% of these being performed in freestanding units. The 2001 Audit Commission report for England and Wales showed day surgery rates between 10% and 80% for different Trusts, the median rate being about 45%. Performance even varied between procedures within the same Trust.

Today the Department of Health estimates that with good organisation 75% of all surgical procedures could be undertaken as day cases in the UK.

## TERMS AND DEFINITIONS

- **Day Case Surgery.** An operation or investigation performed on a planned non-resident basis, where the patient requires either full theatre facilities or facilities for recovery or most often both. Does not include minor procedures like toenail removal or skin biopsy. May not include endoscopy. May not include many pain procedures.

- **23-Hour Stay Surgery.** An operation or investigation requiring more prolonged recovery or even overnight care, provided the discharge home occurs within 24 h.

- **Short Stay Surgery.** Includes both true day case surgery and 23-h stay surgery.

- **Ambulatory Surgery.** The American term for day case surgery.

- **Office-Based Surgery.** An operation or investigation performed on a planned non-resident basis that can take place in the physician's office. May include some true day case surgery as well as more minor procedures.

## ORGANISATIONAL ASPECTS OF SHORT STAY SURGERY

### Unit Design

Day care facilities can be categorised as follows:

- **Hospital-Integrated.** In this situation day case patients are managed through the same facilities as the inpatients, although some of the processes of management may be different. Generally, this results in care of variable quality, which can be less efficient as it is more likely to be influenced by the inpatient workload.

- **Hospital-Based.** This is a separate unit located within the hospital, but with dedicated facilities for day case and short stay surgery. It may share some equipment and personnel with the hospital in special circumstances. All recommendations for day care suggest that dedicated units are the ideal.

- **Freestanding.** The unit is separate from the hospital, fully integrated and self-contained, and is dedicated to day surgery alone. Audits have shown that more rigorous patient selection criteria have to be applied to stand-alone units.

■ **Office-Based.** There may be some limited operating and recovery facilities in conjunction with physician's offices.

There are some general principles that hold for the design of day surgical facilities. Any design must promote maximum efficiency in processing patients, whether for assessment or surgery. If possible the distance patients have to travel should be kept to a minimum and they should not retrace their steps. A circular flow of patients is ideal. Patients receiving assessment should not mix with those undergoing surgery, and patients recovering from surgery should not mix with those waiting for their operations. The environment should be comfortable and friendly, and should preserve privacy and dignity without compromising clinical need. Car parking and pick-up arrangements should be as near to the unit as possible.

Dedicated units should contain a reception with its own office, an admissions area with private consulting rooms, operating theatres and first stage recovery both of the same specification as the equivalent inpatient facility, and a step-down recovery area from which patients are discharged. There should also be enough office and storage space, a kitchen for patients and one for staff, changing rooms, lavatories and a rest area for staff.

Unit design alone is not enough to ensure efficient patient flow. Careful pre-assessment and pre-operative preparations are essential, with all the information readily available to the clinical staff. On the day of surgery, either patients can be admitted in batches at the beginning of each session or their admission times can be staggered. The advantage of the patients arriving together is that the immediate pre-operative preparations can all take place prior to the start of the operating session, leaving clinical staff free to stay in theatre once operating has started. The disadvantages are an increased pressure on space, and that some patients may be required to wait 4 or 5 h for their treatment. As most day case patients do not receive sedative pre-medication, it is perfectly feasible for them to walk to the operating theatre, thus avoiding complicated transfers. Anaesthetic rooms are not always needed. They can be useful in specific circumstances, such as when parents accompany their children at induction. An anaesthetic room will speed turnover only if there is sufficient anaesthetic support. Having clear routines and good communication is essential for efficient patient flow.

## Staffing

The quality of the care that patients receive is dependent on the quality of the people looking after them. These people are the most expensive part of any short stay surgical unit. This makes careful planning of staffing levels and skill mix very important. Multi-skilling is an important concept in short stay surgery. It provides flexibility within the staffing pool, special status to the day case practitioner, and an understanding of the work of others in the team and the process as a whole. Competence is needed in pre-operative assessment, in the pre-operative and post-operative ward area, in theatre and in recovery. A senior nurse most often provides day-to-day coordination of the unit. Published documents offering more detailed guidance are referenced below.

While the nursing staff provide day-to-day consistency, the surgeons and anaesthetists may come and go. This makes a medical clinical lead with a special interest in short stay surgery essential. His or her role lies in planning strategy, operational policy, financial containment, producing clinical protocols, audit, quality and training. All doctors working in the unit should be specially trained in day surgery techniques and be experienced enough to offer speedy, complication free anaesthesia and surgery.

High quality clerical personnel are essential for a day unit to operate effectively. Their role is one of liaison and may include preparation of operating lists, arranging appointments, finding short notice replacement patients, obtaining and collating information and notes, handling telephone enquiries, and preparing audit and research data.

Other staff include operating department practitioners, health care assistants, community nurses, pharmacists, secretaries, receptionists, porters and housekeepers.

A management group, who meet on a regular basis, should represent the interests of all the staff working in the unit.

**Table 1**

| American Society of Anesthesiologists (ASA) physical status grade |
|---|
| 1. Healthy patient. Localised surgical pathology with no systemic disturbance |
| 2. Mild to moderate systemic disturbance (the surgical pathology or other disease process). No activity limitation |
| 3. Severe systemic disturbance from any cause. Some activity limitation |
| 4. Life-threatening systemic disorder. Severe activity limitation |
| 5. Moribund patient with little chance of survival |

**Table 2**

| Discharge criteria following day case surgery |
|---|
| • Stable vital signs for more than 30 min |
| • No new signs or symptoms after the operation |
| • No active bleeding or oozing |
| • Minimal nausea or emesis for more than 30 min |
| • Able to tolerate oral fluids |
| • Pain controlled with oral analgesics |
| • Able to self-care, dress and mobilise |
| • Able to pass urine after genito-urinary intervention, hernia repair, anal surgery or caudal anaesthesia |
| • No evidence of swelling or impaired neurological or circulatory function after extremity surgery |
| • Orientation to person, time and space |
| • A responsible escort and adult carer for 24 h |

## Patient Selection

Successful short stay anaesthesia and surgery depends on careful patient selection and preparation. Pre-operative assessment reduces operative risk, short notice cancellations and unexpected hospital admission. In assessing the patient domestic, surgical and medical criteria should be considered.

All patients undergoing same day surgery must have a responsible adult who will accompany them home and care for them over the following 24 h. They should have access to a telephone and adequate bathroom facilities. Those having more complex surgery should live not more than one hour's journey from the hospital. If the assessment staff experience difficulties in communicating with the patient or their carer, the patient should be looked after in hospital.

The following surgical considerations are made when selecting suitable short stay patients. Intrathoracic, intracranial and intra-abdominal operations are generally not suitable unless undertaken by minimally invasive techniques. Patients' pain should be controlled by oral or rectal analgesics. There should be no continued requirement for intravenous fluids. The risk of complications such as bleeding or ischaemia should be negligible. Patients should be ambulatory. With improved anaesthesia, duration of surgery is no longer an issue as long as the patients are able to meet prescribed discharge criteria. Published lists of suitable procedures are listed on the BADS (British Association of Day Case Surgery) web site referenced at the end of this chapter.

Medically, patients should be either American Society of Anesthesiologists (ASA) grades 1 or 2, but stable ASA grade 3 patients are being increasingly considered for general anaesthesia (Table 1). Any underlying medical condition should be well controlled and the patient should have a reasonable cardio-respiratory reserve. Day surgery patients should have no previous or family history of an adverse anaesthetic outcome, and they should have no major mobility problems. Both anaesthetic and surgical complications are increased in obesity, and these patients require especially careful assessment. Recently published guidance suggests that patients with a BMI of up to 40, who are otherwise healthy, may be considered for day case surgery. Patients with documented sleep apnoea should probably be monitored in hospital overnight after a general anaesthetic. Neonates may also need apnoea monitoring post-operatively. Age, as such, is no bar to day surgery, providing all the criteria outlined above are fulfilled. Detailed, locally agreed guidelines for the selection process should be freely available and should be regularly reviewed.

The timing of assessment should be such that there is opportunity to optimise any underlying condition before surgery, yet should not be so far in advance that any underlying condition is likely to have changed. Three months is usually about right. A date for surgery should be agreed only after assessment, bearing in mind that those patients who are offered a choice of dates will be less likely to cancel.

## Patient Preparation

Once the patient has been selected for same day surgery they will require careful preparation. All patients undergoing general anaesthesia or regional blockade should be starved. Evidence suggests that patients should not eat for 6 h before anaesthesia, but that it is safe to drink clear fluids for up to 2 h beforehand. Organising pre-medications and take home analgesia well in advance will avoid delays on the day of surgery. Pre-medications may include analgesia and anti-emetics, β-agonists or medications for aspiration and DVT prophylaxis. Sedative pre-medication is rarely used in day surgery, although it may be useful in children and in adults with special needs. Take home medicines may commonly include analgesics, antibiotics, antiemetics and dressings.

Providing adequate, accurate written and verbal information is very important to the success of day case surgery as patients will be expected to take a lot of responsibility for their own welfare. Every effort should be made to ensure that both the patient and the home carer understand what to expect at each stage of treatment. Written patient information should contain a simple description of the operation, the risks and side effects accompanying the operation, clear descriptions of the preparation needed before surgery and of the aftercare, including a description of the likely duration of the various stages of recovery. Patients should be given a realistic idea of the amount of pain they could expect, but this should not be exaggerated and should be accompanied by reassuring instructions on how it can be controlled. Many bodies offer guidelines and assistance in developing effective patient information: The Patient Information Forum and The Plain English Campaign, to name but two. Information of varying quality is also available on the Internet.

Increasingly, pre-operative assessment and preparation is being undertaken by nursing staff. With training, clear protocols and ready medical back-up, nurses can perform this task extremely well. Patients are more likely to receive an authoritative and efficient service if the assessor has a good understanding of the entire care pathway. Pre-operative assessment and preparation can be achieved using a varie-

**Table 3**

| Features of the ideal short stay general anaesthetic |
|---|
| • Safety with minimal cardiovascular and respiratory depression |
| • Good operating conditions |
| • Rapid, smooth induction |
| • Rapid recovery |
| • Minimal early post-operative complications |
| • Reliable, safe, prompt discharge |
| • Minimal delayed post-operative morbidity |

**Table 4**

**Characteristics of the intravenous induction agents**

| Induction agent | Half time | Comments |
|---|---|---|
| Propofol | $\alpha$ 2.5 min | Antiemetic |
| | $\beta$ 35–45 min | Good laryngeal relaxation |
| | Elimination 4 h | Rapid recovery |
| | | Suitable for infusion |
| | | Pain on injection |
| Thiopentone | a 4 min | Prolonged hangover effect |
| | Elimination 11.5 h | Unsuitable for infusion |
| Methohexitone | Elimination 4 h | Excitatory effects, especially in unpremedicated patients |
| | | Pain on injection |
| Etomidate | Elimination 1.25 h | High incidence of PON+V |
| | | Adrenal suppression |

ty of methods, the gold standard being a dedicated, fully equipped clinic attended by all patients. Other ways of offering assessment may be by telephone, or by questionnaire. Best efficiency would probably use a combination of methods dictated by the degree of surgery and type of anaesthesia. By far the most time consuming part of this process is the information giving, but allowing sufficient time to do this well helps to prevent problems on the day of surgery and after discharge.

## Consent

Competent patients must give their informed consent before any examination or treatment. Giving and obtaining consent is a process which starts when the decision to operate is made. It must be given voluntarily, and with as much discussion as possible in a form the patient can understand. Ideally, the actual person treating the patient should obtain consent. In day surgery this often means the consent is formally obtained very shortly before the procedure. The validity of consent can be greatly aided by patients having had the opportunity to receive accurate information including copies of the consent forms well before their surgical date. All organisations performing surgery should have a consent policy commensurate with the law of the land.

## Discharge and Follow-up

Patients must fulfil established discharge criteria before they go home. After their procedure, every patient should be seen by his or her anaesthetist and surgeon. The nursing staff may take the responsibility for the final assessment of street fitness, provided they follow clear protocols (Table 2).

Patients (and carers) should receive verbal and written instructions before discharge. They should be supplied with analgesics and any other medications they will need during their recovery. They should have clear instructions as to how to obtain help should an unexpected post-operative complication occur and any follow-up arrangements should be made at this time. A telephone call to all patients on the day following surgery will help to reassure and pre-empt problems, as well as provide the unit with valuable audit information.

Early communication with the patient's primary care physician by facsimile or telephone is essential. A discharge summary that includes the nature of the anaesthetic, surgery and any medications provided should be compiled before the patient is discharged. Copies can be given to the patient, to be available in case of an immediate emergency.

## Quality Assessment

The main measures of good day surgery management are DNA rates (patients who did not attend without giving notice), short notice cancellation rates (cancellations for whatever reason, resulting in unfilled operating slots), and unplanned in-patient admission rates (day case patients that have to be unexpectedly transferred to an inpatient facility rather than go home). These three figures are expressed as a percentage of all day case patients. DNA rates can be reduced to less than 1% by careful liaison with patients over their surgical date, together with confirmation, 2 or 3 days before surgery, of their intention to attend. Careful pre-operative selection and assessment reduces both cancellations and unplanned admission rates. Meticulous anaesthetic and surgical technique also reduces unexpected admission rates, which in the best units run at less than 1%.

Some of the advantages for patients of short stay surgery are that they are less subject to cancellation, are provided with clear information, should be ensured of a senior anaesthetist and surgeon, are less exposed to hospital acquired infections, benefit from early mobilisation, and may suffer less disruption of domestic and working life. Disadvantages include the patient and carer being responsible for post-operative pain control and early recognition of other possible anaesthetic or surgical complications.

Disadvantages can be minimised by robust protocols for pain control, and assessment of patients by telephone after discharge. All of these aspects of patient care should be regularly audited. Methods for this include patient satisfaction surveys, patient focus groups and take home diaries to monitor complications and interventions that may have occurred after the patient has been discharged home.

## Economic Containment

The drive for short stay surgery has mostly been financial. It is important to provide value for money, and this means containing costs while maintaining an excellent quality of service. It is beyond the scope of this chapter to detail how this can be achieved, but the following are some brief pointers.

**Table 5**

**Characteristics of the volatile anaesthetic agents**

| Volatile agent | Blood/gas coefficient (low number indicates fast onset and elimination) | Comments |
|---|---|---|
| Halothane | 2.4 | Hepatotoxic<br>Arrhythmias<br>Cheap |
| Enflurane | 1.9 | Little to choose between enflurane and isoflurane |
| Isoflurane | 1.46 | |
| Sevoflurane | 0.63 | Smooth induction<br>Haemodynamically stable<br>Expensive |
| Desflurane | 0.4 | Pungent<br>Smooth induction is difficult in unpremedicated patients<br>Expensive |

■ **Personnel.** The right skill mix in a unit will mean that highly qualified staff can undertake the skilled tasks, leaving less trained staff for the more routine work. Multi-skilling gives both flexibility and job satisfaction within the workforce. Ongoing training reduces risk, and a supportive working environment retains staff and minimises sickness levels.

■ **Theatre Utilisation.** Pre-operative preparation is key. Those who understand the clinical priorities as well as the capabilities of surgeon and anaesthetist should compile the operation lists. Complex operations should not take place late in the day, and very minor operations should take place in the outpatient department or office. Routes and methods for transporting patients around the unit should be as simple as possible, avoiding bottlenecks.

■ **Supplies and Equipment.** It is important to have a named individual in each section accountable for ordering and costs. Stock levels should be minimised. All equipment should be regularly maintained. Those using the equipment should understand how it works and feel ownership of it.

■ **Drugs.** Evidence-based guidelines for drug use should be readily available and regularly updated. A committee should review the need for all new drugs.

■ **Risk Management.** The unit should have a risk management team led by a named individual with overall responsibility. Critical incidents and morbidity should be documented, discussed and the outcomes disseminated to all staff.

## ANAESTHETIC ASPECTS OF SHORT STAY SURGERY

### General Anaesthesia

Almost any anaesthetic technique is available to short stay surgical patients; a good result is obtained by careful consideration of all factors and attention to detail (Table 3). Choice of anaesthesia is dictated by the underlying condition of the patient, the surgery, the need for early mobilisation and the need to minimise post-operative complications. The most important of these are pain and post-operative nausea and vomiting. Improvements in anaesthetic technique have made short stay surgery available to patients with more complex underlying disease, and the presence of these patients in the day unit has in turn further driven the development of anaesthesia.

### Induction

Propofol is established as the intravenous induction agent of choice in day surgery (Table 4). Although many studies have shown that the early recovery time after propofol induction is shortened when compared with other induction agents, its main advantage is that it has anti-emetic properties. This will be apparent only if care is taken to avoid emesis during the rest of the anaesthetic technique. Propofol also causes a degree of respiratory inhibition that allows easy placement of a laryngeal mask. The main disadvantage of propofol is that up to 30% of patients experience pain on injection. Newer preparations, which reduce the concentration of propofol in the aqueous phase, have been shown to decrease this phenomenon.

A gas induction may be especially useful in special needs patients and in children. The smoothest and fastest gas induction is produced by sevoflurane. Volatile agents cause more post-operative nausea and vomiting than propofol.

### Maintenance

The advantages of propofol are maximised when it is also used to maintain anaesthesia. Total intravenous anaesthesia (TIVA) provides a balanced anaesthetic technique using the intravenous route alone. TIVA allows just as rapid control of the depth of anaesthesia as the volatile agents, and is less polluting. Despite the advantages of TIVA for short stay surgery, it is still not widely used. Some of the reasons for this include: lack of familiarity and training in the technique, the need for reliable infusion devices, and concerns about awareness and cost. The detailed practicalities of TIVA are referenced at the end of this chapter.

Sevoflurane is probably the most clinically acceptable volatile agent for short stay anaesthesia maintenance, but it is expensive (Table 5). Nitrous oxide is very cheap, has good analgesic properties and a rapid onset and offset. Although it is not potent enough to use as a sole anaesthetic agent, it significantly reduces the MAC (minimum alveolar concentration) of the volatile agents. Some studies have shown that it increases the incidence of post-operative nausea and vomiting, although others suggest this does not occur if propofol is used for induction. The advantages of nitrous oxide in reducing the dose, and therefore the side effects of the volatile agents, should be balanced against this disadvantage in individual patients.

Table 6

Characteristics of the short-acting opioid drugs

| Short-acting opioid | Half times | Comments |
|---|---|---|
| Fentanyl | α 1–2 min | Plasma-brain level lag time, 5 min |
| | β 10–30 min | Highly lipid soluble |
| | Elimination 2–4 h | Cardiovascular stability |
| | | Respiratory depression with infusions |
| Sufentanil | α 1.4 min | Highly lipid soluble |
| | β 17.7 min | |
| | Elimination 2.7 h | |
| Alfentanil | α 1–2 min | Plasma-brain level lag time, 2 min |
| | β 4–17 min | Less lipid soluble |
| | Elimination 1.6 h | |
| Remifentanil | α 0.5–0.9 min | Least lipid soluble |
| | β 5.8–9.5 min | Hydrolysed by non-specific esterases |
| | Elimination 10–25 min | Half-life not context sensitive |
| | | Easy titration |
| | | Respiratory depression |

## Intra-operative Analgesia

In the absence of local anaesthesia, short acting opioid drugs provide intra-operative analgesia in ambulatory surgery. Fentanyl and sufentanil are usually given by bolus, alfentanil by bolus or infusion and remifentanil by infusion (Table 6). Fentanyl has the longest duration of action, and so can provide some analgesia into the early post-operative period. Small boluses of 25–50 μg may be given intermittently and still maintain adequate spontaneous respiration. Alfentanil has a similar pharmacokinetic profile to propofol and so has been used for TIVA. Rarely, prolonged use of alfentanil by infusion has resulted in recurrent respiratory depression, which is a worry in the context of ambulatory surgery. Remifentanil as an infusion is ideal for day case anaesthesia. It has a short half-life and zero-order kinetics so recovery is very rapid and independent of the duration of the infusion. This feature of remifentanil means that post-operative pain will ensue unless an appropriate analgesia strategy has been employed. Spontaneous respiration is only possible at low remifentanil infusion rates.

## Muscle Relaxants

Many procedures in short stay surgery do not require muscle relaxants, but their use is increasing as surgical techniques become more complex. The depolarising agent suxamenthonium should be avoided wherever possible. It has a relatively high incidence of anaphylaxis, is associated with malignant hyperpyrexia, but most of all causes post-operative myalgia, which is worse in the day case surgical population. Its only indication may be for rapid sequence induction in those patients at risk of aspiration, but even this is challenged with newer fast acting non-depolarising agents such as rocuronium, and the excellent intubation conditions that can be obtained by combining propofol and alfentanil or remifentanil.

In short stay surgery, the choice of muscle relaxant lies between the shorter acting agents (Table 7). Ideally the muscle relaxant should have a rapid onset, a short duration, should be easily reversed, have no side effects and be inexpensive.

## Fluids

Some studies have shown real benefits of peri-operative intravenous fluids in short stay surgical patients. Intravenous fluids can reduce the incidence of drowsiness, dizziness, thirst and nausea after all types of surgery. They also reduce the need for early oral intake, which can provoke vomiting. Intravenous fluids are inexpensive, and should probably be used in all patients, but especially in those having longer or more invasive surgery and those who have had long periods of pre-operative starvation.

## Regional and Local Anaesthesia

Whether used alone or in combination with general anaesthesia, a local anaesthetic technique should be part of the multimodal analgesia plan for every short stay surgery patient. Local anaesthetic techniques used alone are often the simplest, safest, cheapest, have the fewest side effects and result in fewer unexpected hospital admissions. Local or regional anaesthetic techniques can afford short stay surgery to some patients who would normally be considered medically unfit for general anaesthesia in this context. These techniques may also enable some procedures to be undertaken in the outpatient department or office rather than in the day surgery unit. Patients undergoing regional anaesthesia should be prepared and monitored as carefully as those having a general anaesthetic.

## Local Anaesthetic Agents

All local anaesthetic drugs have a narrow therapeutic margin. Toxicity depends on several factors including the vulnerability of the patient. Longer acting local anaesthetics tend to have a higher toxicity (Table 8). Plasma levels are higher following injections into vascular areas of the body. Every care should be taken to avoid inadvertent intravascular injection. All clinicians using these agents should understand how to calculate appropriate doses and dilutions of local anaesthetic, and should be familiar with the symptoms, signs and treatment of toxicity. A 1% local anaesthetic solution will contain 10 mg/ml.

## Regional Blocks

Virtually every regional anaesthetic technique can be used in day case surgery (Table 9), and they can offer several advantages. Patients benefit from enhanced post-operative analgesia, less nausea and vomiting, increased alertness and shorter discharge times. Factors that have to be considered in planning regional anaesthesia are: the patient's ability to understand and cooperate with the procedure, the possibility of a longer preparation time and the risks associated with a numb extremity. Choice of agent is dictated by the duration of surgery, and considerations of toxicity.

**Table 7**

| Characteristics of the shorter acting muscle relaxants | |
|---|---|
| **Muscle relaxant** | **Comments** |
| Atracurium | Onset 2–3 min. May not need reversal after 45 min, but can be difficult to reverse after much shorter operations. Histamine release |
| Cisatracurium | Similar to atracurium, but less histamine release |
| Vecuronium | Onset 3 min. Longer duration than atracurium, but lower dose may be used for shorter procedures, when it may be easier to reverse |
| Mivacurium | Onset 3 min. Short duration of action. May not need reversal, as metabolised by plasma cholinesterase |
| Rocuronium | Onset 1–2 min. Similar duration to vecuronium. Expensive |

**Table 8**

| Toxic doses of common local anaesthetic drugs | |
|---|---|
| **Local anaesthetic** | **Toxic dose in mg/kg** |
| Prilocaine | Plain: 6<br>With epinephrine: 8 |
| Lignocaine | Plain: 3<br>With epinephrine: 7 |
| Ropivacaine | Plain: 2.5 |
| Bupivacaine | Plain: 2<br>With epinephrine: 2 |

With the widespread use of small-gauge, pencil-point needles, spinal anaesthesia can be safely and successfully used for day surgery. Spinal anaesthesia is associated with a higher incidence of urinary retention, especially in patients undergoing anal or penile surgery, and so is probably best reserved for those patients who have a positive indication for it. Over-distending the bladder will increase the risk of urinary retention. This can be avoided by ensuring that the patient passes urine just before surgery, and by minimising the height of the sympathetic block, thus limiting the amount of intravenous fluid needed to control hypotension. In addition to bladder function, patients who have undergone spinal or epidural anaesthesia will have to be carefully assessed for their ability to walk before discharge home. A good indication of this is the ability to evert the foot, demonstrating the return of S1.

## Sedation

Sedation is used to treat anxiety, not pain. It is important to differentiate the two as pain is treated with local anaesthetic techniques or short onset analgesics such as fentanyl, and anxiety with reassurance and anxiolytics such as midazolam. Sedation falls on a conscious level continuum between fully conscious and anaesthetised. The margin for error can be quite narrow, and the poor safety profile attributed to sedation is largely because those without basic anaesthetic skills, such as airway management, have administered it.

Patients undergoing sedation should be prepared and starved as for general anaesthesia. Minimum standards of monitoring include pulse oximetry, ECG and blood pressure. The person administering the sedation should not be involved in the procedure so that they are able to pay full attention to the patient's conscious level. Patients will vary widely in their response to sedative drugs. This makes careful titration essential. Using a single agent for sedation is safest, but if combinations of opioids and sedatives are needed, particular caution is required, with the opioid given first and allowed to become maximally effective before the sedative is given. Oxygen supplementation should be given to all patients. Recovery facilities and discharge criteria are also the same as those for general anaesthesia.

## Post-operative Pain Control

Good post-operative pain management in day surgery starts with pre-assessment. Every patient needs to give a detailed drug history including allergies and contraindications, especially as many patients will already be using analgesics.

A peri-operative analgesia plan should be formulated in cooperation with the patient. A multimodal approach to pain management is important. Prophylactic use of analgesics, especially NSAIDs, will help to ensure that adequate drug levels are present immediately after recovery from anaesthesia. Local anaesthesia is key to patients waking up comfortable and should be employed wherever possible.

Pain assessment scales, such as the verbal rating scale, should be used in first stage recovery. Patients should have reasonable pain control before they are transferred into the second stage ward area. Long acting opioids are better avoided. When they are occasionally required they should always be accompanied by antiemetic treatment.

Oral analgesics are the mainstay of pain relief after discharge home. Take home analgesia should be prescribed according to protocol, thus avoiding any individual's misconception as to how painful a procedure may be. Again a multimodal approach is best, although the more simple the regime the easier and safer it is for the patient. A combination of paracetamol and a NSAID is most often used. Other common analgesics include codeine and tramadol. Patients should be instructed to take their painkillers regularly. Those who have received a regional block should be told when to anticipate the return of sensation and treat any pain early. All patients should be provided with verbal and written information about any medications they are given, including their main side effects.

## SELECTED REFERENCES

Audit Commission (2001) Acute hospital portfolio: day surgery report. http://www.audit-commission.gov.uk

British Association of Day Case Surgery (1999) Basket and trolley of procedures. www.bads.co.uk

Chung F (1995) Recovery pattern and home-readiness after ambulatory surgery. Anesth Analg 80 : 896–902

Department of Health (2002) Day surgery: operational guide. www.doh.gov.uk/daysurgery

NHS Estates (1993 and 1996) Accommodation for day care: day surgery unit. Health Building Note 52, vol 1 (and Suppl)

NHS Management Executive (1991) Day surgery: making it happen. HMSO, London

National Good Practice Guidance on Pre-operative Assessment for Day Surgery (2003): NHS Modernisation Agency. www.modern.nhs.uk/theatreprogramme/preop

Padfield NL (ed) (2000) Total intravenous anaesthesia. Butterworth-Heinemann, Boston, MA

**Table 9**

**Some common regional blocks used in day surgery**

| Common regional anaesthetic techniques in day case surgery | Indications |
|---|---|
| Ilioinguinal and iliohypogastric block | Inguinal hernia repair |
| Spinal | Lower limb or abdominal surgery |
| Caudal epidural | Perineal surgery. Orchidopexy and hernia repair in children |
| Penile block | Circumcision |
| Interscalene or supraclavicular block | Shoulder and upper limb surgery |
| Axillary block | Hand surgery |
| Bier's block | Hand and lower arm surgery |
| Digital ring blocks | Finger and toe surgery |
| Ankle block | Foot surgery |
| Peribulbar and retrobulbar blocks | Anterior chamber eye surgery |
| Dental blocks | Teeth extraction |

CHAPTER 2

# Basic Surgical Techniques

William E.G. Thomas

## INTRODUCTION

Short stay surgery, however efficient and effective the environment and organisational arrangements, is particularly dependent upon good surgical technique and attention to detail. It is undoubtedly the case that the greater the requirement for the shortest stay possible after surgery, the greater the need for a more experienced surgeon and anaesthetist. It is for this reason that day surgery units are commonly staffed and served by consultants rather than trainee surgeons and anaesthetists, although the nature of the surgery may actually be fairly straightforward and uncomplicated. Therefore it is essential that safe and sound surgical technique is an integral part of the consideration of any 'short stay' facility and although the subsequent chapters in this book will deal with the specific techniques required for individual procedures, this chapter is devoted to the basic techniques that will be utilised in all operative procedures.

The procedures that are suitable for consideration as 'short stay surgery' are particularly suitable as training procedures, and yet the demands of short stay surgery indicate that a senior surgeon (and anaesthetist) be present. However to exclude surgical trainees from this environment would be to exclude them access to a vast number of procedures that are particularly suitable to their training needs and requirements. This chapter will therefore assist them in describing and emphasising the safe and sound basic surgical techniques that are required in the short stay surgical unit, and once embraced will allow trainees to actively participate in this practice under the guidance and tutorship of their consultant educational supervisor. However it must be emphasised that these basic surgical techniques are not just important for trainees but must be embraced by *all* surgeons working in this sphere of surgery. Safe and sound basic surgical technique is the underpinning of any short stay facility and any short cuts will cause such a unit to fail.

## SUTURING AND SUTURE MATERIALS

The suturing of any wound or anastomosis needs to take into consideration the site and tissues involved, and the suture material and technique should be chosen accordingly. Furthermore, the correct choice of technique and material will never compensate for inadequate operative technique and so for any wound closure there must be a good blood supply and no tension. The ideal suture for all situations has yet to be produced. However many of the desired characteristics are as listed in Table 1 [1]. Certain procedures require specific characteristics of the suture material, e.g. vascular anastomoses require a smooth, non-absorbable and non-elastic material, while biliary anastomoses require an absorbable material that will not promote tissue reaction or stone formation. For absorbable material the time in which wound support is maintained will vary according to the tissues in which it is inserted. Furthermore, certain tissues require wound support for longer than others such as muscular aponeuroses as compared with subcutaneous tissues. It is therefore crucial for the surgeon to select the suture material and suture technique that will most effectively achieve the desired objective for each wound closure or anastomosis.

■ **Suture and Ligature Materials.** For any suture material, there are five specific characteristics to be considered.

## Table 1

Table 1 lists the characteristics of the perfect suture that unfortunately does not as yet exist.

## Figure 1: Physical Structure

Suture material may be monofilament or multifilament. Monofilament suture material is smooth and tends to slide through tissues easily without any sawing action but is more difficult with regard to knot formation. Such material can be easily damaged by gripping it with a needle holder or forceps and this can lead to fracture of the suture. Multifilament or braided sutures are much easier to knot, but the suture material is no longer smooth. Such material has a surface area several thousand times that of monofilament sutures and thus has a capillary action and interstices where bacteria may lodge and be responsible for persistent infection or sinuses. In order to overcome some of these problems, certain materials are produced as a braided suture which is coated with silicone in order to make it smooth.

## Table 2: Strength

The strength of a suture material depends upon its thickness, the material it is made of and its behaviour in the tissues. This strength can be expressed as the force required to break it when pulling the two ends apart. This is known as its tensile strength but is only a useful approximation as to its strength in the tissues, as what really matters is the material's in vivo strength. Absorbable sutures show a decay of this strength with the passage of time and although a material may last in the tissues for the stated period in the manufacturer's data sheet, its tensile strength cannot be relied on in vivo for this entire period. Materials such as catgut have a tensile strength of only about a week while polydioxanone (PDS) will remain strong in the tissues for several weeks. Even non-absorbable sutures do not maintain their strength indefinitely. Non-absorbable materials of synthetic origin such as polypropylene probably retain their tensile strength indefinitely and do not change in mass in the tissues. However it is possible for them to fracture. Non-absorbable materials of biological origin such as silk however will definitely fragment with time and lose their strength. Such materials therefore should never be used in vascular anastomoses for fear of late fistula formation.

**Table 1**

| |
|---|
| Adequate strength retention, with secure wound support throughout the critical healing period |
| Rapid absorption |
| High uniform tensile strength, permitting use of finer sizes |
| Pliable for ease of handling and knot security |
| Minimal tissue reaction |
| Predictable performance |
| Sterile |
| Consistent uniform diameter |

**Figure 1**

**Structure of suture material**

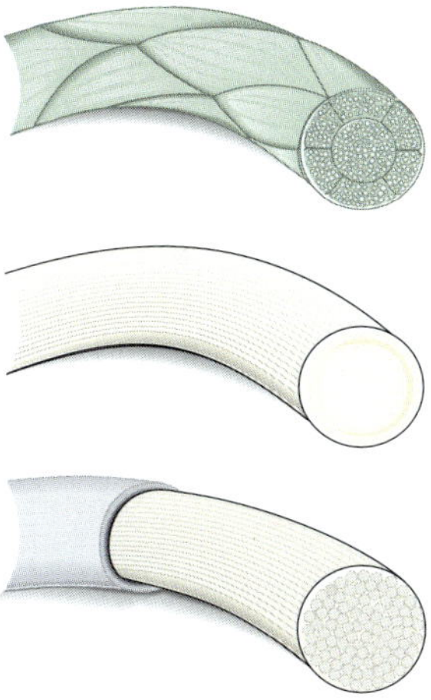


**Table 2**

| Metric (Eur Ph) | Range of diameter (mm) | USP ("old") |
|---|---|---|
| 1 | 0.100–0.149 | 5-0 |
| 1.5 | 0.150–0.199 | 4-0 |
| 2 | 0.200–0.249 | 3-0 |
| 3 | 0.300–0.349 | 2-0 |
| 3.5 | 0.350–0.399 | 0 |
| 4 | 0.400–0.499 | 1 |
| 5 | 0.500–0.599 | 2 |

## Figure 2: Tensile Behaviour

Suture materials behave differently depending upon their deformability and flexibility. Some may be elastic in which the material will return to its original length once the pull is released, or they may be plastic in which case this phenomenon does not occur. Sutures may be deformable in that a circular cross section may be converted to an oval shape or they may be more rigid or have the somewhat irritating capacity to kink and coil. Many synthetic materials demonstrate 'memory' in which they keep curling up in the pattern in which they were packaged. A sharp but gentle pull on the suture material helps to diminish this 'memory' but the more 'memory' a suture material has, the less is the knot security. Therefore knotting technique also plays a significant role in the tensile strength of any suture line and it is important to recognise that sutures lose 50% of their strength at the knot.

## Table 3: Absorbability

Suture materials may be absorbable or non-absorbable and this property should be taken into consideration when choosing suture materials for specific sites. Sutures for use in the biliary tract or urinary tract need to be absorbable in order to minimise the risk of stone production. However a vascular anastomosis requires a non-absorbable material and it is wise to avoid braided material as platelet adherence may predispose to distal embolisation. Non-absorbable materials tend to be preferred where persistent strength is required and, as an artificial graft or prosthesis never heals fully or integrates into a host artery, a persistent monofilament suture material such as polypropylene is universally used.

## Figure 3: Biological Behaviour

The biological behaviour of suture material within the tissues depends upon the origin of the raw materials. Biological or natural sutures such as catgut are proteolysed but this involves a process that is not entirely predictable and can cause local irritation. Manmade synthetic polymers are hydrolysed and their disappearance in the tissues is more predictable. However, the presence of infection, urine or faeces influences the final result and renders the outcome once again unpredictable. There is also some evidence that in the gut, cancer cells may accumulate at sites where sutures persist possibly giving rise to local recurrence. For this reason, synthetic materials that have a greater predictability and elicit minimal tissue reaction, may have an important non-carcinogenic property.

■ **Suture Techniques.** There are four frequently used suture techniques [2].

Figure 2

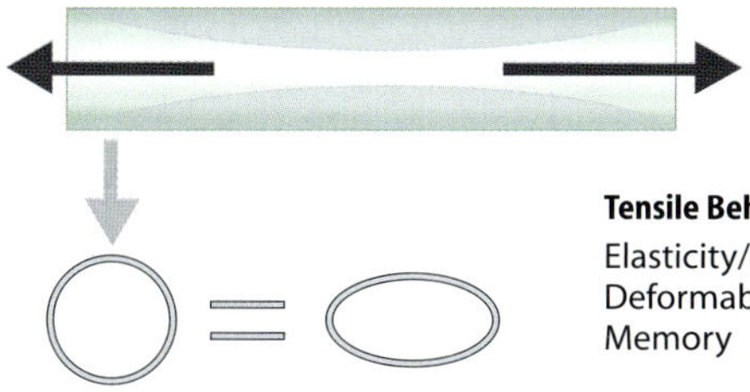

**Tensile Behaviour**
Elasticity/Plasticity
Deformability/Flexibility
Memory

Table 3

| Material | Type | 50% loss of tensile strength | Dissolution |
|---|---|---|---|
| Polyglycolic acid (Dexon) | Braided | 14–18 | 90–120 |
| Lactomer 9-1 (Polysorb) | Braided, coated | 14–18 | 50–70 |
| Polyglactin 910 (Vicryl) | Braided, coated | 18 | 70–90 |
| Glycomer 631 (Biosyn) | Mono-filament | 21 | 90–110 |
| Polyglyconate (Maxon) | Mono-filament | 28 | 180 |
| Polydioxanone (PDS II) | Mono-filament | 35 | 180 |

Figure 3

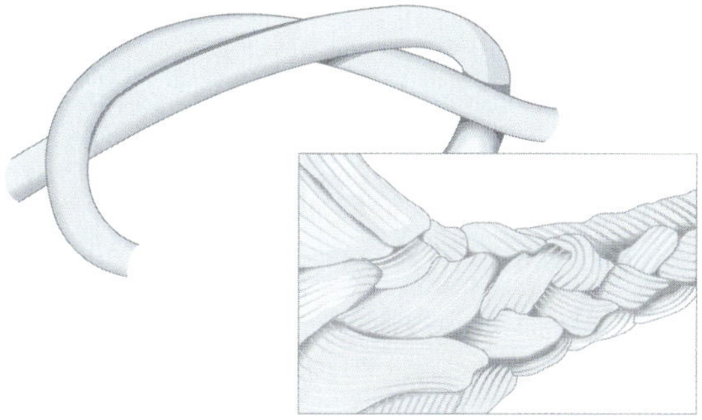

## Figure 4A, B: Interrupted Sutures

Interrupted sutures require the needle to be inserted at right angles to the incision and then to pass through both aspects of the suture line and exit again at right angles. It is important for the needle to be rotated through the tissues rather than to be dragged through for fear of unnecessarily enlarging the needle hole. As a guide, the distance from the entry point of the needle to the edge of the wound should be approximately the same as the depth of the tissue being sutured, and each successive suture should be placed at twice this distance apart (Fig. 4B). Each suture should reach into the depths of the wound and be placed at right angles to the axis of the wound. In linear wounds it is sometimes easier to insert the middle suture first and then to complete the closure by successively inserting sutures, halving the remaining deficits in the wound length.

## Figure 5: Continuous Sutures

For a continuous suture the first suture is inserted in an identical manner to an interrupted suture but the rest of the sutures are inserted in a continuous manner until the far end of the wound is reached. Each throw of the continuous suture should be inserted at right angles to the wound and this will mean that the externally observed suture material will lie diagonal to the axis of the wound. It is important to have an assistant who will follow the suture, keeping it at the same tension in order to avoid either 'purse-stringing' the wound by too much tension, or leaving the suture material too slack. There is more danger of producing too much tension by using too little suture length than there is of leaving the suture line too lax. Post-operative oedema will often take up any slack in the suture material. It has been estimated that for abdominal wall closure the length of the suture material should be at least 4 times the length of the wound to be closed. At the far end of the wound, this suture line should be secured either by using an Aberdeen knot or by tying the free end to the loop of the last suture to be inserted.

**Figure 4A, B**

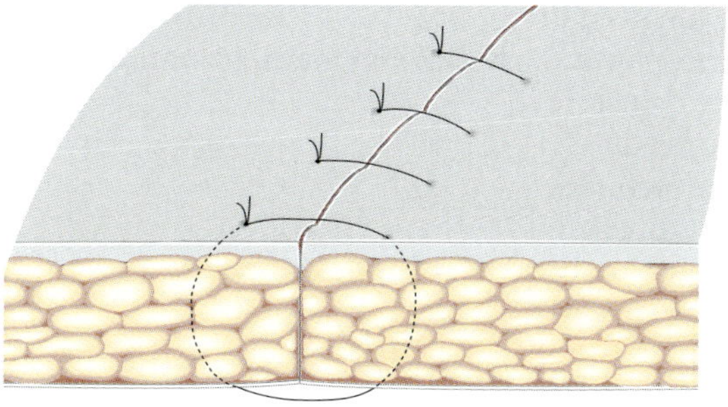

A

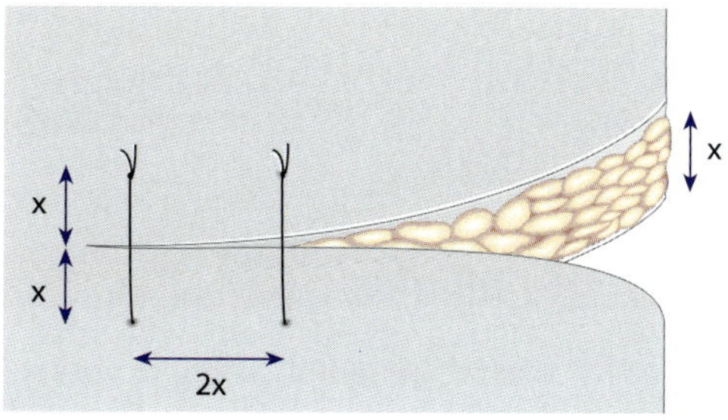


B

**Figure 5**

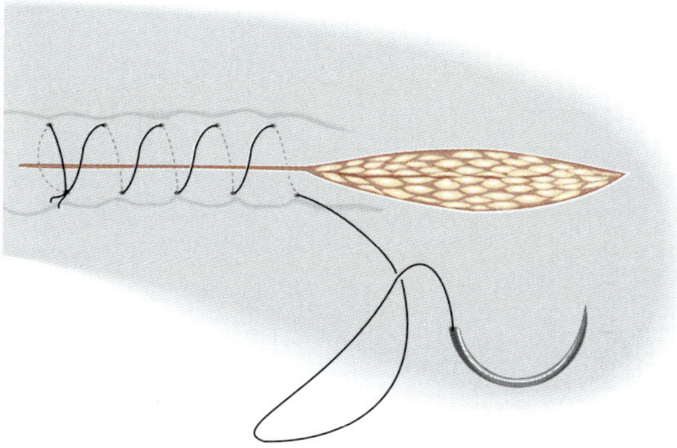

## Figure 6A, B: Mattress Sutures

Mattress sutures may be either vertical or horizontal and tend to be used to produce either eversion or inversion of a wound edge. The initial suture is inserted as for an interrupted suture but then the needle either moves horizontally or vertically and traverses both edges of the wound once again. Such sutures are very useful in producing accurate approximation of wound edges, especially when the edges to be anastomosed are irregular in depth or disposition.

Fig. 6a is a vertical mattress suture while 6B is a horizontal mattress suture.

## Figure 7A, B: Subcuticular Suture

This technique is used in skin where a cosmetic appearance is important and where the skin edges may be approximated easily. The suture material used may be either absorbable or non-absorbable. For non-absorbable sutures the ends may be secured by means of a collar and bead, or tied loosely over the wound. When absorbable sutures are used the ends may be secured using a buried knot. Small bites of the subcuticular tissues are taken on alternate sides of the wound and then gently pulled together thus approximating the wound edges without the risk of the cross-hatched markings of interrupted sutures.

**Figure 6A, B**

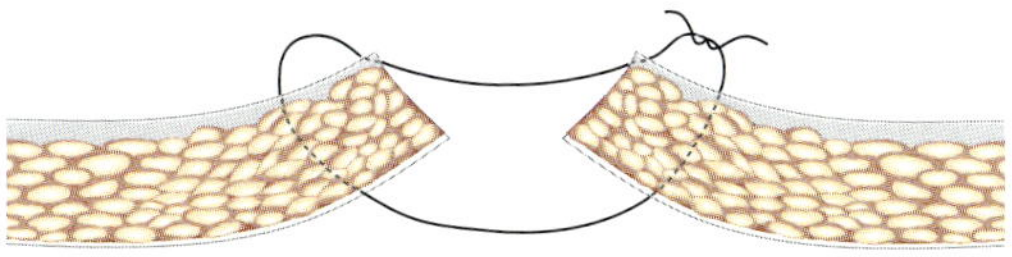

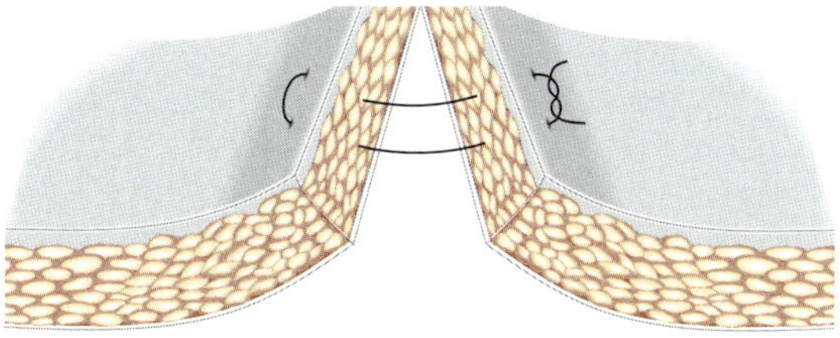

**Figure 7A, B**

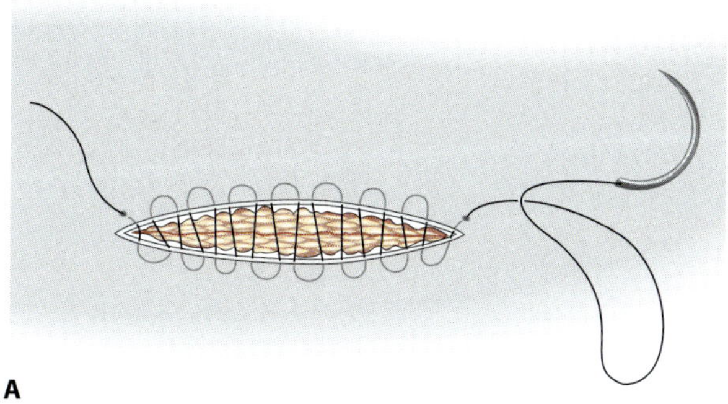

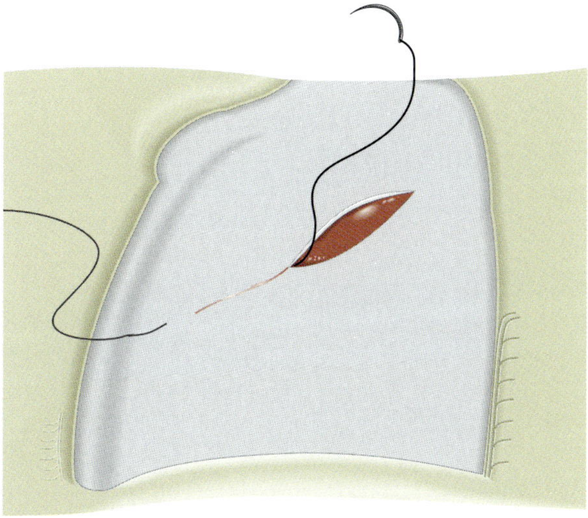

## Figure 8A, B: Alternative Techniques to Sutures

Several alternatives to standard suture materials are now available for the closure of wounds. For the skin, self adhesive tapes or Steristrips (Fig. 8A) may be used in situations where there is no tension or too much moisture. Tissue adhesive or glue is also available based upon a solution of *n*-butyl-2 cyanoacrylate monomer. When it is applied to a wound it polymerises to form a firm adhesive bond but once again the wound needs to be clean, dry and under no tension. Staples of stainless steel may also be used (Fig. 8B), and such devices have the advantage of being quick and easy to use but the disadvantage of being more expensive. Furthermore it is vital for the surgeon to be familiar both with the principles and the practice behind each stapling device that is used.

Figure 8A, B

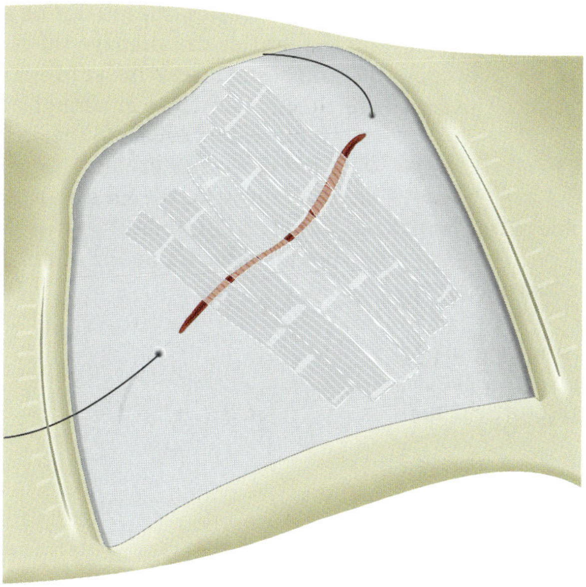

A

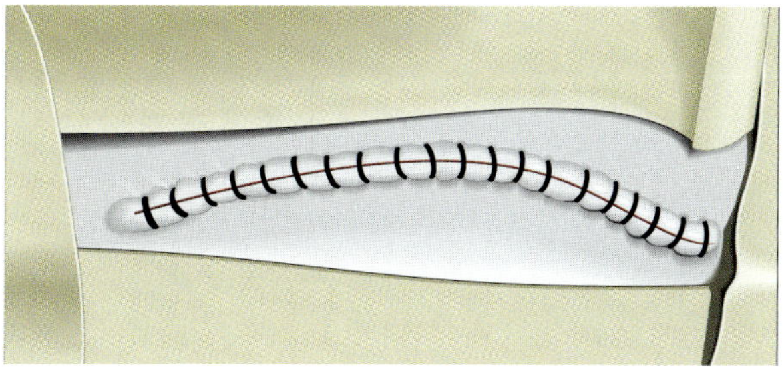

B

## Figure 9A, B: Knot Tying

Knot tying is one of the most fundamental techniques in surgery and yet is often poorly performed [3]. Time taken to perfect one's knot tying technique is time well invested and requires practice. The general principles include:

- The knot must be firm and unable to slip (e.g. a reef knot)
- The knot must be as small as possible to minimise implanted foreign material
- The suture material should not be 'sawed' during tying as this weakens the material
- The suture material itself should not be grasped by a needle holder or artery forceps (except at the free end) as this weakens and can fracture the material
- Excess tension should not be applied during ligation as this can damage the structure being ligated or even break the suture material. Correct application of tension should always be applied at 180° or else damage to the structure being ligated will follow (Fig. 9)
- Each throw of the knot must be applied correctly (square knots) and 'bedded down' accurately using the index finger or thumb as appropriate

Figure 9A, B

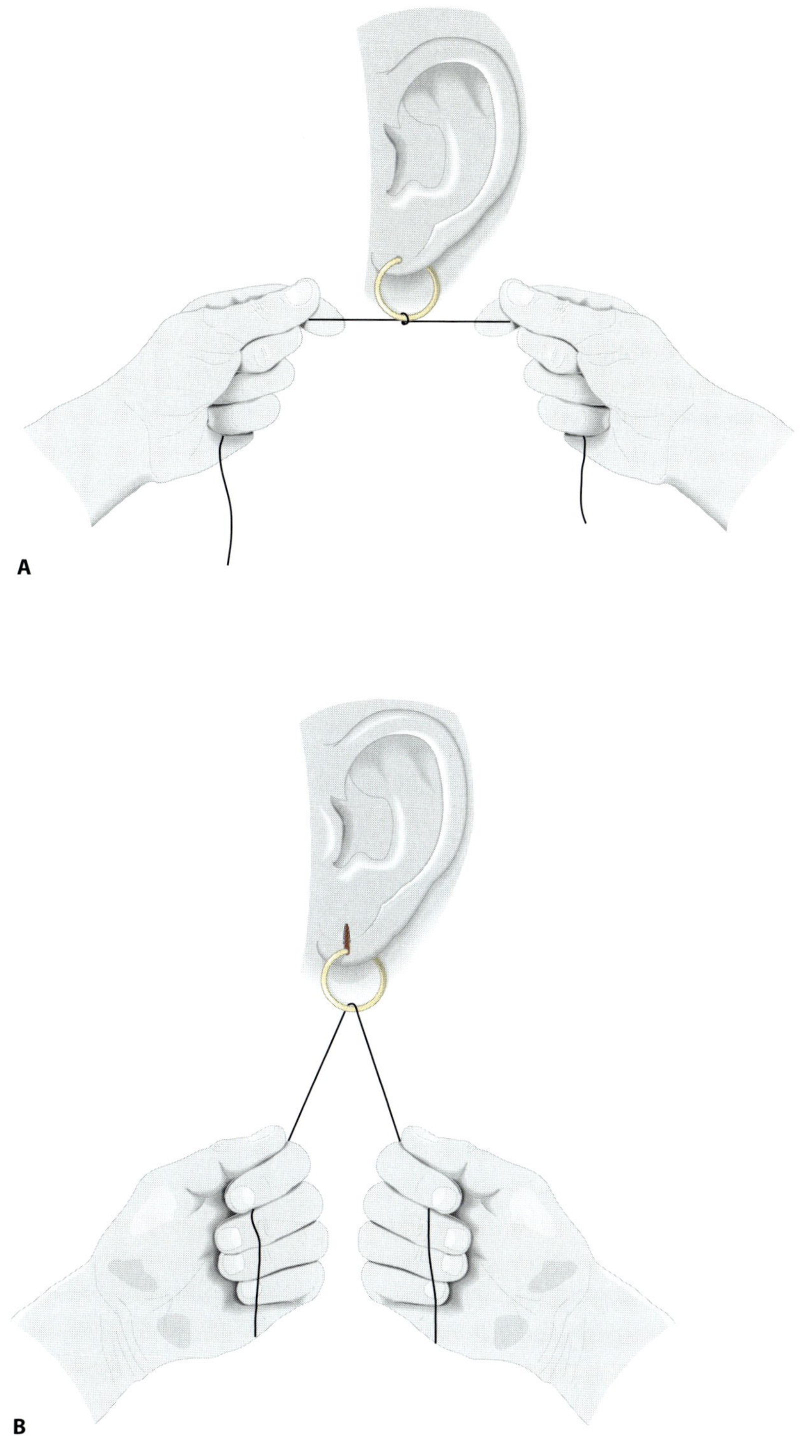

## Figure 10A–C: The One-Handed Reef Knot

This is a very versatile and useful technique. It is valuable to be able to tie this knot using the non-dominant hand as this allows an instrument to be 'palmed' in the dominant hand.

- Grasp the short end of the suture between the thumb and middle finger of the non-dominant hand (left) with the loop over the extended index finger. The remainder of the suture material is held in the dominant hand (right) (Fig. 10A). Bring the remainder of the suture material in the right hand over the left index finger by moving the right hand away from the operator (Fig. 10B). Use the distal phalanx of the left index finger to pass under the thread held in the left hand (Fig. 10C) and then pull it through the loop grasping it between the left index finger and middle finger, drawing the left hand towards the operator and the right hand away from the operator.

**Figure 10A–C**

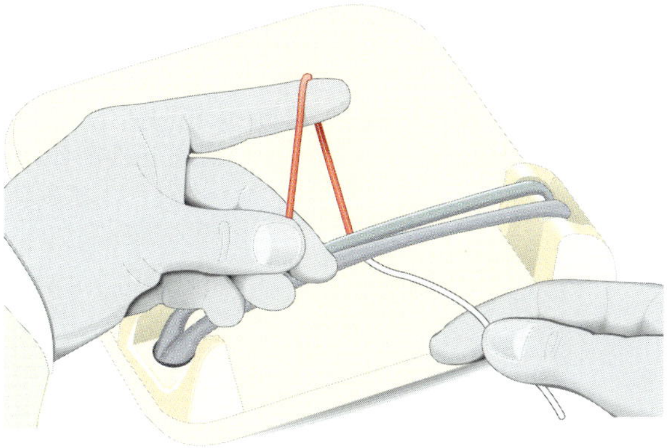

A

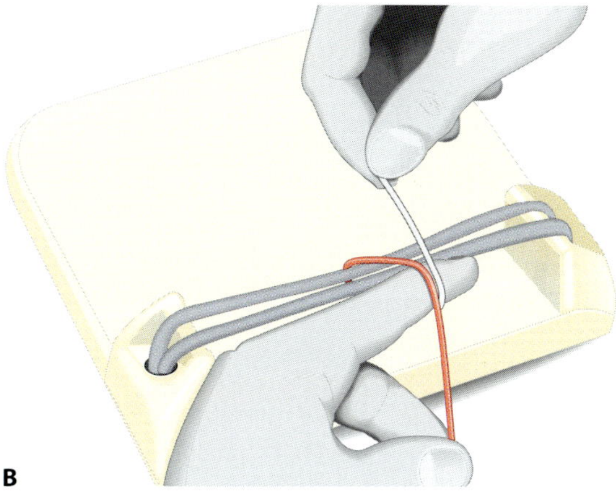

B

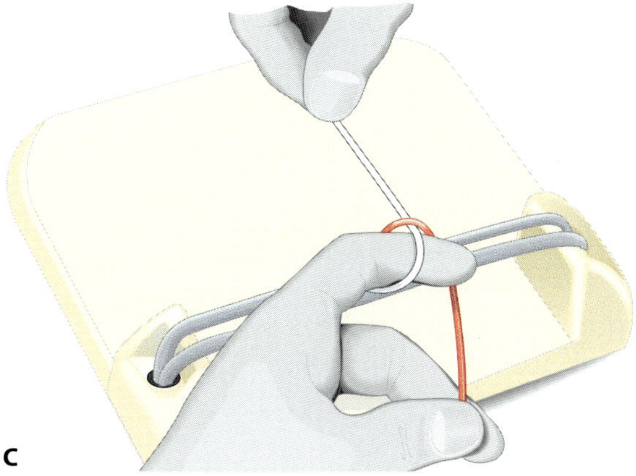

C

## Figure 11A–C: The One-Handed Reef Knot

- Complete the first throw ensuring that the knot is 'bedded' down correctly (Fig. 11A). Thus the hands have been crossed and the first throw of a reef knot completed. Continue to hold the short end between the thumb and index finger of the left hand, looping the rest of the thread around the other three fingers (Fig. 11B). Bring the suture material held in the right hand across the middle, ring and little fingers of the left hand thus crossing over the left handed thread (Fig. 11C).

Figure 11A–C

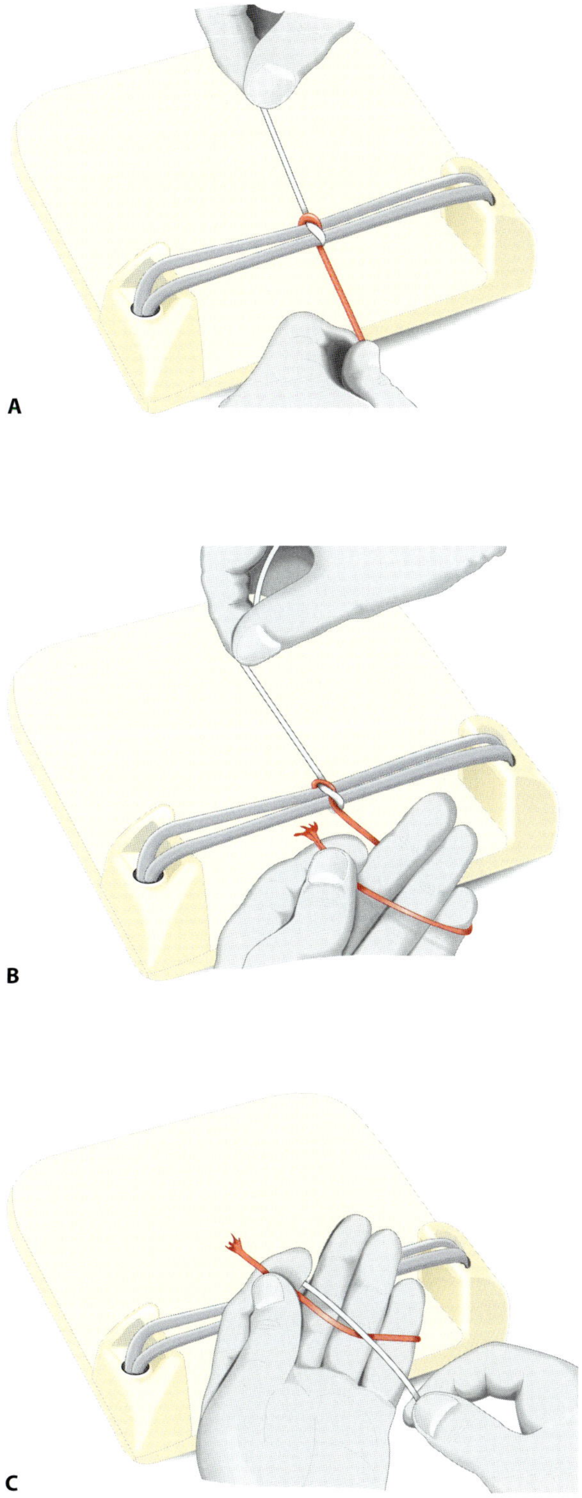

## Figure 12A–D: The One-Handed Reef Knot

- The distal phalanx of the left middle finger should then be inserted under the left handed thread (Fig. 12A) and used to bring this under the right handed strand grasping it between the middle and ring fingers. This throw is then completed by drawing the right hand towards the operator and the left hand away from the operator (Fig. 12B). Completion is confirmed by 'bedding' the throw down well and the classical configuration of a reef knot can be seen (Fig. 12C). For security another throw is performed using the initial 'index finger' technique. Three throws are usually adequate for multifilamentous material but if a monofilament material such as polypropylene is used, multiple throws are required or a surgeon's knot technique used (see below).

**Figure 12A–D**

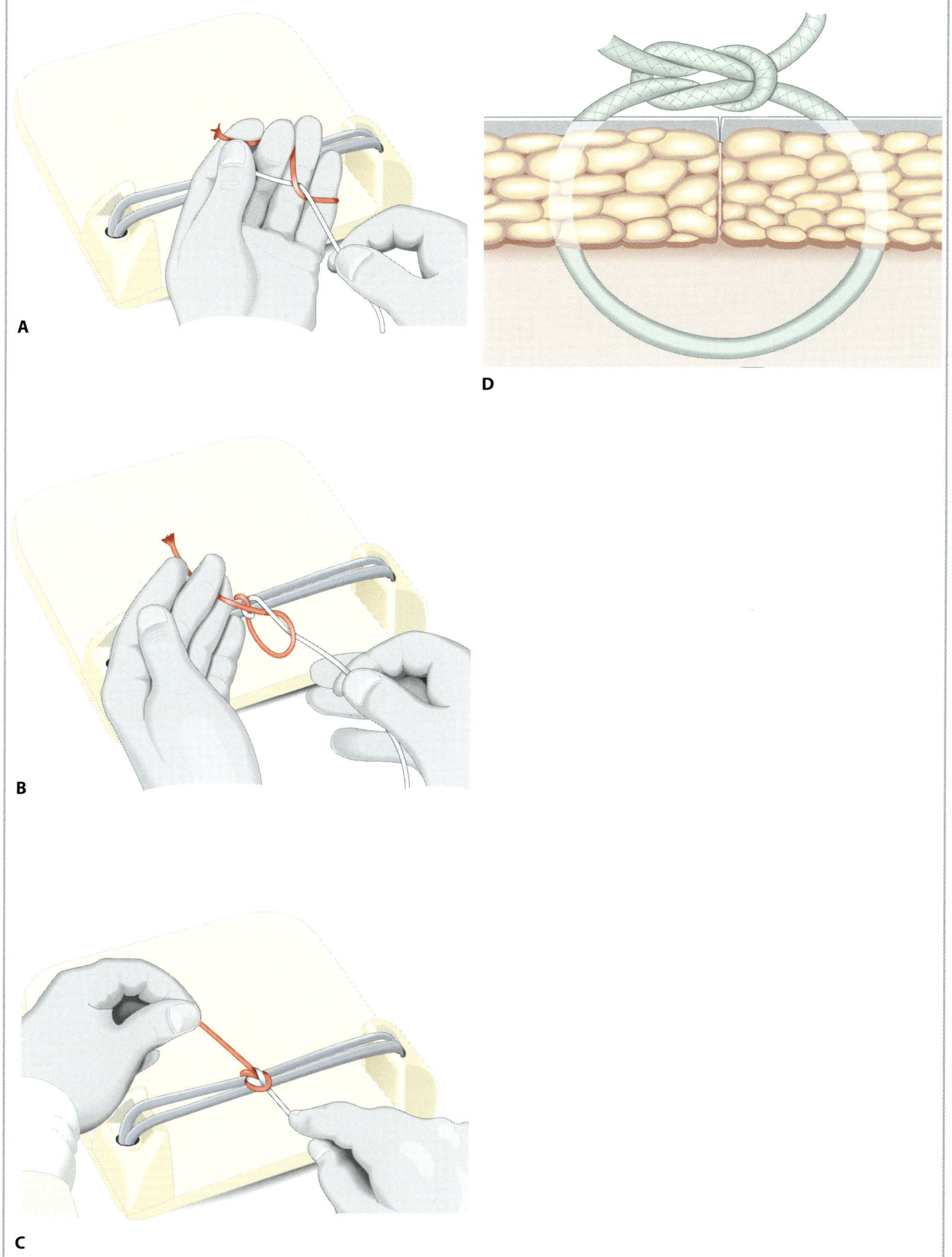

## Figure 13A–C: The Instrument Tied Reef Knot

This is a useful technique especially if the suture material length is a little short.

- Loop the long end of the suture material around the instrument, the instrument being placed over the thread (Fig. 13A). Grasp the short end right at its free end within the jaws of the instrument (Fig. 13B) and pull it through the loop and complete the first hitch (Fig. 13C). Ensure that this first throw is 'bedded' down correctly.

Figure 13A–C

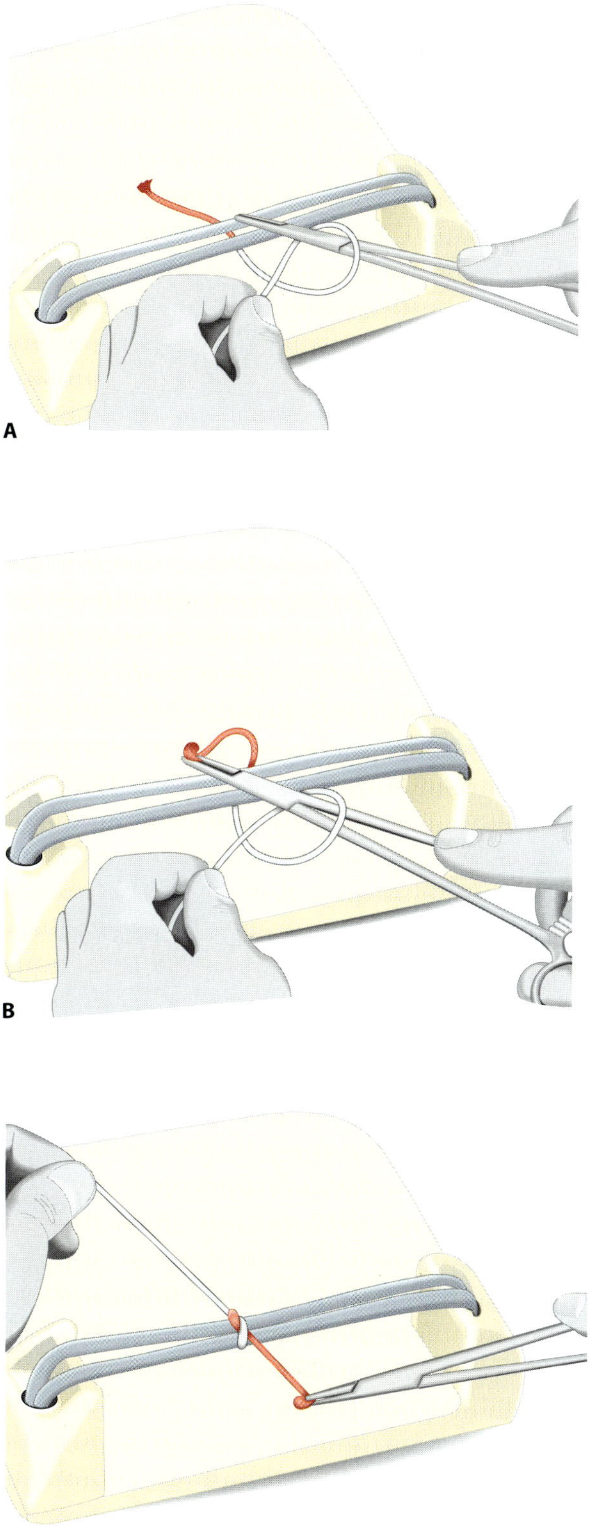

A

B

C

## Figure 14A–C: The Instrument Tied Reef Knot



- Now form a similar loop around the instrument again placing the instrument over the distal thread (Fig. 14A), draw it towards the operator and grasp the free end of the short end again (Fig. 14B) pulling it through to complete the classical reef knot (Fig. 14C). For security three throws should be used for multifilament material but several throws are required for monofilament material. Indeed for vascular anastomoses using fine polypropylene up to seven throws have been advocated.

Figure 14A–C

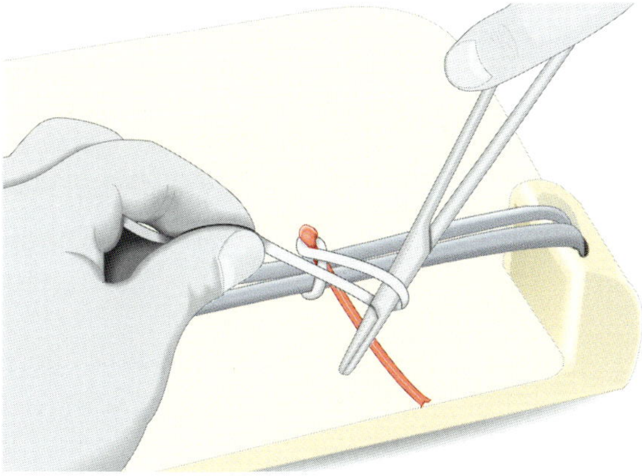

A

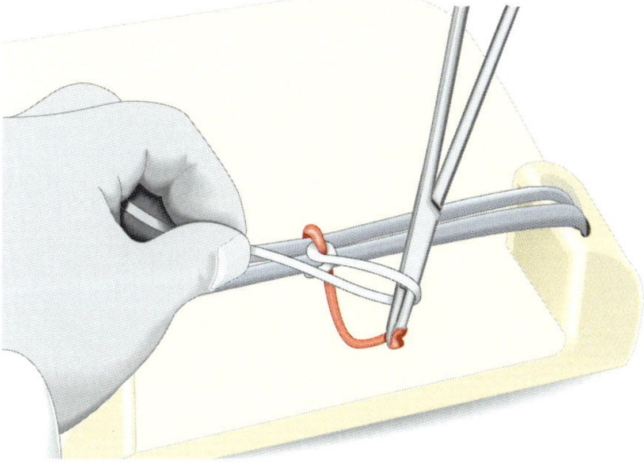

B

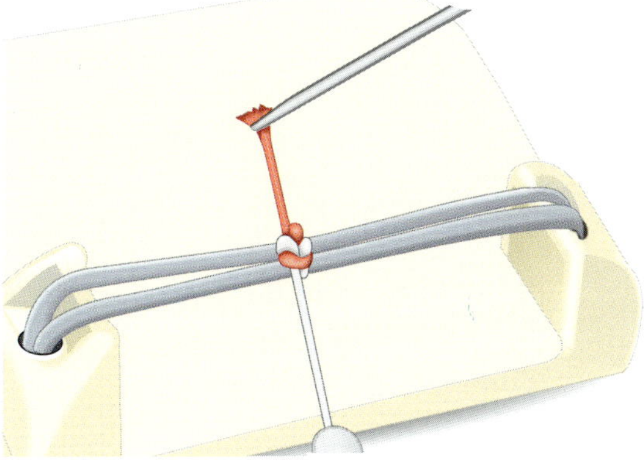

C

## Figure 15A–C: The Surgeon's Knot Technique

This is a very secure knot and involves two throws for each hitch. It looks very cumbersome in the illustrations as such thick thread is used for clarity. However it is a very useful technique when a highly secure knot is required.

- A single throw is formed using a one or two handed technique (Fig. 15A). However before this is 'bedded' down a further throw is made in the same manner (Fig. 15B) and then this is tightened in the conventional manner taking care not to exert any tension on the structure being ligated (Fig. 15C).

**Figure 15A–C**

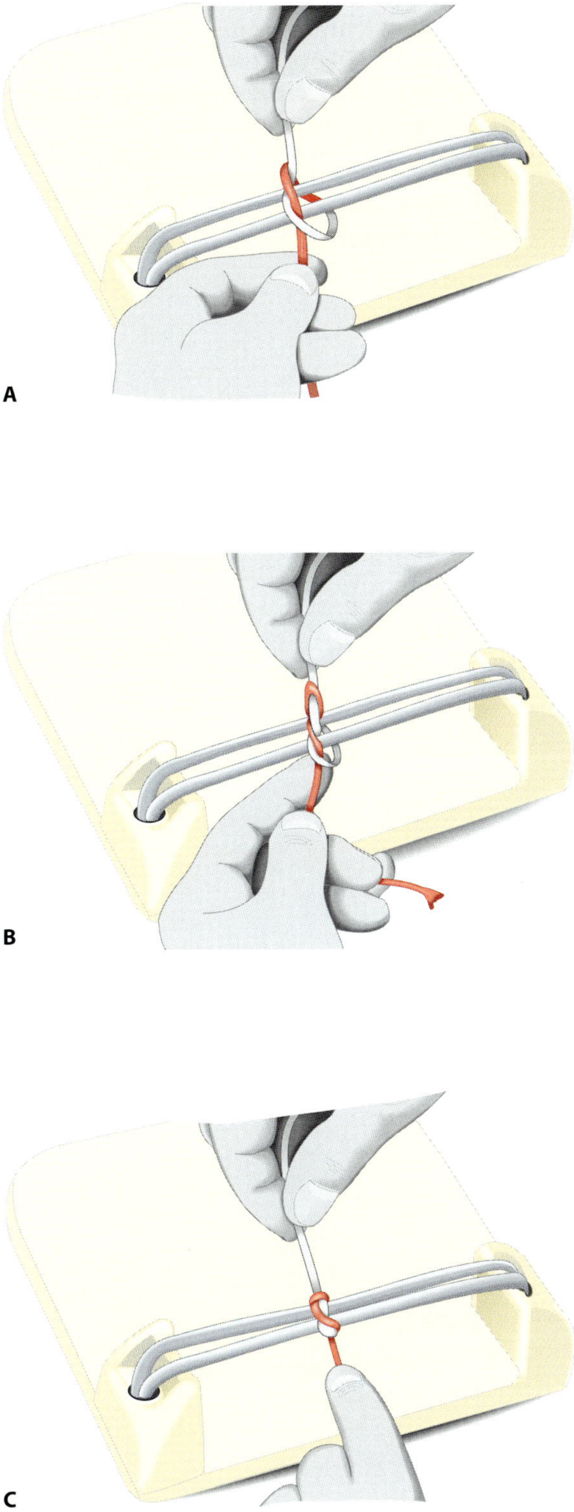

A

B

C

## Figure 16A–D: The Surgeon's Knot Technique



- A further throw is now fashioned in the same manner as for a reef knot (Fig. 16A) but again this is not tightened at this stage. A similar throw is again fashioned producing a double throw as before (Fig. 16B) and this is then tightened down. The resulting knot does not look exactly elegant (Fig. 16C) but it is very secure as long as the final throw is tightened as horizontally as possible. Although two throws of a surgeon's knot are very secure, convention dictates that three throws are often used.

Figure 16A–D

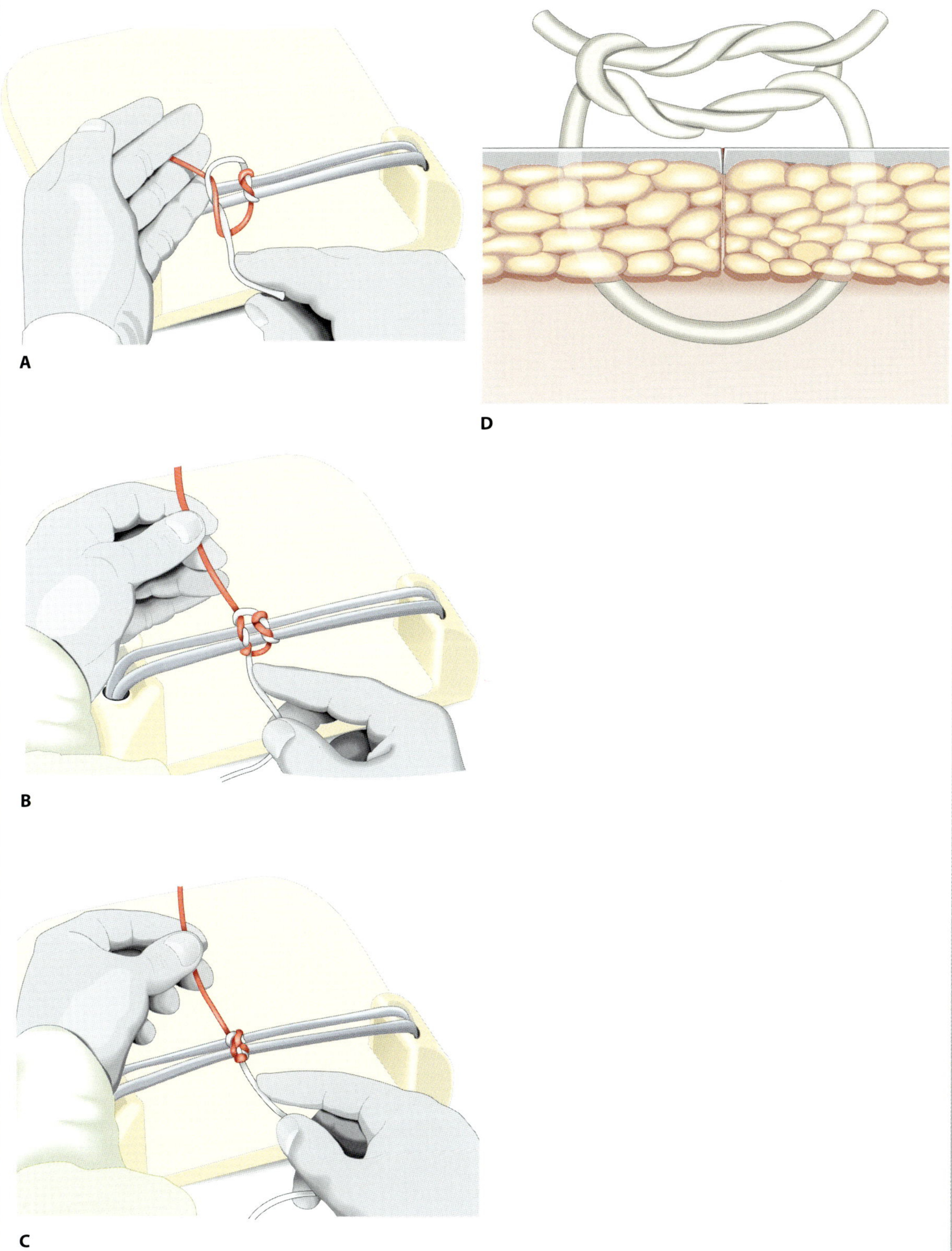

## Figure 17A–C: The Aberdeen Knot Technique

This is a useful technique, when having finished a continuous suture line, the surgeon is left with a loop and a free end (Fig. 17A).

- Display the loop between the index finger and thumb of the left hand, making the loop as small as possible by pulling on the other end of the thread with the right hand (Fig. 17B). Grasp the free end of the suture material held in the right hand between the index finger and thumb of the left hand and draw it through the loop, and by releasing the right hand thread and tightening the new loop, the old loop is eliminated and a new loop is formed (Fig. 17C).

**Figure 17A–C**

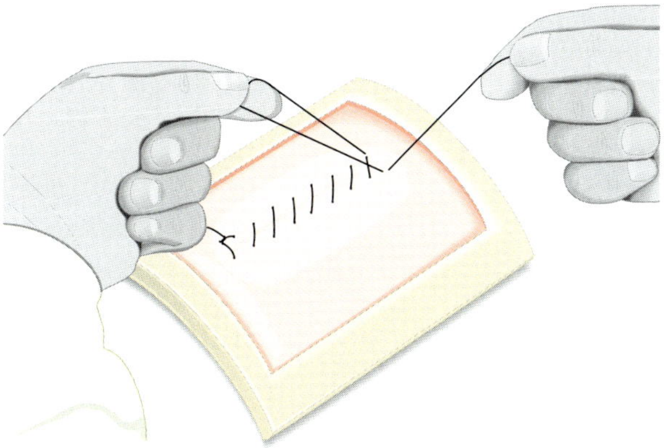

A

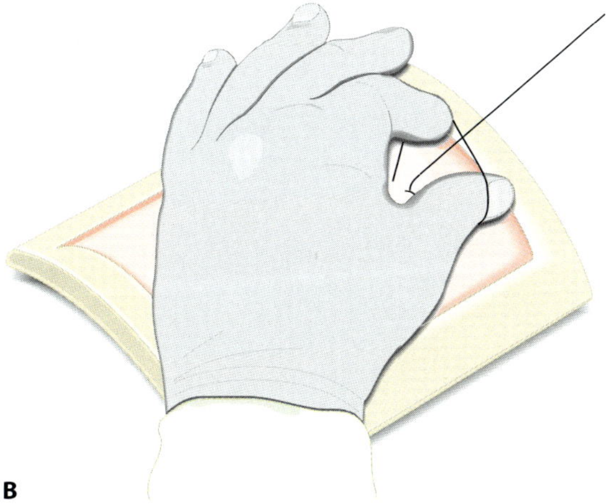

B

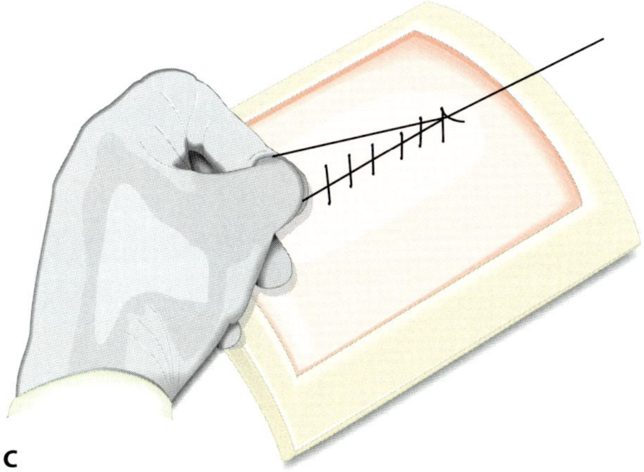

C

## Figure 18A–C: The Aberdeen Knot Technique

- Once again make the new loop as small as possible by pulling on the right hand thread and repeat the process (Fig. 18A) tightening each time using a type of 'see-saw' movement. This process is repeated about 6–7 times. Finally pass the free end entirely through the loop (Fig. 18B) and tighten down (Fig. 18C). The thread can now be cut ensuring a suitable length is left to prevent the knot from unravelling.

Figure 18A–C

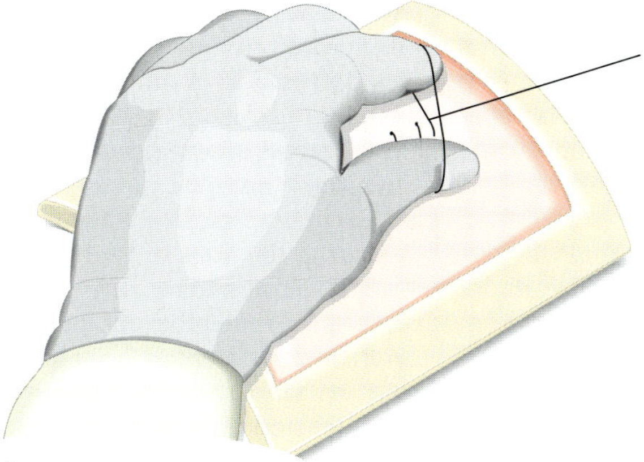

A

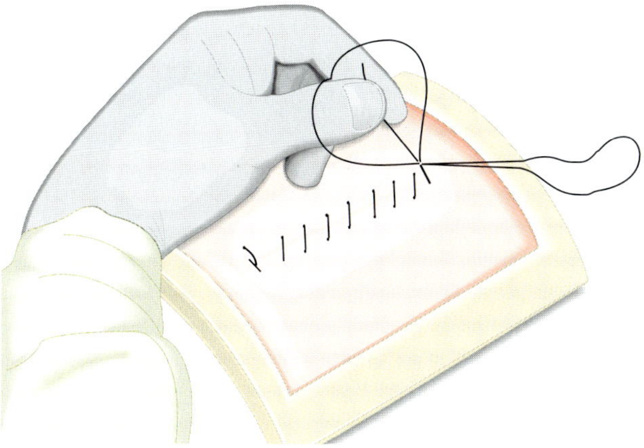

B

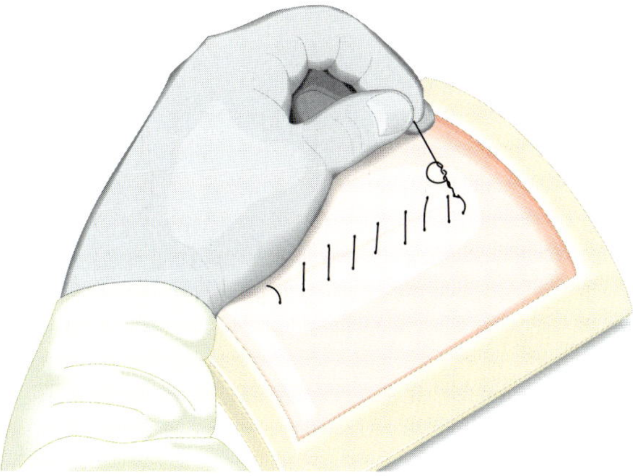

C

## Figures 19A, B: Incisions



The aims and requirements for any incision are to provide adequate access for the necessary procedure, to heal well with a low failure rate and to be as cosmetically acceptable as possible. Each incision therefore requires planning. Similar principles apply when considering port sites for laparoscopic surgery as is considered below.

The correct choice of incision is one that will give the best access for the particular procedure under consideration. Once the type of incision has been chosen then, to obtain the most favourable cosmetic outcome, the line of skin creases and Langer's lines should be considered (Fig. 19A). In general, an incision parallel to skin creases or along Langer's lines tends to result in a more satisfactory scar. At times this may be difficult to ascertain and then attempts to pick up the skin in different directions may indicate the lines of tension. Occasionally it may be appropriate to excise a skin lesion with a circular incision when these lines are not apparent and then observe as the circular incision is converted to an ellipse thus indicating the lines of tension. This then allows the circular incision to be converted into a formal elliptical incision remembering the 'rule of thumb' that *'an elliptical incision must be at least three times as long as it is wide'* [4] for the wound to heal without too much tension (Fig. 19B).

Figure 19A, B

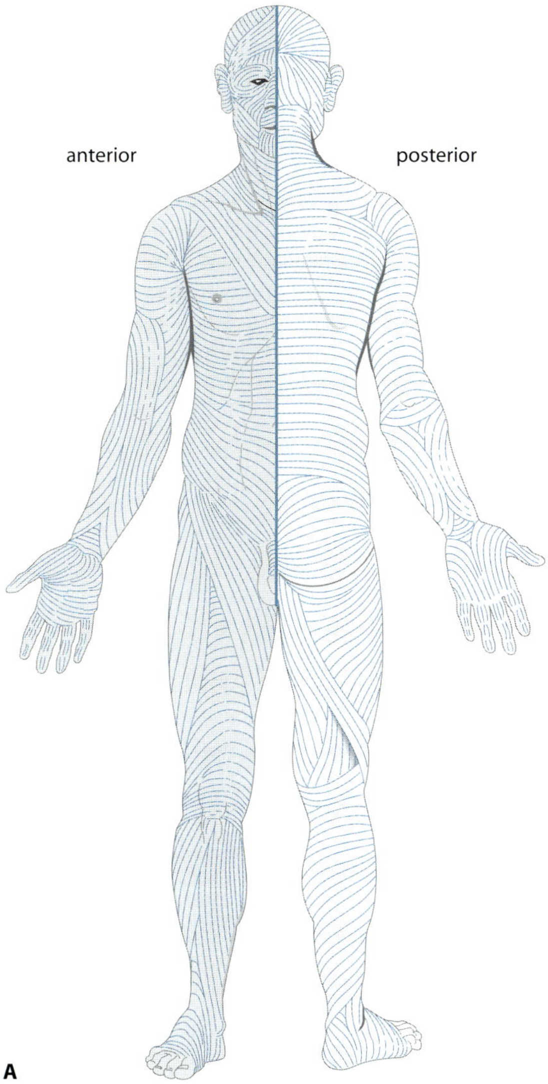


A

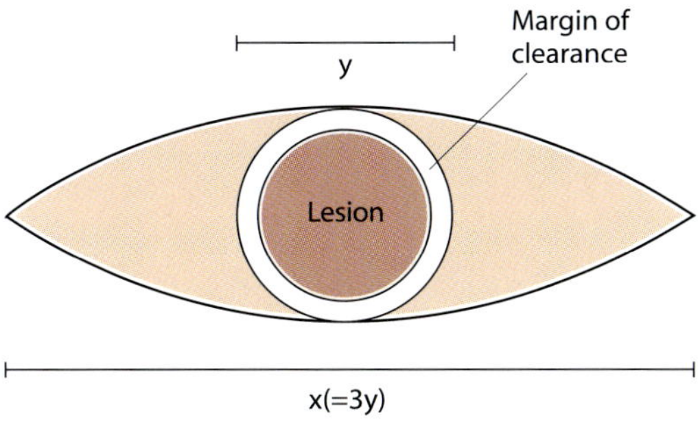


B

## Figures 20A, B: Incisions



Occasionally 'dog-ears' remain in the corner of elliptical incisions in spite of adequate care having been taken during formation and primary closure of an elliptical wound. In these situations it is advisable to pick up the 'dog-ear' with a skin hook and excise it as shown in Fig. 20A [5]. This allows for a satisfactory cosmetic outcome. However, despite optimal management and great care during closure, certain areas of the body such as the shoulders, anterior chest wall, lower neck and back (Fig. 20B) are prone to hypertrophic, widened and keloid scars. It is therefore vital that patients are warned of this possibility prior to surgery and wherever possible this risk factor should be recorded on the consent form. Finally it is always important when planning skin incisions to consider the anatomical location of important subcutaneous nerves as it is crucial to avoid injuring these structures, e.g. the mandibular and cervical branches of the facial nerve during submandibular and parotid salivary gland surgery.

Figure 20A, B

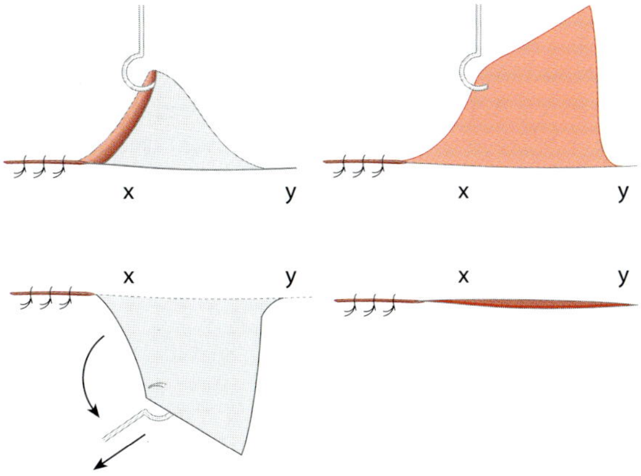


A

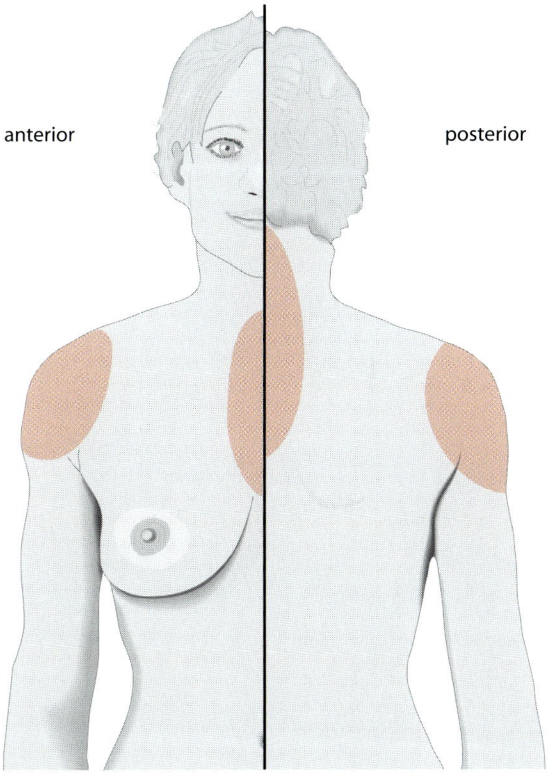


B

## Figure 21: Incisions in Common Use

Abdominal incisions depend upon the procedure being performed. A midline incision has the advantage that it provides rapid access, has minimal blood loss, can be extended up and/or down in an emergency situation and is easy to close. It is for these reasons that it is commonly used in an emergency situation, being initially centred around the umbilicus and extended appropriately depending upon the operative findings. Paramedian incisions take longer to perform and close and are associated with a slightly higher blood loss. However they have a low complication rate and reputedly have a lower incidence of incisional hernia. Transverse incisions are said to be associated with a lower incidence of chest infections (fewer dermatomes are involved), have better skin healing and allow good direct access, but they involve muscle cutting, are associated with a higher blood loss and in some series are associated with a greater incidence of incisional herniation.

Figure 21

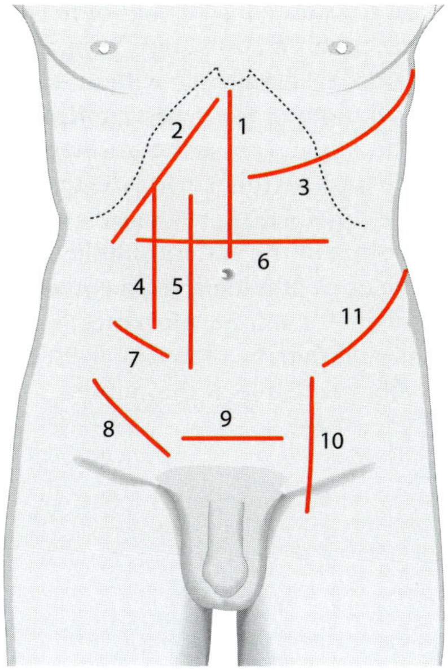


1 Midline
2 Kocher's
3 Thoracoabdominal
4 Rectus split
5 Paramedian
6 Transverse
7 McBurney's gridiron
8 Inguinal
9 Pfannenstiel
10 McEvedy
11 Rutherford Morrison

## Figure 22A, B: Laparoscopic Access

Port siting for laparoscopic surgery follows the same principles as for incisions in open surgery. The port sites should allow for maximum access and good vision to allow safe surgical manipulation. In deciding the best port sites for access, it should be borne in mind that the most efficient working conditions are achieved when the optical axis-to-target viewing angle approximates to 90° (Fig. 22A) and any diminution in this angle results in a less efficient performance. It should be recognised that if an oblique viewing endoscope is used (e.g. 30°), then there is a visual field change whenever the scope is rotated. When inserting the ports, the working angles must be considered. Maximal efficiency is achieved when the 'manipulation angle' (Fig. 22B) is between 45° and 75° (ideal being 60°) with an equal 'azimuth angle' on both sides of the camera port. As with the 'manipulation angle', the optimum 'elevation angle' is 60° and the best performance is seen when these two angles are equal. Furthermore, when considering port sites, the size of the patient should be taken into account as the optimum intra:extra corporeal shaft ratio for the most efficient performance is 2:1. The VDU monitor should then be placed in front of the surgeon preferably in the line of the camera.

Figure 22A, B

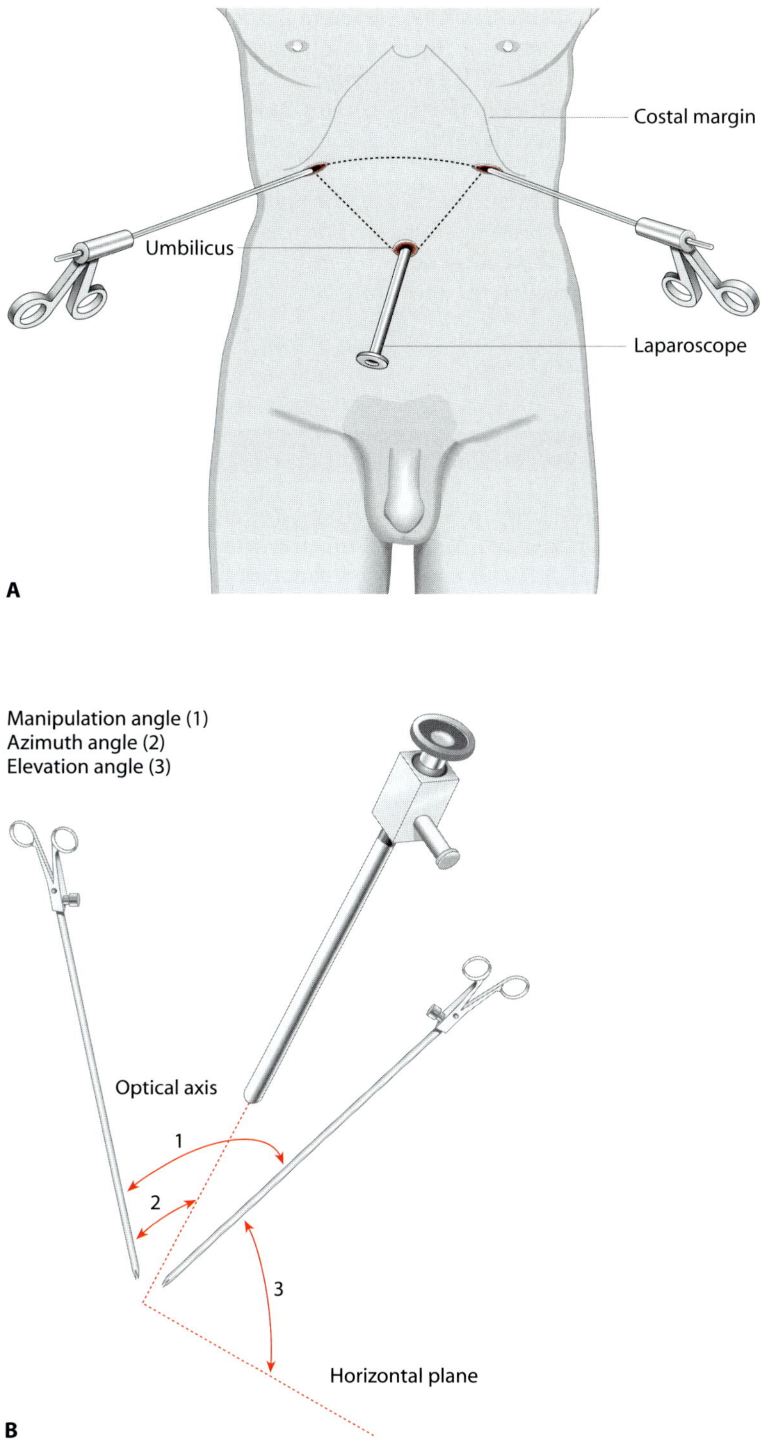
Costal margin
Umbilicus
Laparoscope
A
Manipulation angle (1)
Azimuth angle (2)
Elevation angle (3)
Optical axis
1
2
3
Horizontal plane
B

## DIATHERMY

Short wave diathermy is a most valuable and versatile aid to surgical technique in securing haemostasis by means of coagulation. However by varying the strength or wave form of the current produced, it can also result in a cutting effect and both these effects have been used in open surgery as well as in laparoscopic surgery. Although diathermy is a valuable surgical tool, accidents have occurred due to surgeons being unaware of or not fully understanding the principles of its use. It is therefore vital for a surgeon to have a sound understanding of the principles and practice behind the use of diathermy.

■ **The Principle of Diathermy.** When an electrical current passes through a conductor, some of its energy appears as heat. The heat produced depends upon:

1. The intensity of the current
2. The wave form of the current
3. The electrical property of the tissues through which the current passes
4. The relative sizes of the two electrodes

## Figure 23A, B

There are two basic forms of diathermy in use, monopolar diathermy and bipolar diathermy [6]. In monopolar diathermy (Fig. 23A), which is the most commonly used form, an alternating current is produced by a suitable generator and passed to the patient via an active electrode which has a very small surface area. The current then passes through the tissues and returns via a very large surface plate (the indifferent electrode) back to the earth pole of the generator. As the surface area of contact of the active electrode is so small by comparison to the indifferent electrode, the concentrated powerful current produces heat at the operative site. However the large surface area electrode of the patient plate spreads the returning current over a wide surface area, so it is less concentrated and produces little heat. In bipolar diathermy (Fig. 23B), the two active electrodes are usually represented by the limbs of a pair of diathermy forceps. Both forceps ends are therefore active and current flows between them and only the tissue held between the limbs of the forceps heats up. This form of diathermy is used when it is essential that the surrounding tissue should be free from either the risk of being burned or having current passed through it.

Figure 23A, B

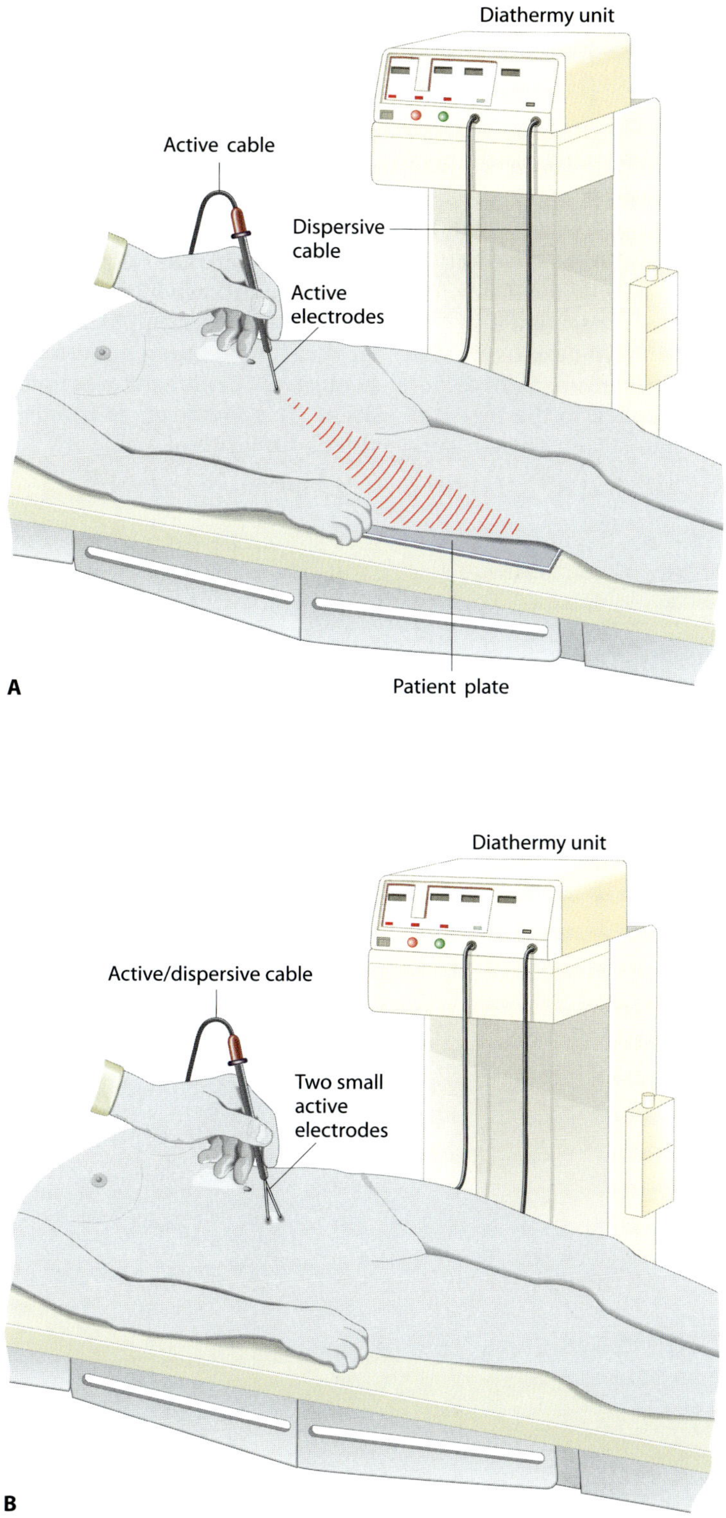
Diathermy unit
Active cable
Dispersive cable
Active electrodes
A
Patient plate
Diathermy unit
Active/dispersive cable
Two small active electrodes
B

2

## Figure 24A–C: The Effects of Diathermy

Diathermy can be used for three purposes:

A Coagulation: the sealing of blood vessels
B Cutting: used to divide tissues during bloodless surgery
C Fulguration: the destructive coagulation of tissues with charring

In coagulation, a heating effect leads to cell death by dehydration and protein denaturation. Bleeding is therefore stopped by a combination of the distortion of the walls of the blood vessel, coagulation of the plasma proteins, dried and shrunken dead tissue and stimulation of the clotting mechanism. Cutting occurs when sufficient heat is applied to the tissue to cause cell water to explode into steam. The cut current is a continuous wave form and the monopolar diathermy is most effective when the active electrode is held a very short distance from the tissues. This allows an electrical discharge to arc across the gap creating a series of sparks which produce the high temperatures needed for cutting. In fulguration the diathermy matching is set to coagulation and a higher effective voltage is used to make larger sparks jump an air gap thus fulgurating the tissues. This can continue until carbonisation or charring occurs. The voltage and power output can be varied by adjusting the duration of bursts of current as well as its intensity to give a combination of both cutting and coagulation. This is known as blended current, and provides both forms of diathermy activity.

**Figure 24A–C**

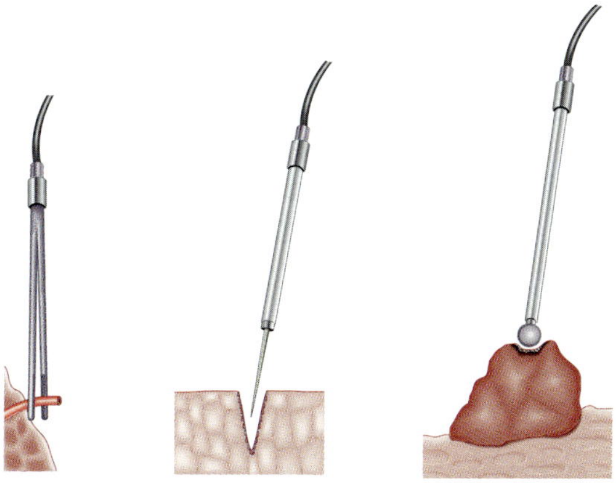

**A** Coagulation **B** Cutting **C** Fulguration

## Figure 25, 26: Complications of Diathermy

1. *Electrocution:* rare with modern well serviced machines
2. *Explosion:* sparks from the diathermy can ignite any volatile or inflammable gas or fluid within the theatre, such as alcohol based skin preparations. Furthermore, diathermy should not be used in the presence of explosive gases, including those which may occur naturally in the colon especially after certain forms of bowel preparation such as mannitol
3. *Burns:* these are the most common type of diathermy accidents in both open and endoscopic surgery. These may occur as a result of:
   a) Faulty application of the indifferent electrode with inadequate contact area
   b) The patient being earthed by touching any metal object, e.g. a leg touching the metal stirrups used in maintaining the lithotomy position
   c) Faulty insulation of the diathermy leads, either due to cracked insulation or instruments such as towel clips pinching the cable
   d) Inadvertent activity such as the accidental activation of the foot pedal, or accidental contact of the active electrode with other metal instruments such as retractors
4. *Channelling:* if current passes up a narrow channel or pedicle to the active electrode, enough heat may be generated within this channel or pedicle to coagulate the tissues (Fig. 25). This can prove disastrous, e.g.:
   a) Coagulation of the penis in a child undergoing circumcision
   b) Coagulation of the spermatic cord when the electrode is applied to the testis
5. *Pacemakers:* pacemakers are designed to be inhibited by high frequency interference, so that the patient may receive no pacing simulation at all while the diathermy is in use. Certain demand pacemakers may revert to the fixed rate of pacing and therefore it would be important for the anaesthetist to have a magnet available so that these can be re-set if necessary. In most cases it is therefore wise to undertake precautions and to use bipolar diathermy wherever possible. If monopolar diathermy is required, then the patient plate should be sited as far away from the pacemaker as possible so that the path of the current does not pass through the heart or the vicinity of the pacemaker.
6. *Laparoscopic surgery:* Diathermy burns are a particular hazard of laparoscopic surgery due to the nature of the visibility of the instrumentation and the actual structure of the instruments used. Such burns may occur by:
   a) Diathermy of the wrong structure because of lack of clarity of vision
   b) Faulty insulation of any of the laparoscopic instruments or equipment
   c) Intraperitoneal contact of the diathermy with another metal instrument
   d) Inadvertent activation of the pedal while the diathermy tip is out of vision of the camera
   e) Retained heat in the diathermy tip touching susceptible structures such as bowel
   f) Capacitance coupling (Fig. 26)

This is a phenomenon in which a capacitor is created by having an insulator sandwiched between two metal electrodes. This can be created in situations where there is a metal laparoscopic port and the diathermy hook is passed through it. The insulation of the diathermy hook acts as the sandwiched insulator and by means of electromagnetic induction, the diathermy current flowing through the hook can induce a current in the metal port, which can potentially damage intraperitoneal structures. In most cases this current is dissipated from the metal port through the abdominal wall, but if a plastic cuff is used, this dissipation of current does not occur and the danger of capacitance coupling is significantly increased. Therefore, metal ports should never be used with a plastic cuff. The danger of capacitance coupling can be completely prevented by using entirely plastic ports.

Figure 25

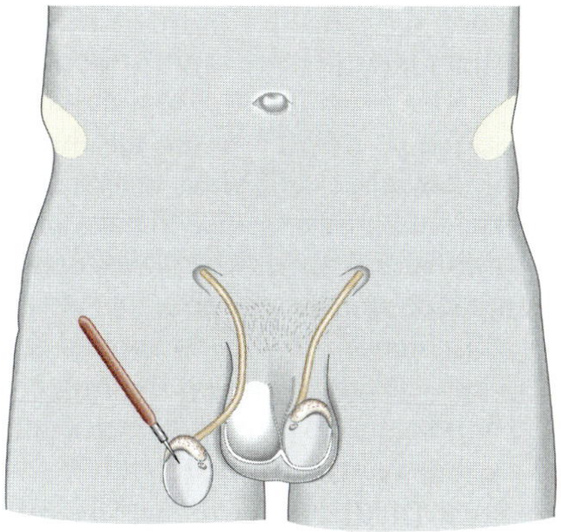

Figure 26

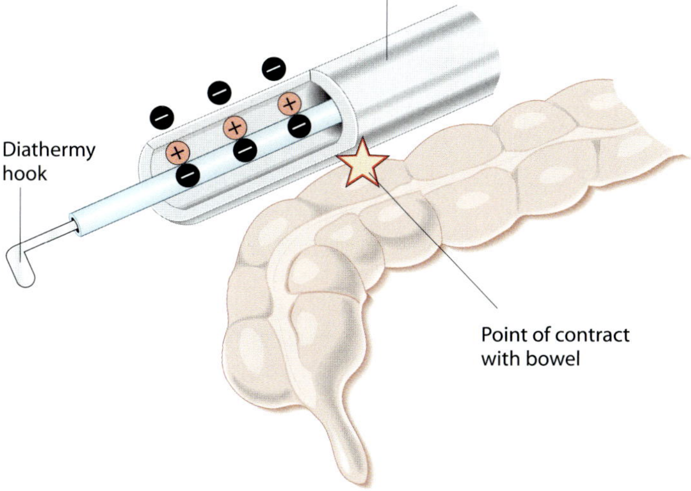

2

## Figure 27, 28: Tourniquets

For certain operations on the limbs, a bloodless field is essential for careful and safe surgery. In these situations it may be advisable to utilise a tourniquet. The principles behind its use include emptying the limb of blood by elevating it for 5 min and then applying a tourniquet around the proximal aspect of the limb over some layers of cotton wool padding or orthopaedic wool. The limb can be further exsanguinated by applying a 3 inch Esmarch bandage (Fig. 27), starting at the tips of the digits and overlapping each turn proximally, thus further emptying the limb of blood. Other sleeve-like appliances are now available to achieve the same purpose. The tourniquet is then inflated to just above systemic arterial blood pressure in the upper limb and to twice the systemic arterial blood pressure for the lower limb. The Esmarch bandage is then unwound. It is important to record the time at which the tourniquet was applied as it is conventional practice to limit tourniquet time to 1 h. If necessary the tourniquet may be released after 1 h and subsequently reinflated if further operative time is required. At the end of the procedure the tourniquet is released before the wound is closed to ensure that all bleeding points have been secured. The use of a tourniquet is contraindicated in limbs affected by vascular disease as this could result in either ischaemia or venous thrombosis. Furthermore tourniquets should be avoided in many cases of trauma in which there is soft tissue injury, infection or bony fractures.

The tourniquet principle is utilised in the technique of a Bier's block for the arm. In this case an intravenous cannula is inserted into a suitable vein of the limb and it is wise to have a similar cannula in the opposite limb for vascular access throughout the procedure. Once a cannula has been sited a double cuff tourniquet (Fig. 28) is applied to the upper arm, the limb elevated and exsanguinated using an Esmarch bandage. The proximal tourniquet is then inflated to above arterial pressure and the Esmarch bandage removed; 30 ml of 0.5% prilocaine may be injected through the intravenous cannula, and once instilled the second distal cuff should be inflated to above arterial pressure, thus allowing some of the prilocaine to have infiltrated below the second cuff, producing a degree of anaesthesia at that site and reducing discomfort for the patient. The double cuff technique is to ensure that if one cuff happened to fail, the prilocaine is not allowed back into the circulation too early. Neither cuff should be deflated in less than 15 min to allow time for the anaesthetic to become fixed within the tissues and the early release of the tourniquet can have disastrous effects causing arrhythmias and even fits. Many surgeons would prefer to keep the cuffs up for 30 min in this situation.

Figure 27

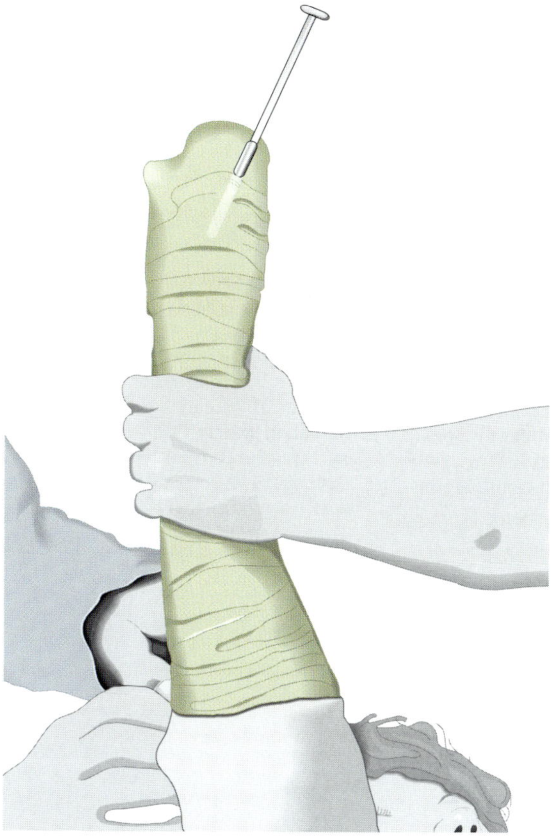

Figure 28

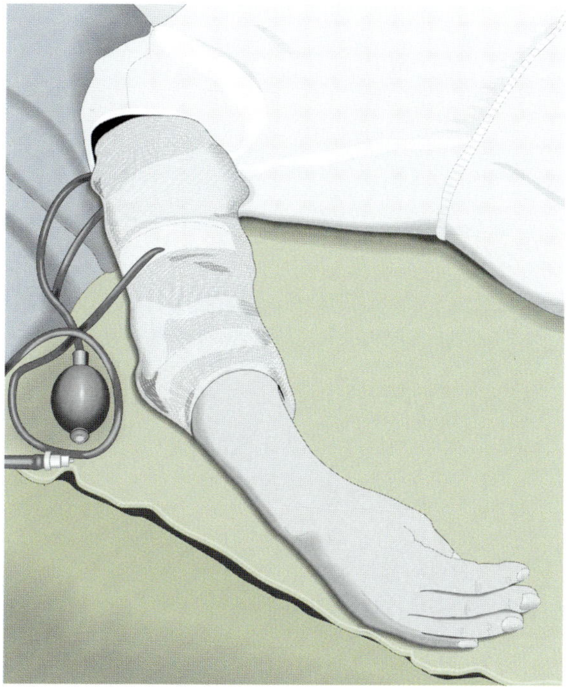

2

## CONCLUSION

In order for short stay surgery to be effective and safe there is no short cut to good results, other than a clear adherence to safe and sound surgical technique. Those described above are certainly not the only safe techniques but represent well accepted approaches that if adopted will result in optimal outcomes. Any departure from sound technique will result in suboptimal results and give short stay surgery a bad name. However if adopted, then short stay surgery can be applied to almost all areas of the body as are described in the subsequent chapters of this book.

## SELECTED REFERENCES

1. Thomas WEG (2002) Sutures, ligature materials and staples. Surgery 20:97–99
2. Thomas WEG (2000) Sutures, staples and knots. In: Tooli J, Russell R, Devitt P, Ingham Clark C (eds) Integrated basic surgical sciences. Arnold, London, pp 714–725
3. Kirk RM (1994) Basic surgical techniques. Churchill Livingstone, Edinburgh
4. Royal College of Surgeons of England (2002) Basic surgical skills – the Intercollegiate Participants Handbook. Royal College of Surgeons of England, London
5. Jaibaji M, Morton JD, Green AR (2001) Dog ear: an overview of causes and treatment. Ann R Coll Surg Engl 83:136–138
6. Jayaweera RLA (2000) Diathermy. In: Tooli J, Russell R, Devitt P, Ingham Clark C (eds) Integrated basic surgical sciences. Arnold, London, pp 726–732

Part II

# Skin and Subcutaneous Tissues

CHAPTER 3

# Plastic Surgery

Jutta Liebau, Norbert Senninger

## INTRODUCTION

A variety of surgical procedures involving skin and subcutaneous tissue can be performed on the basis of short stay surgery. A knowledge of the basic principles and techniques is mandatory for a successful outcome for the patient. This chapter describes the basic techniques in detail for practical use within any surgical discipline. Anatomical details and possible pitfalls are mentioned. We demonstrate the principles of local and distant flaps in reconstructive surgery as well as technical aspects of skin grafts. Lesions such as benign and malignant tumors are included in this chapter as well as scar repair techniques.

3

## Figure 1A, B: Plastic Surgical Procedures

The anatomy of the skin and the vascular perfusion are important for any surgical planning (Fig. 1: A, random pattern flap; B, axial pattern flap). Planning defect closure requires a knowledge of the relaxed skin tension lines (RSTLs), the tissue quality, the amount of skin excess and the anatomical limits. The experienced plastic surgeon plans the procedure taking into account the surrounding tissue, in order to decide on the most appropriate method of defect closure. This whole procedure begins with planning the incision. The majority of surgery on the face and the scalp can be performed on an outpatient basis.

**Figure 1A, B**

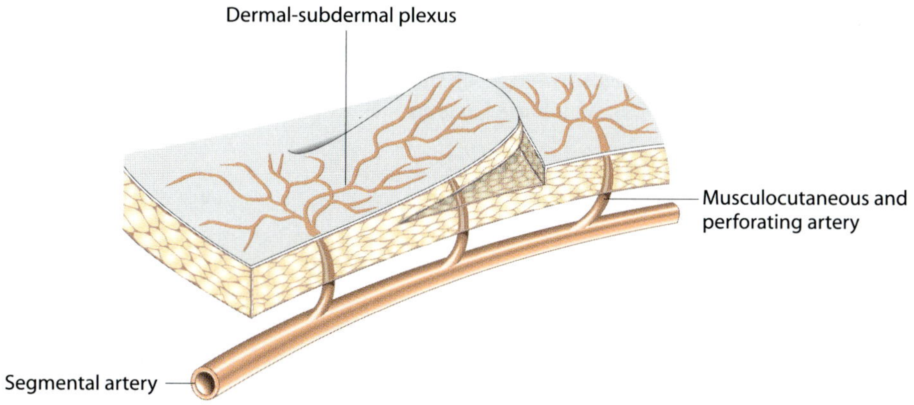
Dermal-subdermal plexus
Musculocutaneous and perforating artery
Segmental artery

**A**

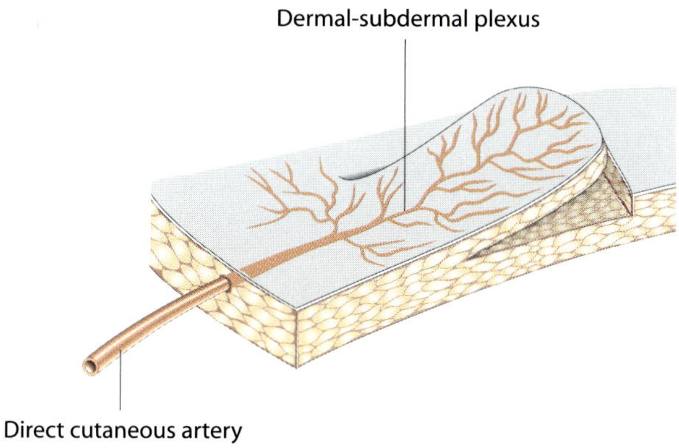
Dermal-subdermal plexus
Direct cutaneous artery

**B**

## Figure 2A–C: Planning the Incision

Planning the appropriate incision is the key to inconspicuous scar formation in plastic surgery. The basis of incision planning is a detailed knowledge of the relaxed skin tension lines (RSTLs), which are lines in the skin that run according to the lines of minimal skin tension (Fig. 2: A, RSTLs and intrinsic muscles of the face; B–G: RSTLs modified from A.F. Borges and B. Konz; B, frontal view; C, dorsal view).

Figure 2A–C

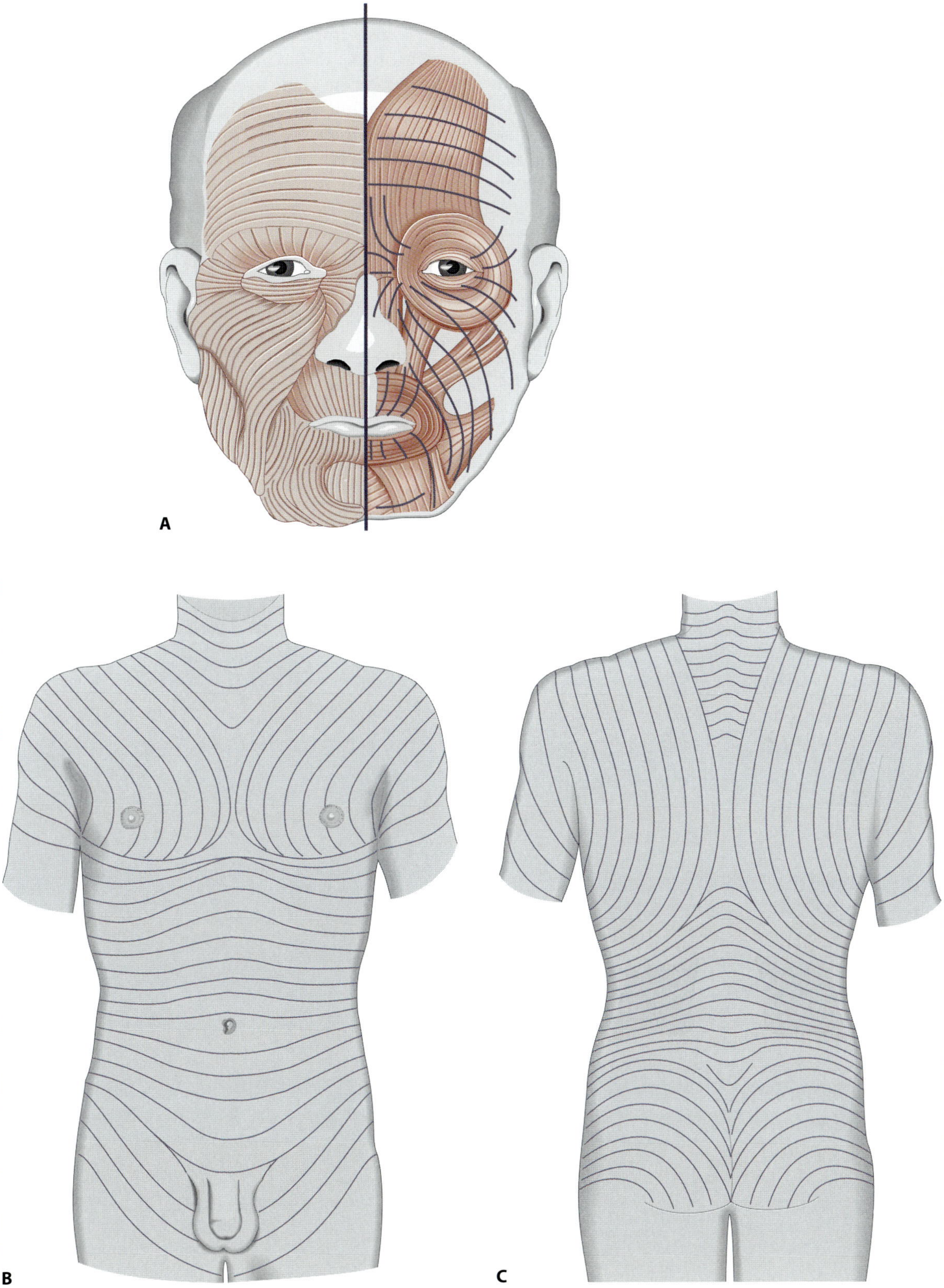

## Figure 2D–G: Planning the Incision

RSTLs modified from A.F. Borges and B. Konz; D, upper extremities; E, lower extremities; F, head, frontal view; G head, side view). In the face particularly, these lines form the basis of surgical planning in order to minimise the degree of scarring. Even simple excision of a skin lesion must take into account the RSTLs at all times. The resulting scar should follow these skin lines in order to be as inconspicuous as possible.

The direction of the actual incision through the skin is also important for primary wound healing and inconspicuous scarring. A 90° incision is usually the appropriate angle for cutting the skin. In the hair bearing region of the scalp the angle must take into account the hair roots. The cut should be parallel to the hair roots in order to avoid alopecia.

Figure 2D–G

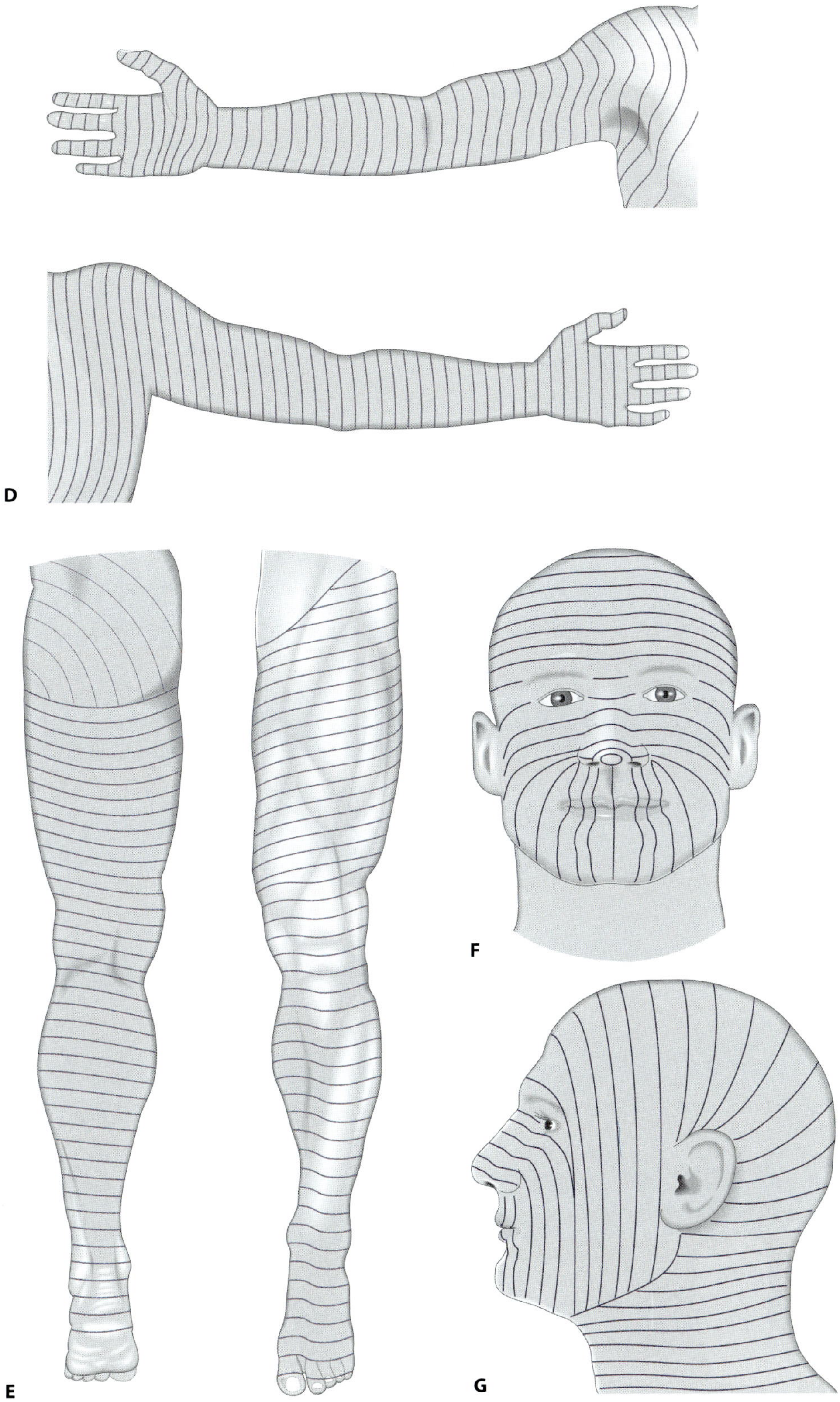

## Figure 3A–C: Suture Techniques

A technically perfect suture technique is the prerequisite for inconspicuous scarring. Depending on the localisation, wound formation and skin tension, different suture techniques are applied

## Figure 3A, B

Fig. 3: A, Running subcutaneous suture and subcuticular suture
Fig. 3: B1, Interrupted sutures
B2, Vertical mattress suture
B3, Intracuticular mattress suture

Figure 3A

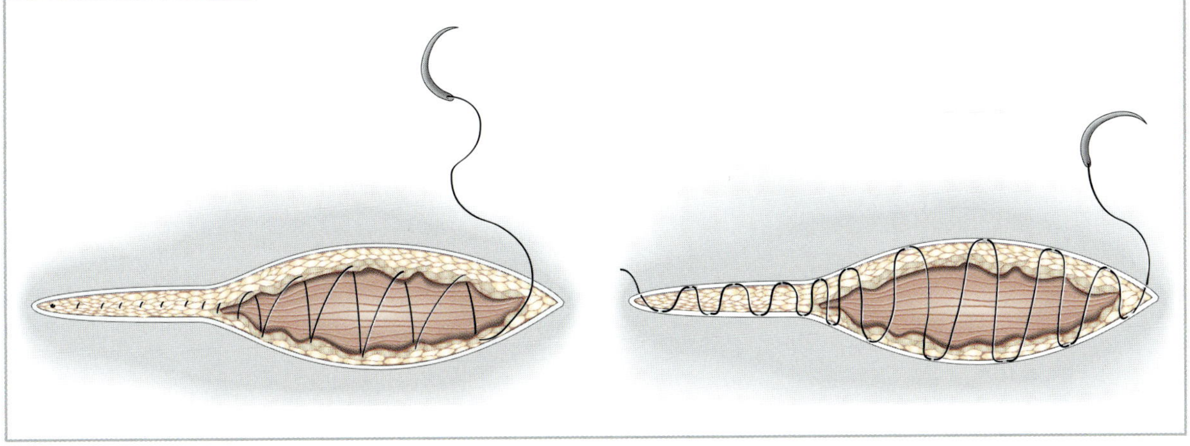

Figure 3B1

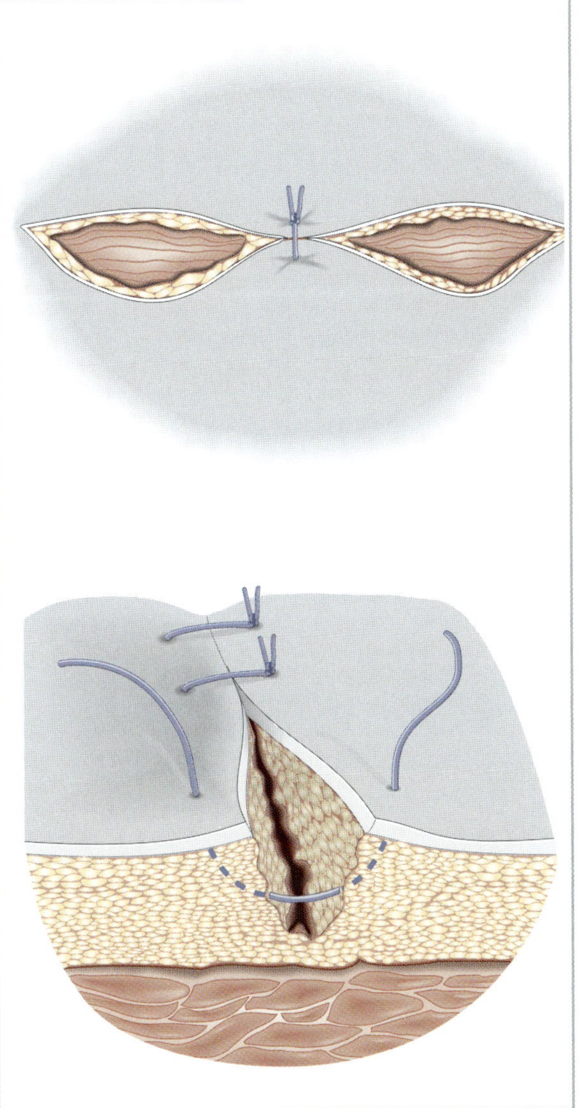

Figure 3B2, 3

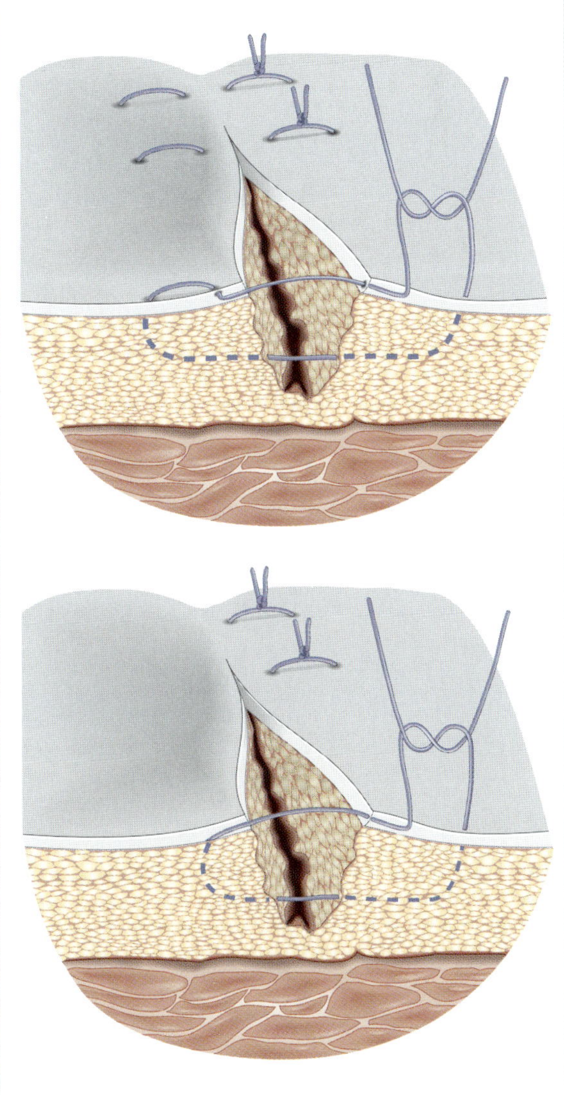

## Figure 3C



Equalisation of different lengths of the wound margin may be achieved by parting the distance into half. Wound closure without tension is the key to satisfactory scar formation. For good wound adaptation a perfect subcutaneous suture with hidden knots is necessary.

Figure 3C1

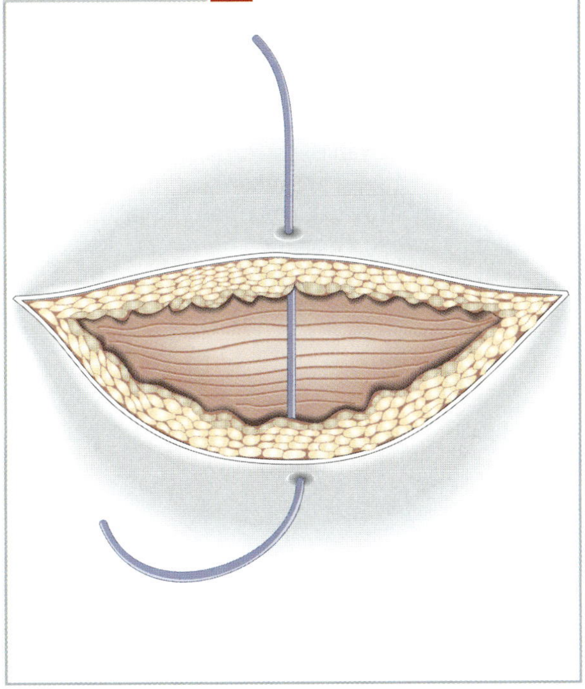

Figure 3C2

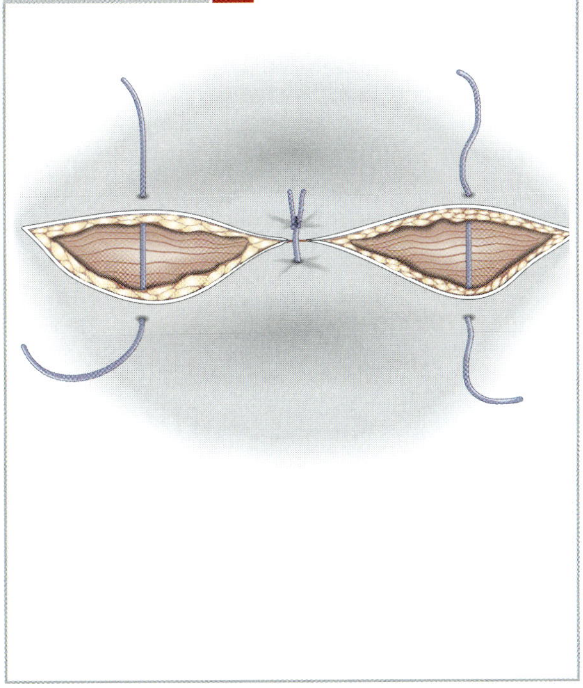

Figure 3C3

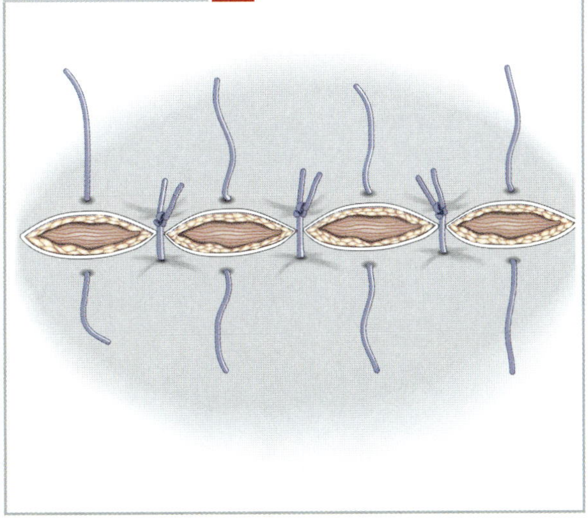

Figure 3C4

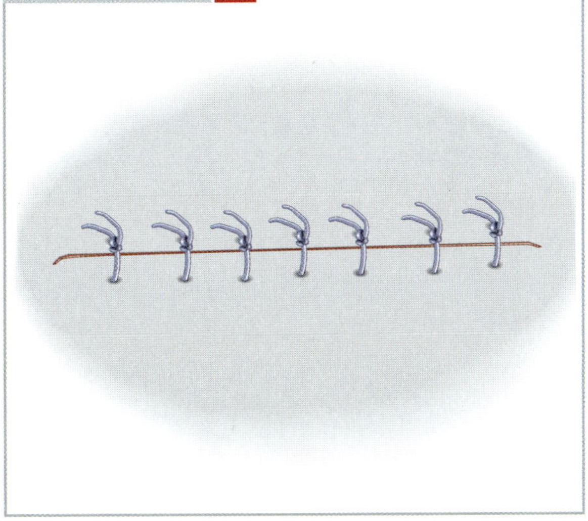

**Figure 4: W-Technique for Dealing with Old Scar**

Depending on the original scar, the RSTLs are evaluated and the scar is excised and broken in a running-w manner in order to cover the old scar line. A running-w is less conspicuous in the long term than the original scar. Initially, however, it might lead to a more visible scar which will fade and become inconspicuous with time.

**Figure 5: Broken-Line Technique**

Scars can also be hidden with the broken-line procedure. This technique is a favoured option for scar corrections particularly in the face. Incisions with different lengths and angles are made that ideally meet in the RSTL. As in all scar corrections, the primary early result may lead to an aggravation of the scar.

Figure 4

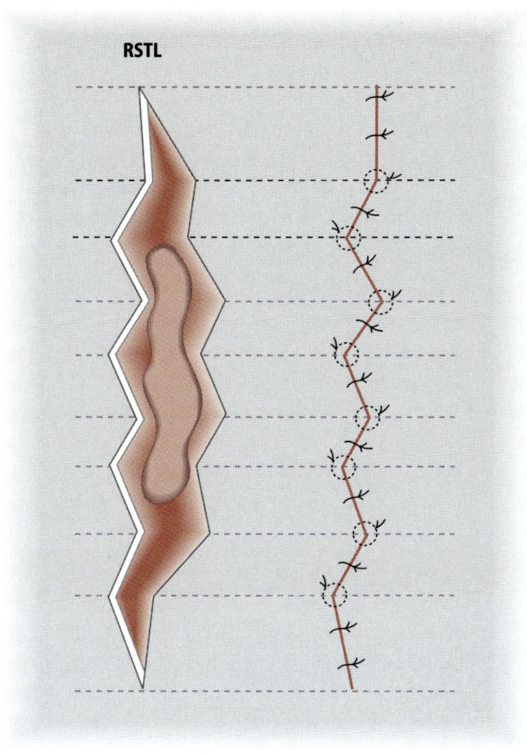


Figure 5

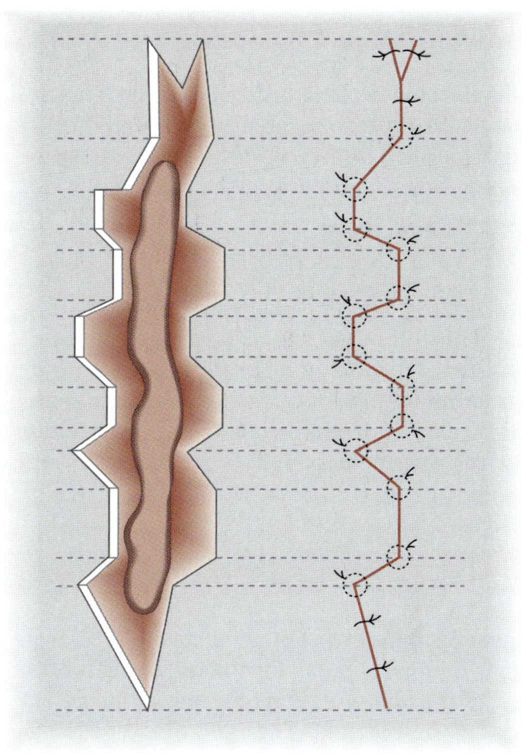

## LOCAL FLAPS AND SKIN TRANSFER

### Figure 6: Z-Plasty

Different gain of length dependant on angles in z-plasty: the bigger the angle the more the gain of length followed by loss of width. The Z-plasty is a frequently used technique in plastic surgery all over the body. If planned at different angles, usually 60°, the Z-plasty reduces the strength of the scar traction (Fig. 6: top, gain in length through loss of width; bottom, different length gains with different cutting angles). This technique can be used in one or a series of Z-plasties depending on the localisation and degree of traction on the scar. One has to take into account that the gain in length is due to the reduction of the transverse diameter.

### Figure 7: VY-Plasty

The YV- or VY-plasty is a technique by which a flap of skin is transferred to cover the defect, leaving a V- or Y-shaped scar (Fig. 7: left, YV-plasty; right, VY-plasty). A combination of these techniques is frequently necessary in order to achieve a satisfactory postoperative result.

## Flap Surgery

In general, different arrangements of vascular perfusion will impact on flap formation. Using this knowledge of the anatomical arrangement, the defect closure can be planned. The type of perfusion determines the type of tissue transfer, and most are random pattern flaps. The procedure is planned according to well defined criteria for the type of tissue to be included. In surgery of the face and scalp, most flap diameters can exceed the recommendet base: length ratio due to the good blood supply in this area.

## Local Flaps

### Figure 8A, B: Rhomboid Flap (Triple Rhomboid Flap)

For square defect closure especially in the scalp region, the rhomboid (Fig. 8A) or triple rhomboid flap (Fig. 8B) can be used. The defect from the flap elevation site can usually be closed without tension.

Figure 6

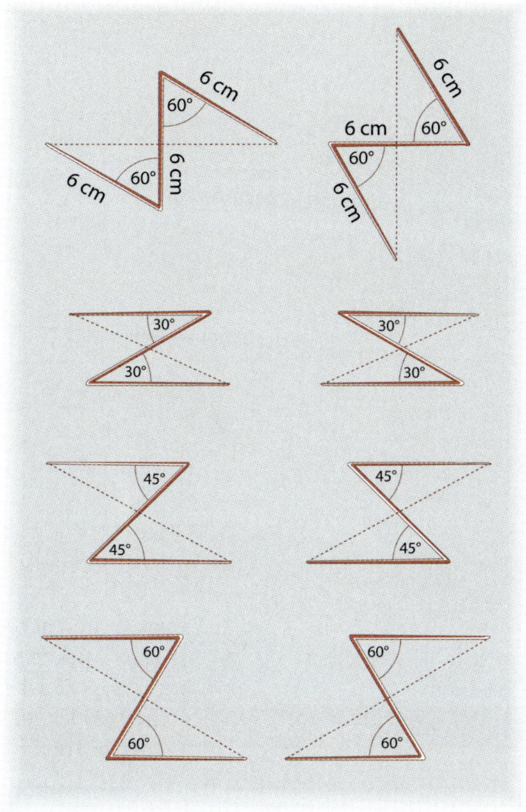


Figure 7

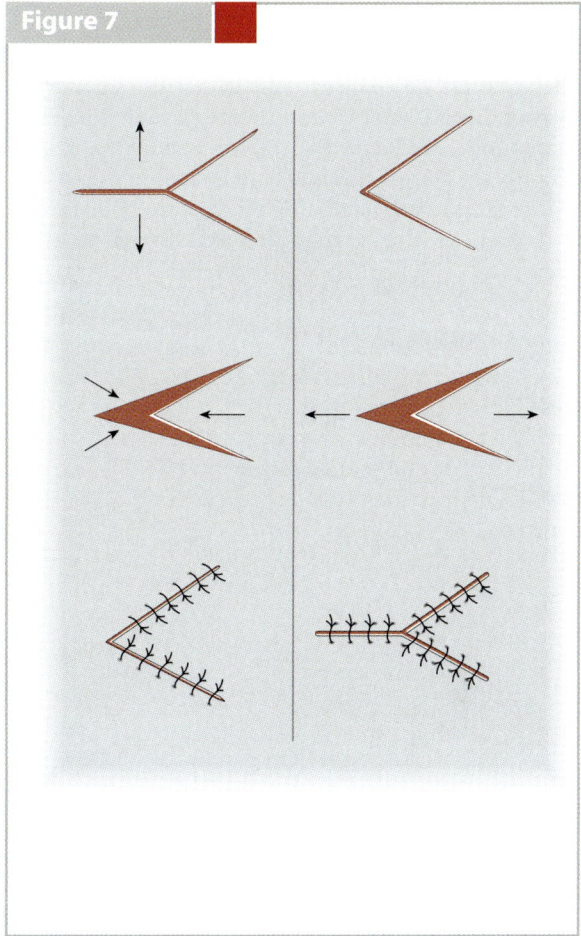

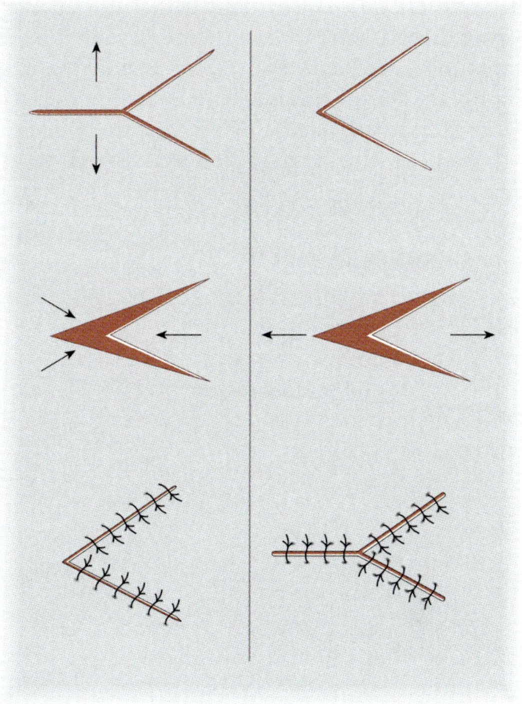

Figure 8A

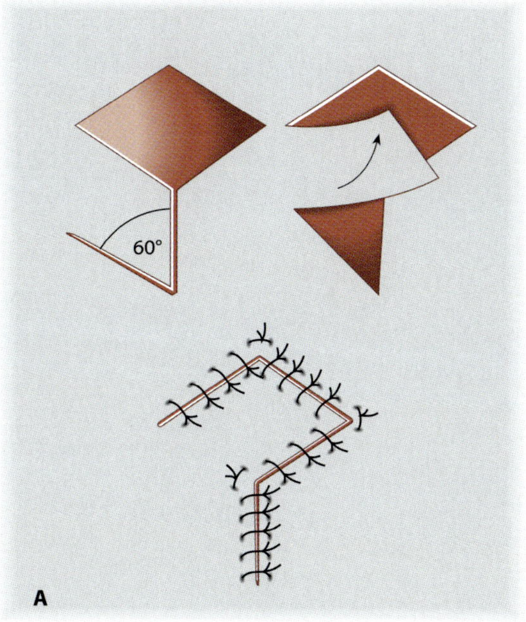


Figure 8B

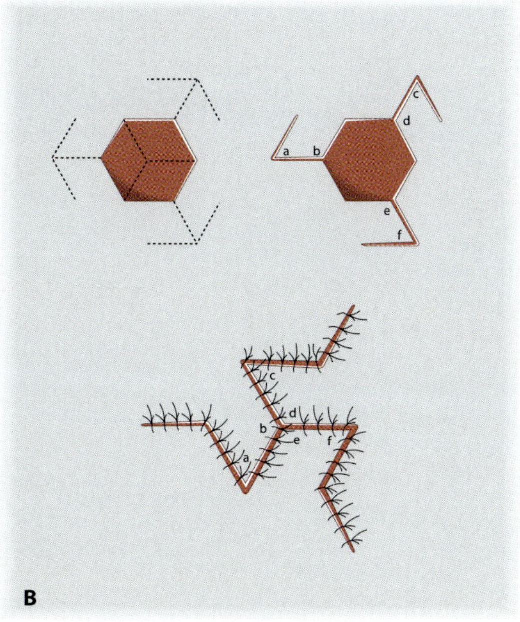

## Figure 9A, B: Rotation Flap

The rotation flap closes defects by mobilising the surrounding tissue in a rotational manner. For ideal adaptation, a back cut (Fig. 9A) or a triangle excision (Fig. 9B: the Burow triangle) can be helpful. This procedure is used especially for the closure of scalp defects, and can also be modified as a double rotation flap.

## Figure 10: Rotation Flap

Double rotation movement according to Webster.

## Figure 11A–C: Bilobed Flap

For small round defects located especially on the nose or cheek, the bilobed flap is an option for defect closure. The angle of rotation of the flaps should be 90–100°, and the area of the second flap should be closed primarily without tension. A Burow triangle must be excised at the base of the defect.

## Figure 12: VY-Subcutaneous Gliding Flap

The VY-subcutaneous gliding flap is a method of tissue transportation suitable in many situations, especially for defects of the nose or the frontal region of the face. It is an island flap with the remaining blood supply at the base of the gliding tissue. Prolonged lymphedema might be a disadvantage of this procedure.

Figure 9A, B

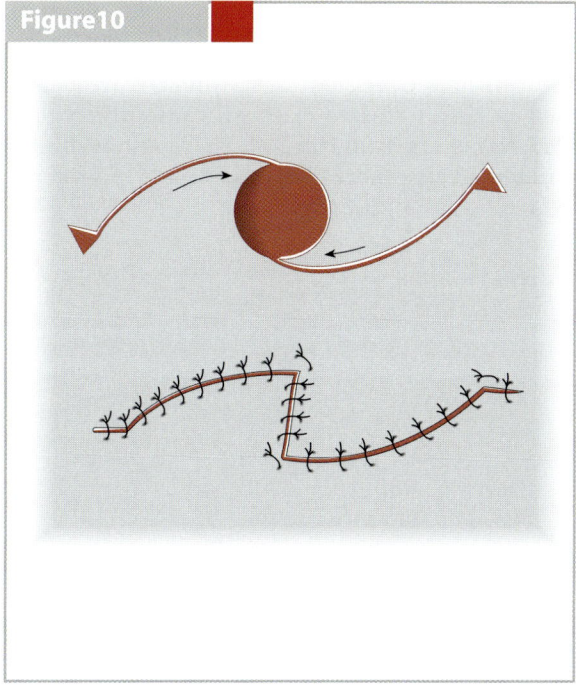

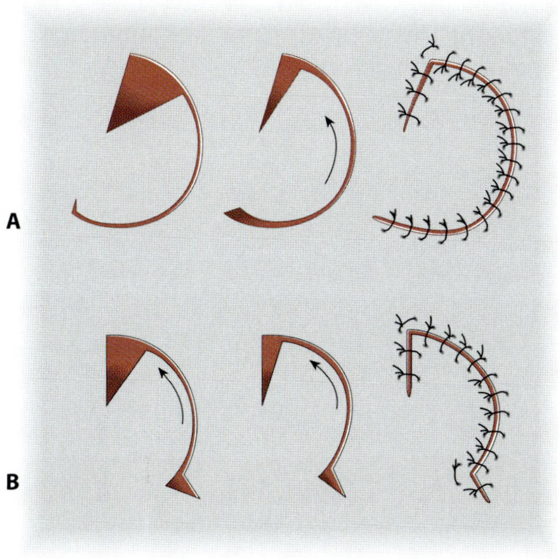


Figure 10

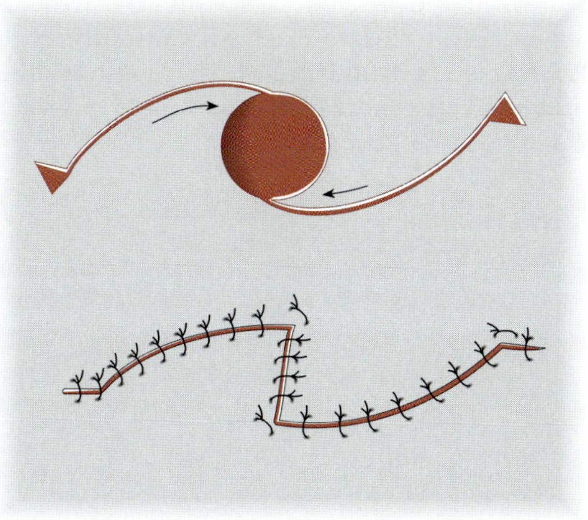

Figure 11A–C

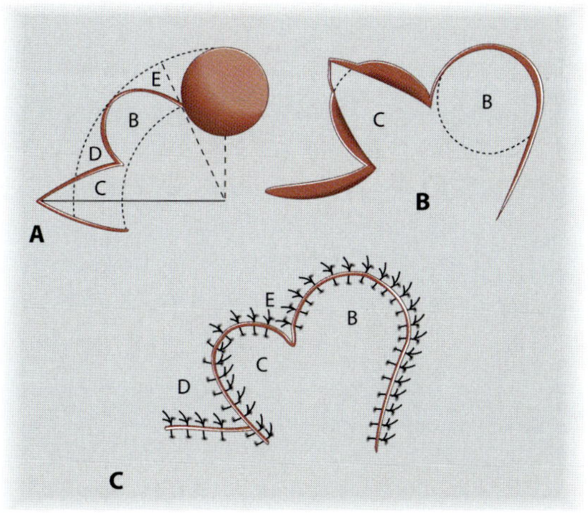


Figure 12

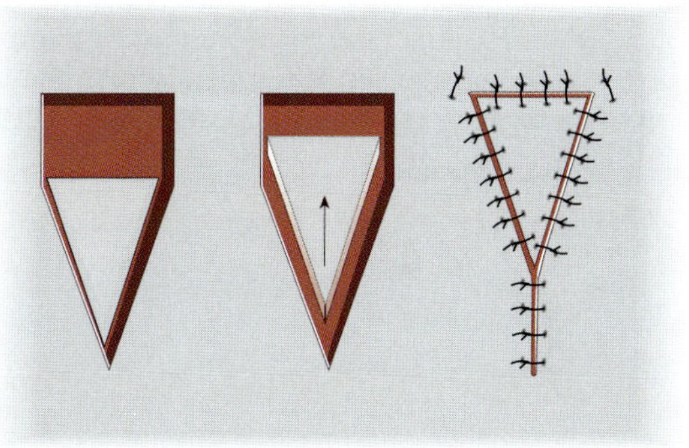

## Figure 13: Transposition Flap

The principle of tissue transposition is frequently used in defect closure (Fig. 13: transposition flap; LMT, line of maximal tension). The length/width ratio should be no more than 2:1. The line of maximal tension must be considered in the planning of this technique. The area of tissue donation must be closed without tension.

## Local Flaps in the Face and Scalp

### Hair Bearing Region

#### Figures 14A–D: Scalp Rotation Flap

In defects of the hair bearing region, a scalp rotation flap may be used to close the defect. Due to the lack of skin excess and the difficulty of mobilising the scalp tissue, the dimension of the rotation must be planned to be of sufficient size, but is frequently planned too small. If necessary, the donor side is closed with a split thickness skin graft.

A Tumor in the scalp area
B Defect after tumor excision
C,D Intraoperative view and defect closure after scalp rotation flap

Figure 13

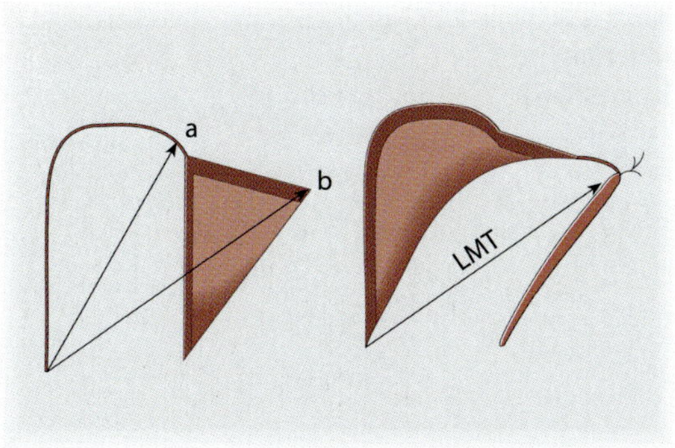


Figure 14A

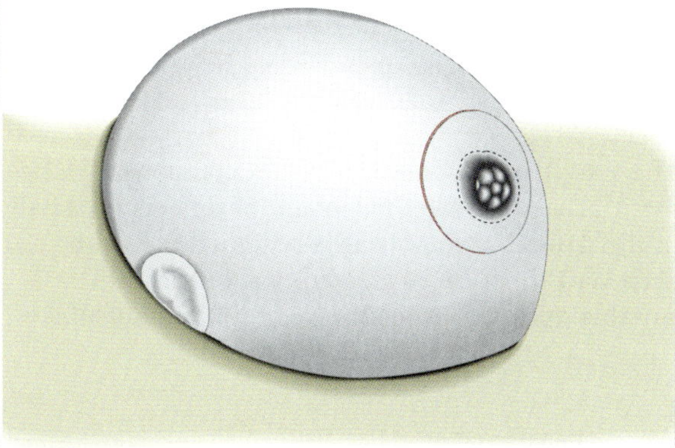

Figure 14B

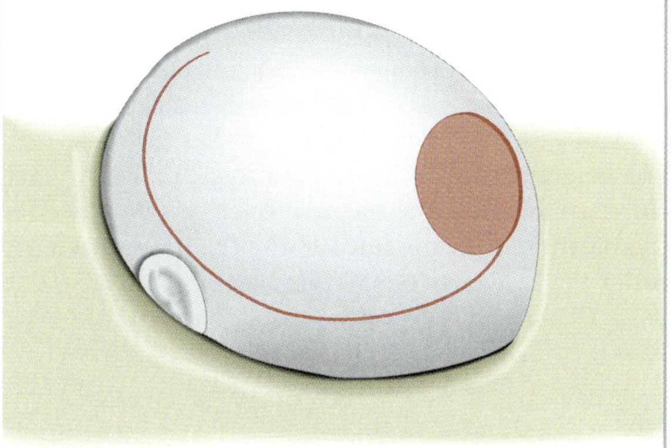

Figure 14C

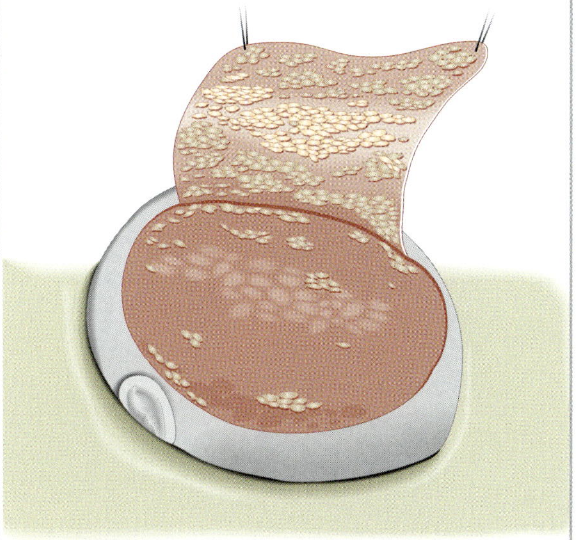

Figure 14D

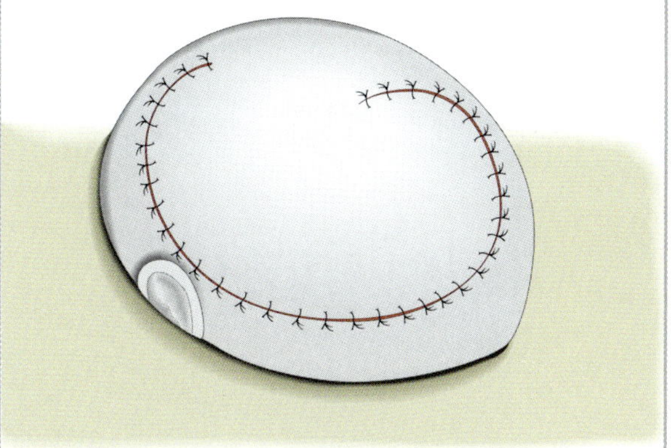

## Figure 15: Scalp Rotation Flap

Double rotation flap with split thickness skin grafts at the donor area. Again the resulting defects may be closed by free skin transfer (indicated by reddish colour).



# Frontal Region

## Figure 16A, B: Burow Excision Kite Flap

For defect closure in the frontal region, Burow excisions are helpful. The incision lines can be placed in the hairline or in the lines of the frontal wrinkles in order to achieve inconspicuous scars.

The kite flap is a double VY-subcutaneous advancement procedure for the closure of defects especially in the frontal region. In this region, the hairline and eyebrows must be respected, so the procedure is a suitable option for the closure of limited defects.

Figure 15

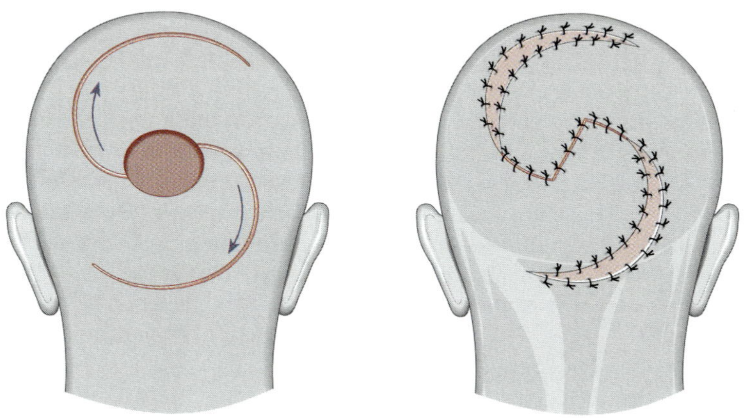

Figure 16A

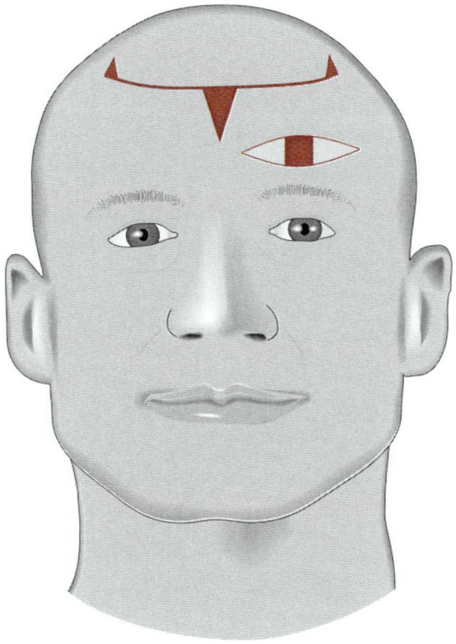

Figure 16B

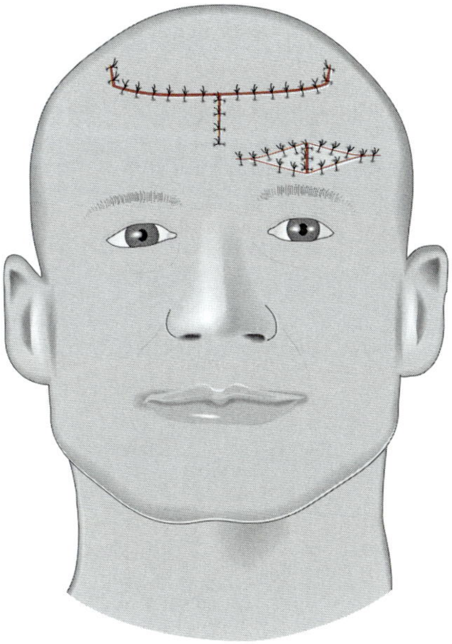

## The Region of the Eye

### Figure 17A, B and Figure 18A, B

3

The eye region is a challenge in plastic surgery. The eyelids with their tarsal support, lateral and medial canthus and lacrimal duct include anatomical structures which have to be conserved in order to achieve a good functional result after reconstruction. A brief overview of this region will give an idea of the complexity of this subject while not seeking to provide a comprehensive review.

Surgery for defects close to the eye depends on the localisation, size and depth of the defect and the anatomical structures involved.

The easiest method of defect closure is the wedge-excision. In defects of more than 6–8 mm, a lateral or medial canthotomy is necessary (Fig. 17: A, skin and orbicularis incised to reveal lateral canthal tendon; B, lid margin and skin incision closed; lateral canthal area closed).

For bigger defects, advancement procedures might be helpful (Fig. 18).

Figure 17A

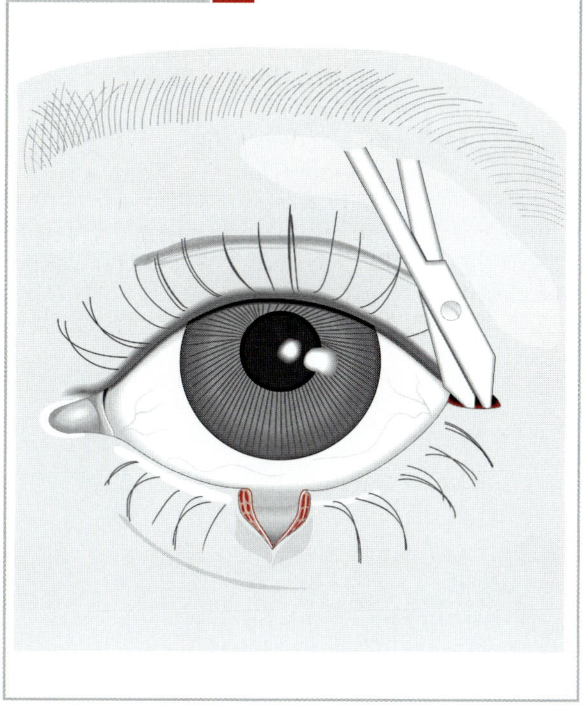

Figure 17B

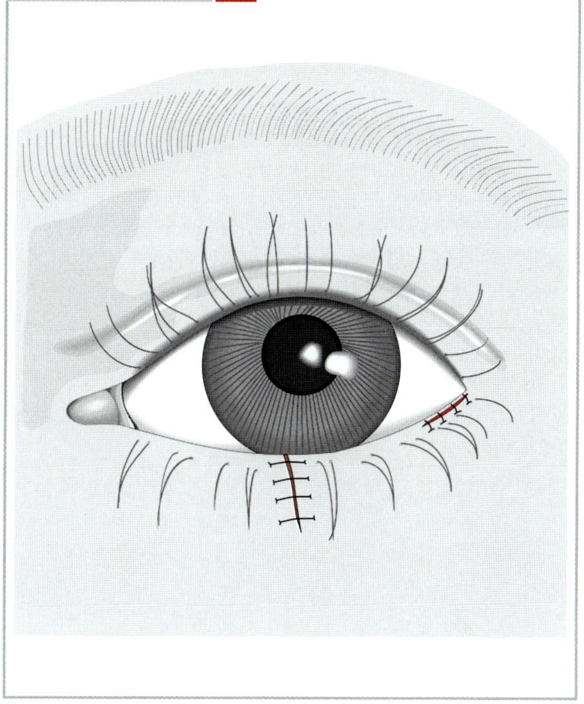

Figure 18A

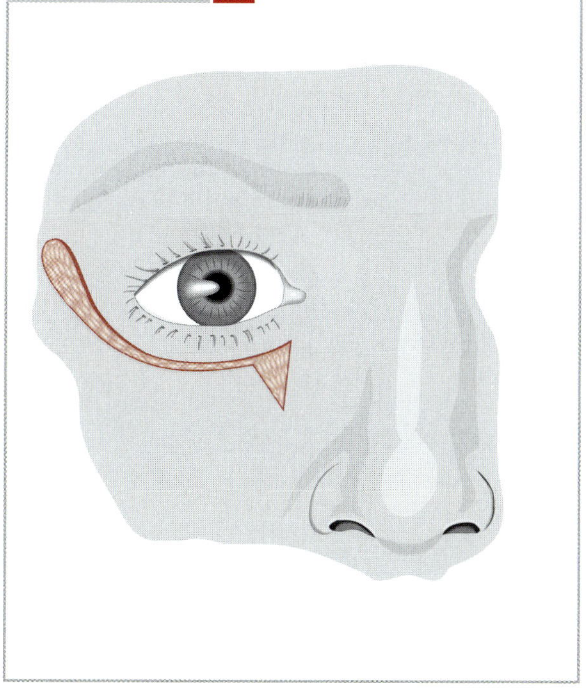

Figure 18B

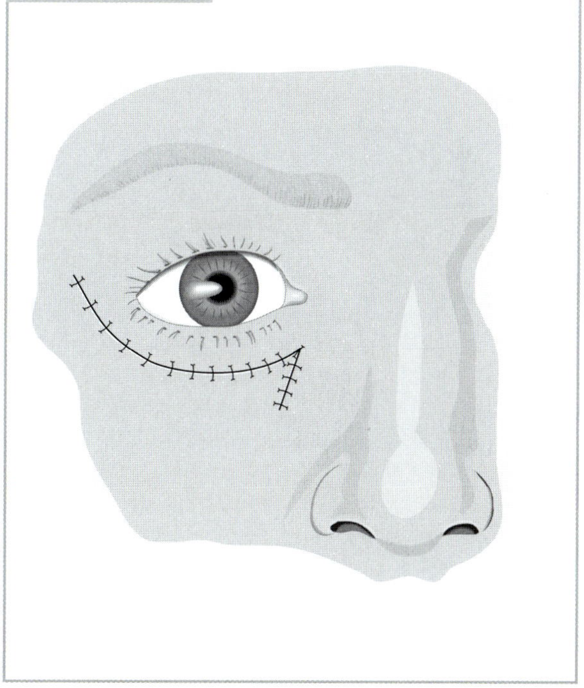

## Figure 19A, B

For extended defects the cheek rotation flap is an option (Fig. 19).

Figure 19A, B

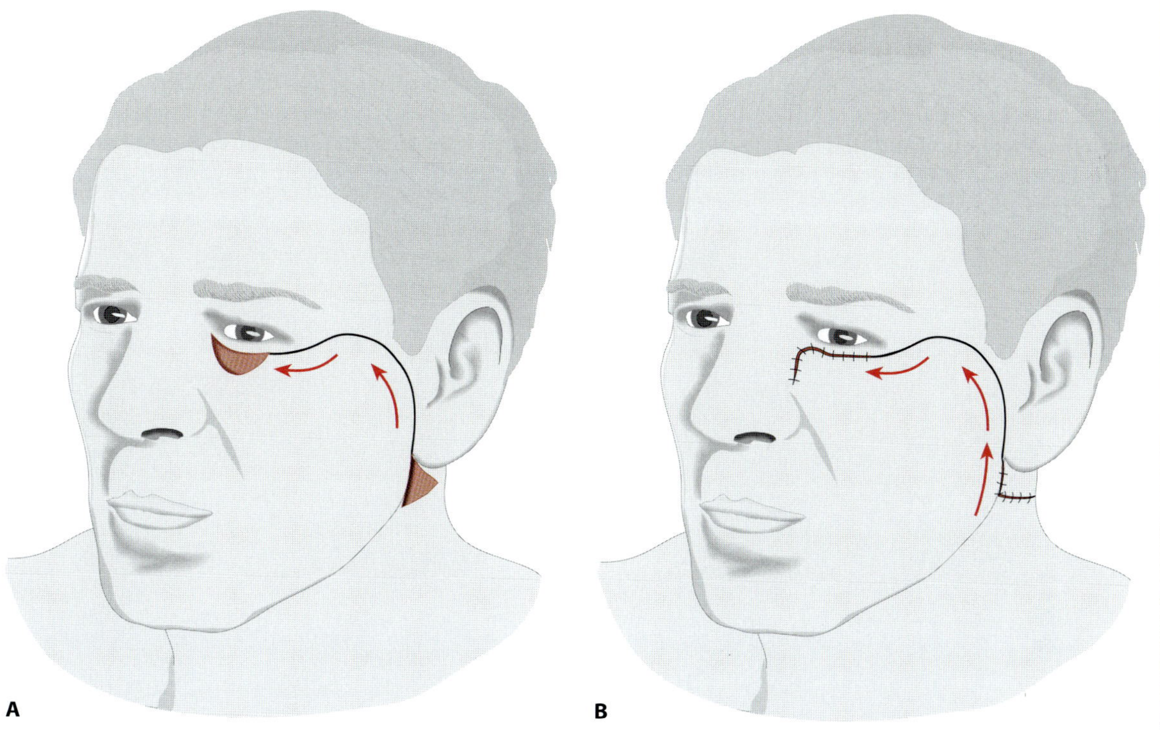

## Figure 20A, B

In the case of tarsal defects the tarsal reconstruction can be performed with tarsomarginal transplants from the other eyelid, and cartilage from the ear or the nasal septum. For a cheek rotation flap the site of incision is important: it should run cranial to the level of the lateral canthus in order to avoid ectropion.

Lateral or medial transposition flaps from the upper lid including the muscle sheet can be used for defect coverage close to the lower lid (Fig. 20: A/B, medial). This is an excellent technique to avoid ectropion. In a second operation after 8–10 weeks the flap base may be released and the contour optimised, if necessary.

Figure 20A, B

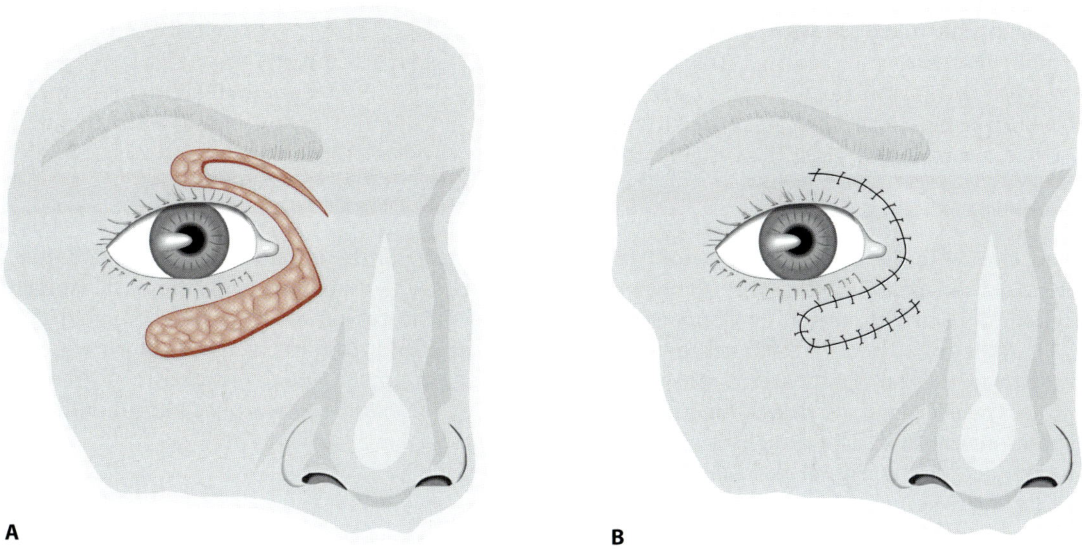

## Nose

The nose is divided into anatomical regions: the dorsum with nasal root, lateral aspect, tip, ala cartilage region and columella.

### Figure 21A–C: Glabella Flap

For defect closure in the area of the nose root and the medial area of the medial canthus, the glabella flap is an excellent option with very little donor site morbidity. The skin excess between the eyebrows is used, and the scar in the donor site area is hidden in the frown line. The eyebrows are drawn together as a result of this manoeuvre. The dimension of this flap can be extended for bigger defects such as an extended glabella flap, where the diameter of the flap reaches towards the hairline.

### Figure 22A–C: Marchac Flap

For defects of the dorsum, the Marchac flap is used. This tissue is mobilised from the nasal dorsum and the glabella region to cover defects up to the nasal tip. In defects close to the nasal tip for which an extended version of this flap is used, a degree of elevation of the nasal tip is a possible side effect of this method.

Figure 21A–C

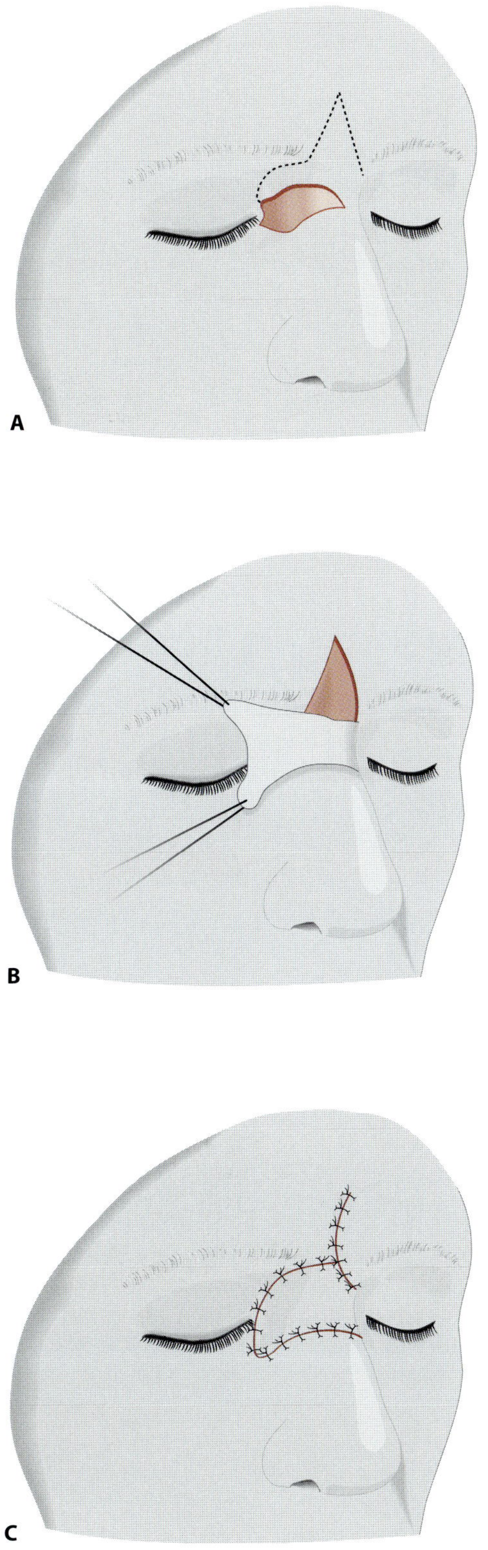


Figure 22A–C

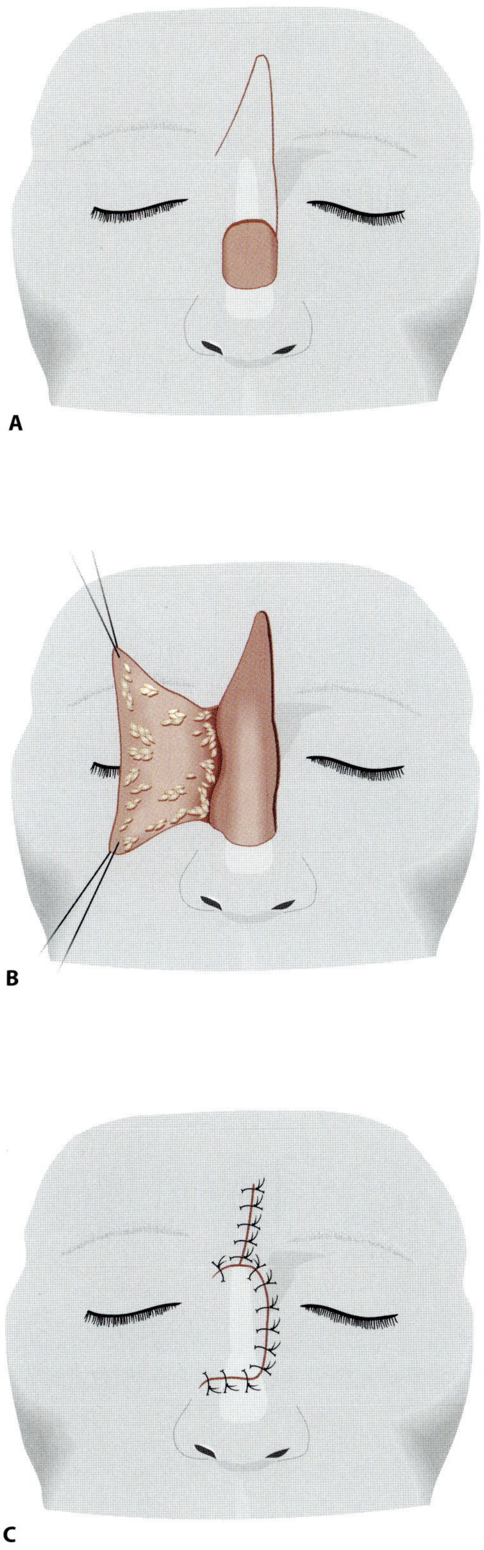

## Figure 23A–C: Nasolabial Flap



The nasolabial flap is an ideal and simple method with variable size and elevation options for defects in the area of the ala region. Its base should be planned depending on the size and localisation of the defect. The flap can be extended in size paranasally towards the cheek for nose reconstruction.

Figure 23A–C

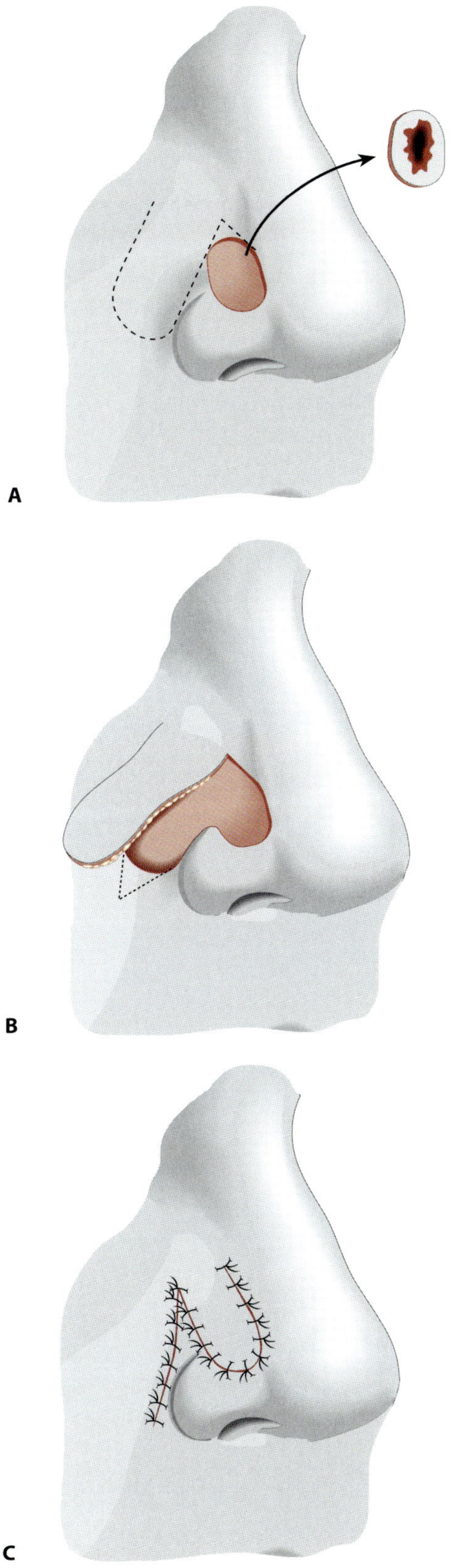

## Cheek Area

In the cheek area, many of the techniques mentioned above are applied: VY-advancement, transposition flap, bilobed flap, rhomboid flap and others.



## Figure 24A–C: Cheek Rotation Flap

For extended cheek defects, the cheek rotation is a valuable flap with a number of variations (Fig. 24: cheek rotation flap according to Esser). The flap design can be extended towards the neck. A back cut extends the radius of the transposition. Important for flap design is the amount of tissue between the defect and the hairline. This distance must be big enough to cover the original defect. The cheek tissue is mobilised cranially and then used to cover the defect using the rotation technique.

Figure 24A–C

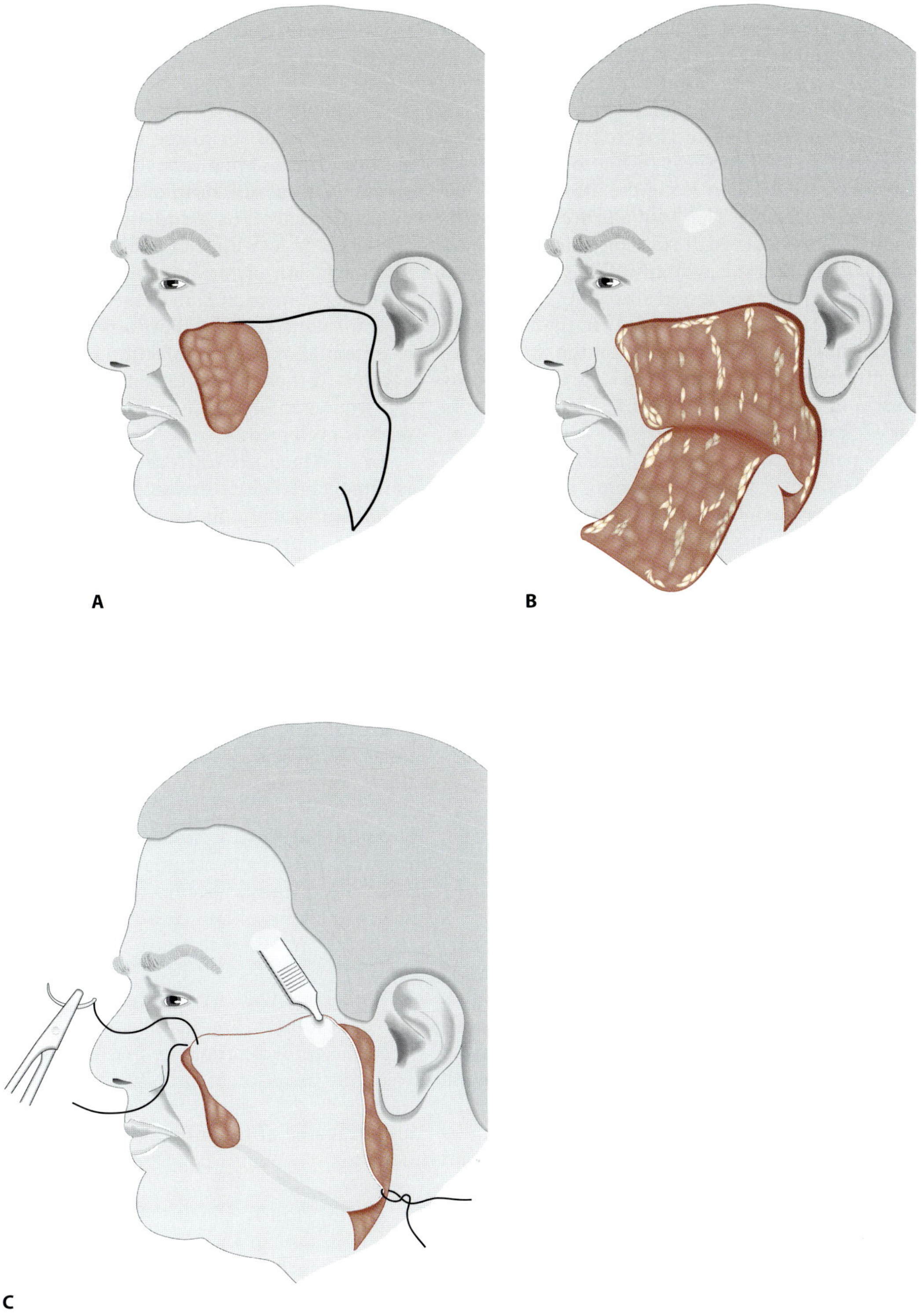

3

### Extremities, Trunk

For reconstruction of defects in the upper and lower extremities and in the trunk, the general principles of plastic surgery and flap design are again applied. The easiest method of defect closure is the mobilisation of tissue around the defect. This technique is limited in its extent. To avoid dog ear formation, a moderate extension of the incision along the axis of the original defect is necessary. The "lazy-S procedure" results in a moderate S-curved formation that should respect the RSTL and the anatomy. With transposition flaps, tissue can be transferred according to the RSTL lines and the amount of tissue laxity in the surrounding area. For sufficient flap perfusion the 2 : 1 length:-base ratio should not be exceeded (Fig. 13). Including the fascia in the flap makes the flap transfer safer in terms of blood supply.

Axial pattern flaps are flaps based on a defined blood vessel. In these flaps the length:base ratio can be extended (Fig. 1). One example is the radial forearm flap known as the fascial or fasciocutaneous flap perfused by the radial artery.

## SKIN GRAFTS

Different sites and thicknesses of skin grafts are available. These can be differentiated into full thickness and split thickness skin grafts, and secondary thick and thin split thickness skin grafts (Fig. 25). The indications for the use of these different skin grafts are dependent on the localisation of the defect, the vascularisation and the degree of contamination of the wound.

■ **Donor Sites.** Full thickness skin grafts can be harvested from the postauricular area, from the neck, the upper eye lids, the arm, the groin and the trunk. The choice of area depends on the size and the localisation of the defect and the colour of the original skin. In full thickness skin grafts the area is limited. The first choice should always be a site close to the defect in order to achieve a postoperative result as inconspicuous as possible concerning colour and texture of the skin graft.

Split thickness skin grafts are harvested from the leg or from all over the body if necessary. The scalp is a favourable donor site with very little donor site morbidity, no pain, rapid epithelialisation and no visible scars. Taken in the appropriate thickness (0.2 mm), the hair growth is not compromised. Split thickness skin transplants can be used in a meshed way to give an enlargement of the area of the skin graft by a ratio of 1:1.5, 1:3 or 1:5. This has the advantage of drainage of wound secretion and the possibility of enlargement of the graft used to cover the wound area, which is especially useful in burn patients.

■ **Recipient Sites.** In general skin grafts show the phenomenon of shrinkage after transplantation. For split thickness skin grafts, this phenomenon is equivalent to about one-third of the surface that was covered originally. For a full thickness skin graft the shrinkage is less than in split thickness skin grafts. The perfusion of the transplanted skin needs to be estimated. The perfusion of the wound bed is the key to transplant survival. Furthermore, the possibility of potential or evident infection should be taken into account. If there is severe wound secretion or potential wound infection, a meshed split thickness skin graft is preferred.

In all skin grafts, the technique of wound coverage is important. Gauze dressings applied to the wound with sutures maintaining some pressure for 5 days if possible, is helpful.

## SKIN LESIONS

### Benign Tumors

A great number of benign tumors occur as skin lesions. Treatment of choice is the radical removal of the lesion.

■ **Epithelial Cyst.** Epithelial cysts may occur after posttraumatic or postoperative injuries of the skin. Clinically a tumor occurs typically close to a skin scar. Treatment of choice is radical surgical removal of the lesion. The recurrence rate is quite high.

■ **Epidermal Cyst.** The epidermal cyst is a tumor of the hair follicle. Frequently inflammatory reaction occurs. Removal should be performed in a situation free from infection in order to avoid impaired wound healing. In the case of acute severe infection, incision and drainage of the inflammatory process are mandatory.

■ **Histiocytoma.** A histiocytoma is a circumscribed fibrous lesion in the skin with a dark appearance. Complete removal is the treatment of choice.

■ **Fibroma.** A fibroma is a connective tissue tumor, often presenting as a soft tissue mass that tends to grow slowly. Treatment is complete removal of the lesion.

Figure 25

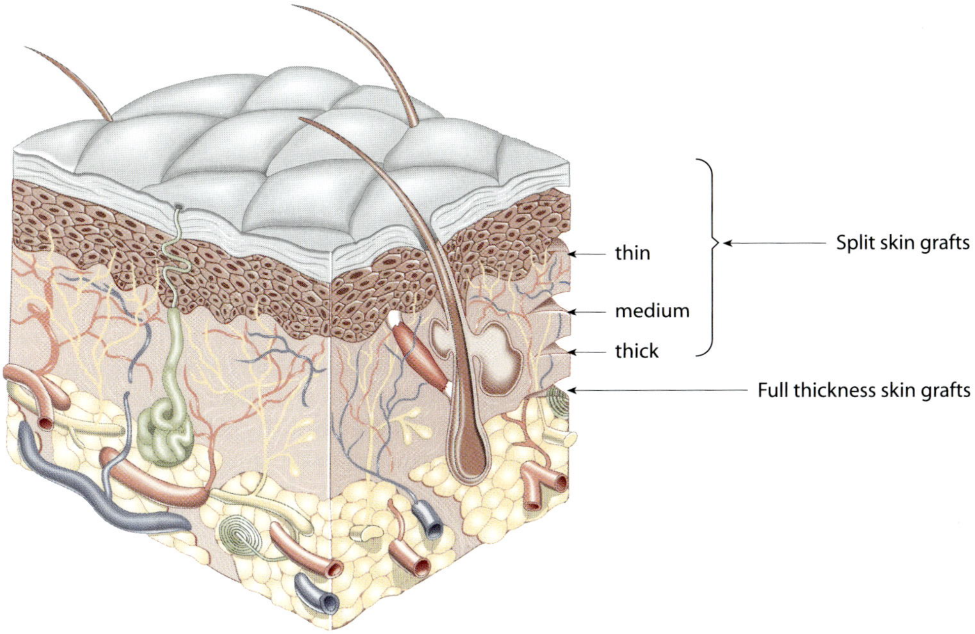


Library
College of Physicians & Surgeons of B.C
400 - 858 Beatty St.
Vancouver BC V6B 1C1

3

## Malignant Tumors

■ **Basal Cell Carcinoma.** Basal cell carcinoma is the most frequent malignant skin tumor with a high local recurrence rate. There is almost no metastatic potential. Treatment is radical excision with excision margins of 2–5 mm from the tumor edge, depending on the site. In the face, secondary defect closure after final histological confirmation of complete tumor excision is advisable. Temporary defect closure is yielded by skin substitutes.

■ **Squamous Cell Carcinoma.** In squamous cell carcinoma a radical excision is required with excision margins of 0.5–1 cm from the tumor edge. Depending on the localisation of the tumor, a primary defect closure, usually with intraoperative histological confirmation of excision, or a second stage procedure is performed.

■ **Bowen's disease.** These skin lesions are an early in situ manifestation of squamous cell carcinoma and are treated in the same way.

■ **Malignant Melanoma.** The thickness of the tumor is an important prognostic indicator for the outcome of patients with malignant melanoma. Excision margins of 1–2 cm from the primary lesion are performed. Tumor staging and examination of the lymph nodes including sentinel node biopsy (SLN) in certain cases, followed by a regional lymphadenectomy in the presence of SLN micrometastases, are part of the standardised therapy regimen.

## Malformations

■ **Vascular Malformations.** Vascular malformations and hemangioma should be examined clinically and radiologically to determine the extent of the lesion. In cases without spontaneous regression treatment such as laser surgery with Nd-YAG laser is used, but the technique needs to be repeated several times to achieve a regression of the malformation. Surgical treatment should be performed in certain situations such as for complications like bleeding and infection and in cases where there is no regression after laser treatment.

■ **Pigmented Lesions.** Depending on the origin and depth of a pigmented lesion, the area should be monitored clinically or excised to avoid the risk of malignant transformation. Surgical removal can be performed depending on the localisation and the size of the nevus. Total excision, serial excision, expander treatment, removal and defect closure with skin grafts are some of the possible surgical interventions.

## Tatoos

The treatment of tatoos depends on the level of the tatoo and the ink used. Tatoos can be removed by surgical excision and laser treatment. In laser treatment, for example, the Nd-YAG laser is applied depending on the colour of the tatoo. In general, nonprofessional tatoos can be removed more easily than professional tatoos, which are frequently placed deeper in the skin. The colour of the tatoo is also relevant when considering laser treatment.

Dermabrasion can be used as a step towards the removal of tatoos but runs the risk of scarring and hypopigmentation.

None of the techniques of tatoo removal are without their sequelae, and in both laser treatment and dermabrasion, hypopigmentation and scarring frequently occur.

Surgical options are simple excision, serial excision of the lesion or tissue expansion of the normal tissue close to the lesion allowing later lesion removal.

## Hyperhydrosis Axillaris

In the case of persistent axillary sweating and following diagnostic iodine testing, conservative treatment using special deodorant, iontophoresis or botulinum toxin may be undertaken. However, the treatment of choice is a limited surgical approach. After iodine testing of the involved region, a local excision of the involved area is performed combined with subcutaneous removal of the sweat glands either using scissors or curettage. Careful hemostasis is important, for bleeding after this procedure is frequent. Drains should be placed to control further bleeding.

## Hidradenitis Suppurativa

Hidradenitis suppurativa is characterised by chronic inflamation of apocrine gland-bearing skin in the axillary, anogenital and rarely the scalp region. Treatment is radical excision of all inflammatory and scarred tissue followed in most cases by secondary wound healing with satisfying functional and aesthetical result.

## Scar Release

Scars can induce functional and/or aesthetic impairment. In regions of joints and in children with the need for physical growth, scar control and corrective procedures demand sophisticated individual planning.

Multiple techniques for scar release can be utilised. Analysis of the underlying problem is the first step towards successful scar treatment. After scar release, further wound closure should be planned carefully with as little skin tension as possible. If necessary, skin grafts, artificial skin and tissue transfer are utilised. Tissue perfusion must be monitored carefully after surgery to ensure tissue survival and a satisfactory postoperative result.

## Subcutaneous Lesions

Subcutaneous lesions should be removed when causing discomfort for the patient. Possible complaints, that will depend on the site and size of the lesion, may include a sensation of pressure, pain, sensory disturbance, or mechanical and aesthetic impairment.

■ **Lipomas.** A lipoma is a soft, pseudofluctuant, well circumscribed, slowly growing tumor that is usually found in the subcutaneous tissues. There is commonly a long history of a slowly growing soft tissue tumor. It can be obscured by surrounding tissue, such as muscle, etc., and if not excised can reach an enormous size. Malignant transformation to a liposarcoma is rare but described in the literature. In this case preoperative radiological examination such as an MRI scan is mandatory. Clinical signs of malignancy are rapid growth with a more solid component to the tumor. Depending on the localisation and size of the lesion, excision can be performed using local anaesthesia on an outpatient basis, but if the lesion is large general anaesthesia may be more appropriate.

■ **Neurofibroma.** Neurofibromas appear like fibromas or even lipomas. They are frequently multiple especially in Recklinghausen's disease. There is often a high recurrence rate after removal, which is usually undertaken for those lesions causing discomfort, in spite of recognising the high recurrence rate and the multiplicity of lesions.

■ **Others.** There are several other soft tissue tumors that can be found in the subcutaneous tissue space such as fibromas, adenomas and cysts. Careful examination should reveal the size of the lesion and its relationship to important structures in the proximity thus allowing a realistic plan to be devised for surgical excision. The nature of the lesion can be revealed by histological examination.

Malignant tumors such as malignant fibrous histiocytoma, dermatofibrosarcoma, and other sarcomas demand preoperative staging and radiological studies, and are in general treated using a definitive surgical approach in hospital, rather than on the basis of short stay surgery.

## Aesthetic Surgery

Rejuvenation is an important facet of plastic surgery. Aesthetic surgery encompasses a wide variety of surgical techniques with a high level of patient expectation. Realistic planning and informed consent from the patient is mandatory for successful outcome in this demanding field. The majority of operations can be performed on an outpatient basis or with a short stay of a very few days.

3

## Face

### Figure 26: Eyelids

One of the most frequently performed surgical interventions in rejuvenation practice is surgery of the upper and lower eyelids. In the case of skin and/or fatty tissue excess, removal of the excess tissue is performed. The aim is the reconstruction of the lid fold and the redistribution of the subcutaneous fat to achieve a rejuvenation effect.

### Figure 27A, B: Ear Correction

Correction of the ear position is a procedure performed predominantly in children. Multiple techniques for the correction of apoptosis otis are described. One reliable technique applicable to the majority of deformities is the technique of remodelling the cartilage of the anthelix fold after a retroauricular incision and removing a small amount of skin.

A Marking the frontal aspect
B Incision from behind, exposure, preparation and positioning of the cartilage

Figure 26

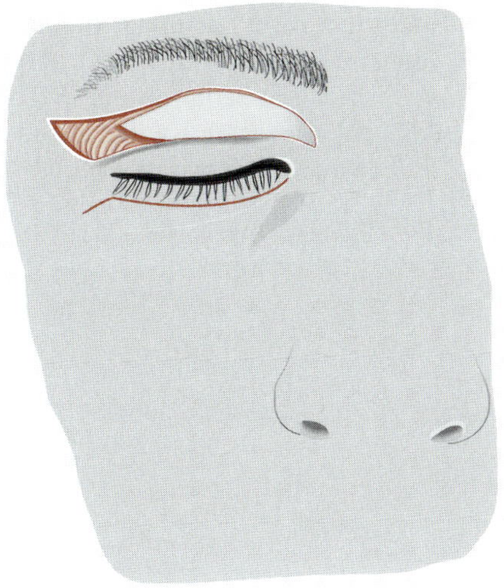

Figure 27A, B

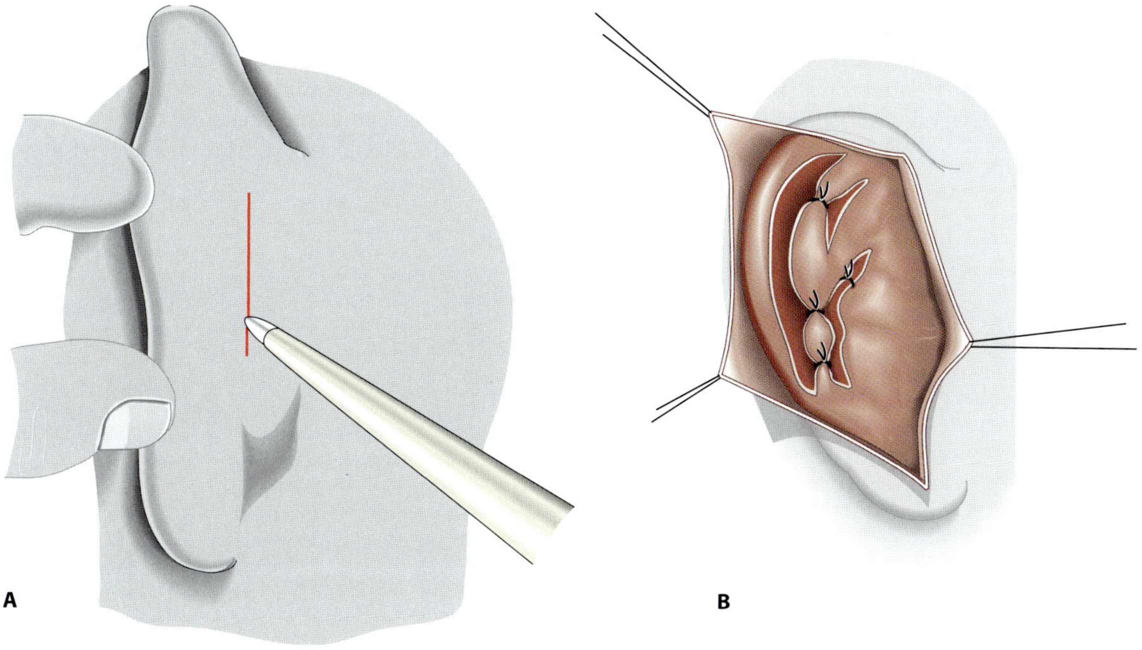

3

### Figure 28: Nose

Nasal deformities can be treated with closed or open rhinoplasty. All bone and cartilage structures of the nose can be treated such as bumps, tip deformities, size and shape of the nose and airway obstruction.

### Figure 29: SMAS Facelift

In the case of skin excess or loosening of the musculoaponeurotic tissues of the face (SMAS), a tightening and repositioning of the soft tissue of the face can achieve a rejuvenation effect. The aim is to achieve a natural appearance without too much tension in order to avoid undesirable sequelae of this treatment.

## Breast Surgery

### Figure 30: Augmentation Mammoplasty

For breast augmentation, implants can be inserted using a submammary, transareolar, axillary or periumbilical approach. The pocket can be created in the submuscular or subglandular position depending on the soft tissue coverage and the patient's expectations.

### Figure 31: Reduction Mammoplasty

For reduction mammoplasty a variety of procedures can be applied depending on the original shape and size of the breast. The inverted T-technique with a vertical and submammary scar is the most popular technique performed in this field. Sufficient blood supply of the nipple areolar complex has to be monitored.

Figure 28

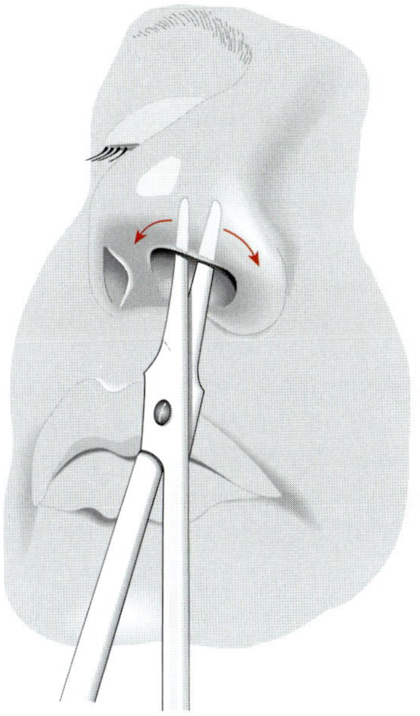

Figure 29

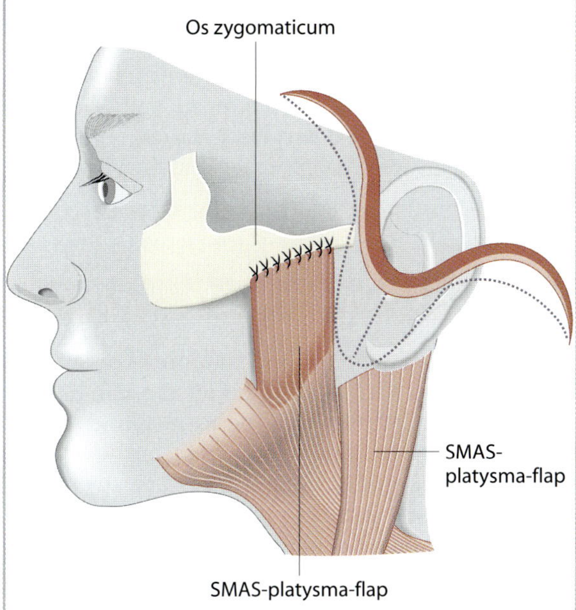


Figure 30

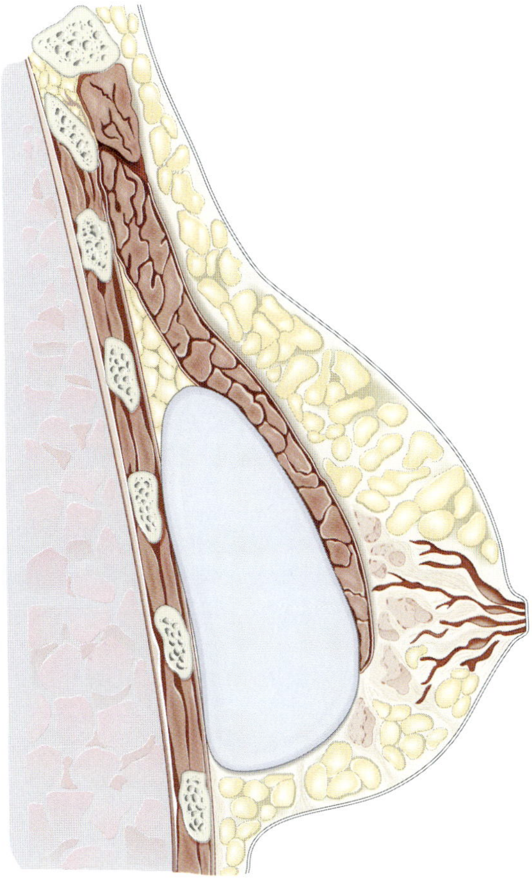

Figure 31

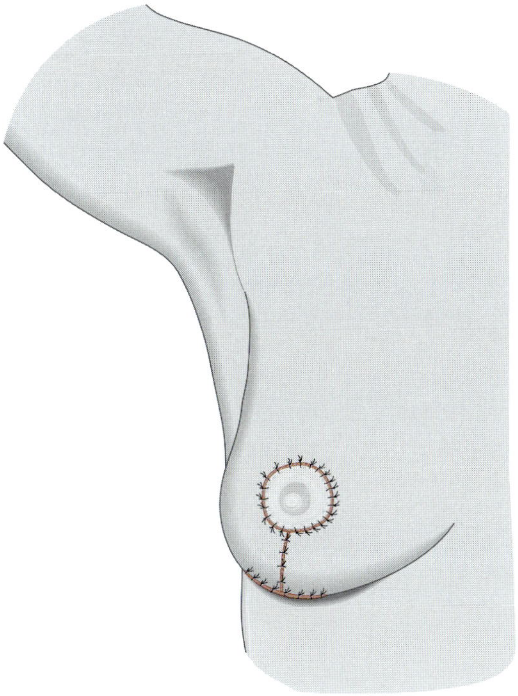

3

## Contour Surgery

■ **Liposuction.** For body contouring, liposuction is a useful technique when the skin retains its elasticity. The aim is not weight reduction but rather correction of any localised fat surplus. Classical regions are the lateral aspect of the upper leg and the abdominal area, but the principles can be applied in any region with a fat tissue surplus. Through small incisions, the fat tissue is removed with a suction cannula after insertion of a tumescent solution.

## Figure 32A, B: Abdominoplasty

For contour correction in the abdominal area when there is skin surplus, an abdominoplasty can be utilised. A suprapubic incision is performed and an epifascial elevation of the skin/subcutaneous fat flap up to the xiphoid is undertaken. If necessary, any diastasis of the rectus muscle can be corrected at the same time. The redundant skin and fat tissue are removed and the umbilicus reinserted into the appropriate site in the skin/subcutaneous flap.

■ **Dermolipectomy.** In any region of the body, removal of any surplus fat and skin can be performed taking into consideration the anatomical landmarks and depending on the amount of redundant tissue, e.g., upper legs, upper arms, the gluteal region and other areas. It is important to suture the superficial scarpa fascia in order to stabilise the result and the scar position.

A Fixation of the umbilicus on the fascia
B Repositioning of the umbilicus in the original position

Figure 32A, B

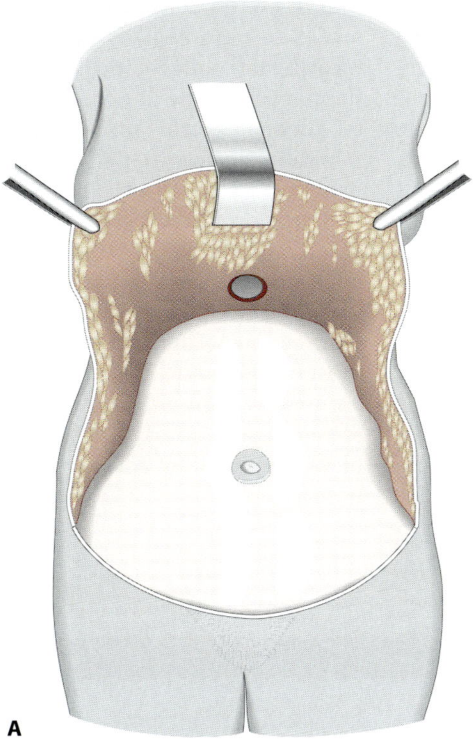


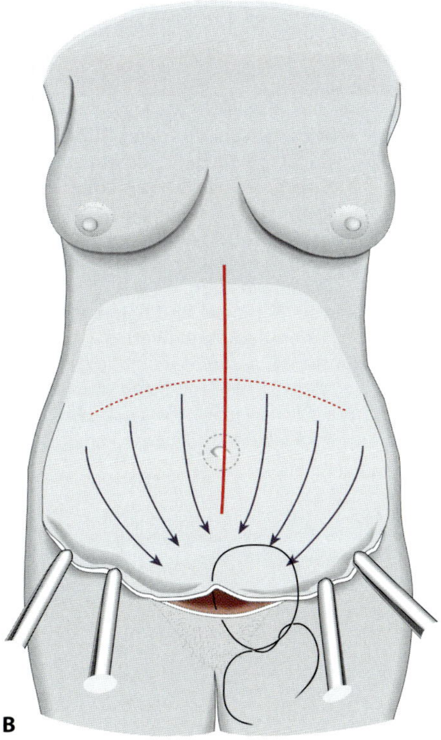

3

## GENERAL PRINCIPLES OF PLASTIC SURGERY

For any defect closure, the principles and techniques of plastic surgery must be applied. Flap surgery and split or full thickness skin grafts are the basic procedures. Flap surgery is divided into local and free flaps. Depending on the demands of the donor site and the contents of the transferred tissue, cutaneous, fasciocutaneous, fascial, muscle, musculocutaneous or osteomyocutaneous flaps can be performed.

A knowledge of the vascular anatomy and tissue perfusion is essential for any plastic surgical intervention.

Local and distant flaps and free microvascular flaps are distinguished. Regarding the blood supply, local flaps are divided into random pattern flaps getting their blood supply from the surrounding skin, and axial pattern flaps deriving their blood supply from a defined axial vessel. In random pattern flaps, the length : width ratio should be in the range of 2 : 1 in order to maintain a sufficient blood supply. In the face, this ratio can be exceeded because of the extraordinary good blood supply of the face. Distant flaps approximate donor and recipient sites to ensure an adequate perfusion, like the pedicled groin flap. Avoiding tension after tissue transfer is an important principle for flap survival.

Throughout the body, anatomical landmarks and vascular perfusion are important for flap design. The anatomical classification of the arterial supply of muscle and musculocutaneous type I–V flaps by Mathes and Nahai (Cormack and Lamberty 1986) must be taken into consideration. In free flaps, different tissues from different body regions can be transferred using clearly defined arterial and venous blood supplies by means of a microsurgical technique.

## CONCLUSION

Many interventions in plastic surgery involving the skin and subcutaneous tissues can be performed as short stay surgery. Prerequisites are an in depth knowledge of anatomy and the principles and techniques of plastic surgery.

## SELECTED REFERENCES

Berger A, Hierner R (2003) Plastische Chirurgie. Springer-Verlag, Berlin Heidelberg

Bostwick J (1990) Plastic and reconstructive breast surgery. Quality Medical Publishing, St. Louis

Cormack GC, Lamberty BG (1986) The arterial anatomy of skin flaps, 2nd edn. Churchill Livingstone, London

Fitzpatrick T et al (2001) Colaratlas and synopsis of clinical dermatology

Haas E (1991) Plastische Gesichtschirurgie. Thieme Verlag, Stuttgart

Krupp S (1994) Plastische Chirurgie. Klinik und Praxis. Ecomed, Landsberg

Lamberty BGH, Healy C (1994) Flaps: physiology, principles of design and pitfalls. In: Cohen M (ed) Mastery of plastic and reconstructive surgery, vol 1. Little, Brown and Co., Boston, pp 56–70

Mathes SJ, Nahai F (1979) Clinical atlas of muscle and musculocutaneous flaps. Mosby, St. Louis

McGregor IA (1972) Fundamental techniques of plastic surgery and their surgical applications, 8th edn. Churchill Livingstone, London

McGregor IA (1989) Plastic surgery. Springer, Berlin Heidelberg New York

Olivari N (2004) Praktische Plastische Chirurgie. Ein Operationsatlas. Kaden Verlag

Smith JW, Aston SJ (eds) (1997) Grabb and Smith's plastic surgery. Little, Brown and Co., Boston

Wcerda H (1999) Plastisch-rekonstruktive Chirurgie im Gesichtsbereich. Thieme Verlag, Stuttgart New York

CHAPTER 4

# Hand Surgery

Martin Langer

## INTRODUCTION: THE ELEMENTS AND GENERAL PRINCIPLES OF HAND SURGERY

The scope of hand surgery is broad, but the majority of injuries and diseases of the hand can be treated in short stay surgery. A complete presentation of these operations is not possible. Here the most important hand surgery procedures are described.

Every operation in hand surgery should be done with the patient under good anaesthesia, using a tourniquet, loupe magnification, and using an atraumatic technique.

Anaesthesia for hand surgery can be provided by various techniques. General anaesthetic techniques do not differ very much from those for other parts of the body, but regional anaesthetic techniques have a special application in anaesthetizing the upper extremity. The most common technique is the brachial plexus block, with blocking of the major nerves at the level of the third part of the axillary artery (axillary block). The simplicity of this technique and the absence of major complications are responsible for its wide acceptance. Blocks around the elbow, the ulnar nerve block at the wrist or the median nerve block are particularly useful for supplementing brachial plexus blocks. The intravenous regional block or the Bier's block is a very simple technique for producing anaesthesia. A dual tourniquet is placed on the upper part of the arm, an intravenous infusion is started on the back of the hand, and the arm is elevated and exsanguinated with an Esmarch bandage, starting from the fingers all the way up to the tourniquet. The proximal tourniquet is inflated and the Esmarch bandage removed. The local anaesthetic solution is then slowly injected through the cannula. The proximal tourniquet is left inflated for 20 min or until the patient notices some discomfort. Then the distal tourniquet is inflated and the proximal tourniquet can be deflated. Because the distal tourniquet is applied over the anaesthetized area, the patient is not likely to experience any discomfort for about 40 min. Even with the use of the double cuff, pain caused by the tourniquet limits the use of this procedure to operations lasting less than 1 h.

■ **Digital Nerve Blocks (Oberst Blocks).** The digits are anaesthetized by subcutaneous infiltration bilaterally at the base of the finger. It is best to inject via the dorsum of the hand rather than through the skin of the palm. The injection should not be made into an infected area and it is important to avoid excessive distension of tissues and the use of epinephrine, either of which may compromise circulation to the fingers.

■ **Tourniquet.** In 1873 Johann Friedrich August von Esmarch introduced the first commonly used rubber bandage to exsanguinate a limb before applying a tourniquet. Sterling Bunnell established the role of the tourniquet in hand surgery. His rhetorical question "*Could a jeweller repair a watch immersed in ink?*" has been a favourite quote of hand surgeons for many years. The goal of the surgeon should be to use the lowest tourniquet pressure compatible with providing a bloodless field. Values range from 250 to 300 mmHg in adults and from 150 to 250 mmHg in children, but slightly higher pressures may be necessary to produce a bloodless field in a patient with an obese arm or with hypertension. Generally 50–75 mmHg higher than systolic will suffice. The absolute maximum tourniquet time is 2 h. Finger tourniquets could be used in performing relatively minor procedures on a single finger. Our preferred method for simultaneous exsanguination of the finger and application of a digital tourniquet is a method using a sterile rubber glove. A finger is cut from the glove, stretched over the digit to be operated on, and rolled proximally to form a ring at the base of the finger after cutting off the tip of the glove. Rubber finger tourniquets are probably safe to use for very short operative procedures, but two distinct hazards must be considered by the surgeon: (1) excessive pressure can easily be produced and (2) the surgeon must not forget to take it off.

■ **Loop Magnification and Atraumatic Technique.** Most professional hand surgeons use loupes in every (major and minor surgery) hand operation. All hand surgeons should be comfortable with loupes ranging from ×2.5 to ×4.5 magnification. The atraumatic technique, introduced by Sterling Bunnell in 1921, has become an essential part of hand surgery. No surgery is truly atraumatic, but refinements in magnification have given us the opportunity to come closer to reaching this goal.

## Figures 1, 2: Carpal Tunnel Syndrome



While this condition did not become known as "carpal tunnel syndrome" until 1947, it was described earlier by several authors under different names and sometimes without a clear understanding of its pathogenesis. The syndrome is caused by sporadic or persistent compression of the median nerve within the carpal tunnel. The cause of the compression is due to a discrepancy between the capacity of the unyielding canal and the volume of its contents.

In the classical case of carpal tunnel syndrome there is a constant sequence of symptoms which often permits the establishment of the diagnosis on the basis of the characteristic history. The patients, the majority of whom are females over 40 years of age, begin to complain of tingling and numbness in the middle finger or in part of the median nerve distribution. This is followed by numbness and pain aggravated by persistent exertion. Frequently the patient is awakened in the middle of the night by pain in the hand, which is relieved by shaking (Flick sign), hanging, massaging, or exercising the hand. More than 70% of patients have a positive Hoffmann-Tinel sign when the median nerve is tapped in the wrist. More than 70% have a positive "Phalen's test" with increased pain and paraesthesia within 1 min of wrist flexion. Splints to wrist and forearm and restriction of activity can produce some relief, and injection of hydrocortisone into the carpal tunnel allays the symptoms temporarily. Non-operative therapy therefore includes splinting the wrist in the neutral position, oral anti-inflammatory drugs in those cases with tenosynovitis, diuretics to reduce oedema, and management of the underlying systemic diseases. However, operative intervention by sectioning the retinaculum flexorum (Figure 1) is the only treatment which permanently corrects severe degrees of median nerve compression.

Use of the two different operative techniques, classic open carpal tunnel release and endoscopic transection of the retinaculum flexorum, are still the subject of some controversy.

The most frequently adopted incision follows the line described by Taleisnik. This incision avoids the multiple cutaneous branches of the median and ulnar nerves (Figure 2).

Figure 1

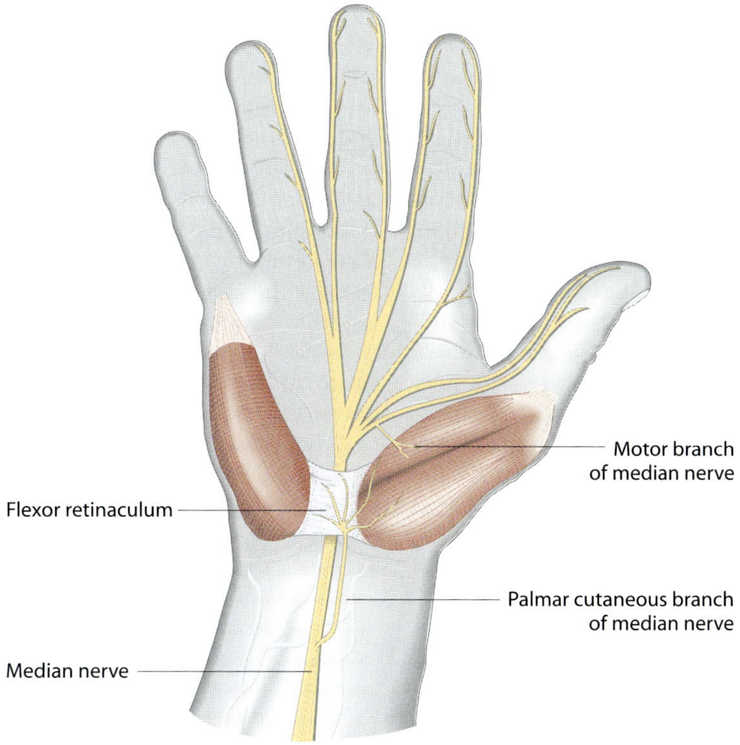
Motor branch
of median nerve
Flexor retinaculum
Palmar cutaneous branch
of median nerve
Median nerve

Figure 2

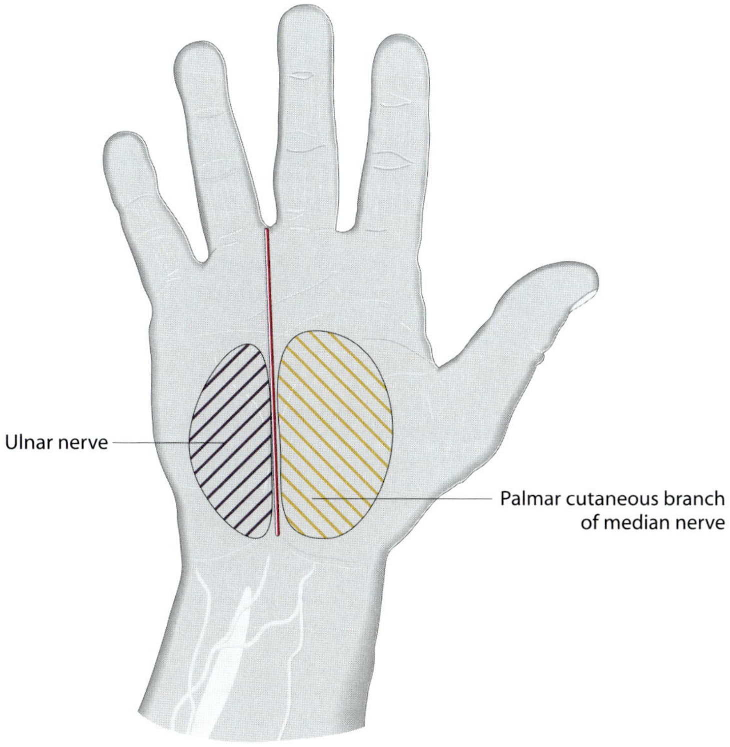
Ulnar nerve
Palmar cutaneous branch
of median nerve

## Figures 3, 4: Carpal Tunnel Syndrome

4

Today the length of the incision in this line is usually about 3 cm placed 1 cm distal to the distal palmar crease. Incisions proximal to the palm tend to result in poor scars. The palmar cutaneous nerves, if identified, should be preserved. The palmar aponeurosis is divided and retracted. The flexor retinaculum, after exposing its entire length, is carefully divided at its ulnar border just beneath the hamulus of the hamate bone. The contents of the canal are inspected and the median nerve is carefully dissected from the thickened tenosynovium. The motor branch of the median nerve is identified as it pierces the radial side of distal end of the flexor retinaculum and is carefully preserved. When the tenosynovium is greatly thickened, the nerve should be retracted radially and the tenosynovium should be excised from around the flexor tendons that occupy the carpal tunnel. It is very important to prevent a scar between the median nerve and the edges of the flexor retinaculum so that the excision of segments of the retinaculum has now been abandoned. Sometimes a reconstruction of the retinaculum is performed. Single layer closure of the wound is followed by a week of wrist immobilization in dorsiflexion by means of a padded palmar plaster splint. Gentle finger motion can be started on the day after operation.

Division of the flexor retinaculum provides immediate, dramatic relief of symptoms. When nerve constriction has been severe, some numbness may persist, although the aching and burning disappear.

In Figs. 1–4, the abbreviations are: A, palmar aponeurosis; R, flexor retinaculum; M, motor thenar nerve; T, sensory nerve to the thumb; I, sensory nerve to radial side of the index finger; I+M, sensory nerve to ulnar side of index finger and radial side of middle finger; M+R, sensory nerve to ulnar side of middle finger and radial side of ring finger.

Figure 3

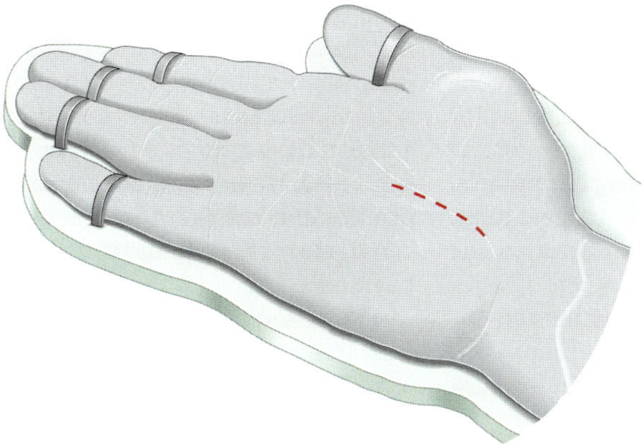

Figure 4

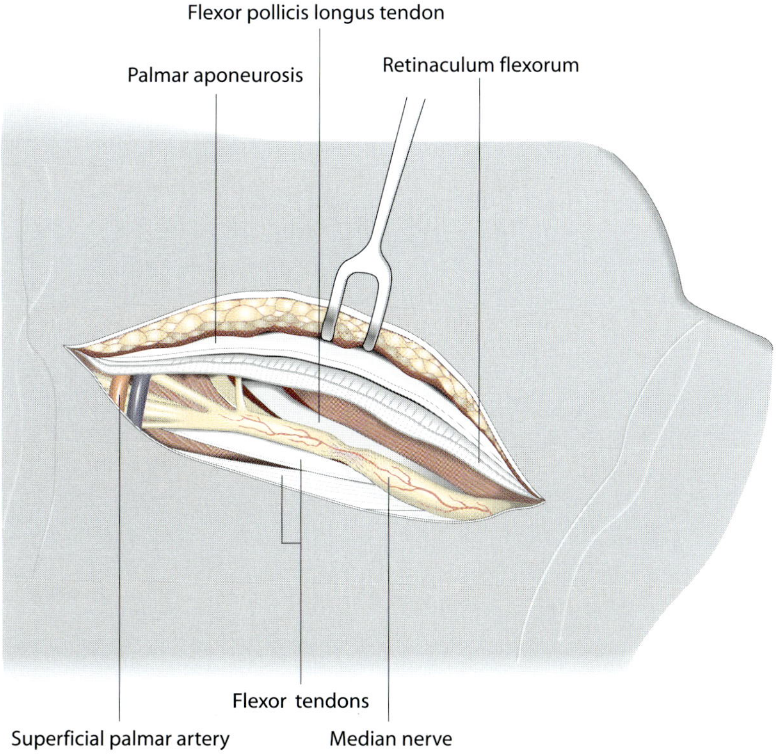

## Figures 5–7: Trigger Finger

Flexor tendon entrapment of the digits is a disorder characterized by snapping or locking of the thumb or fingers (with or without pain). Most cases are secondary to thickening of the digit's A1 pulley, but other pathogeneses include tendon abnormalities at the level of the carpal tunnel, thickening of other pulleys, and abnormalities at the metacarpophalangeal joint. Its historical name, stenosing tenosynovitis of the digits, is inappropriate because histological studies document a lack of inflammation. Flexor tendon entrapment of the fingers is a relatively common, uncomplicated, and non-controversial musculotendinous disorder of the distal upper extremity.

The incision is made parallel to or in the distal palmar crease for release of the index, middle, ring or little fingers. In the thumb the incision in placed in the palmar crease over the metacarpophalangeal joint. The A1 pulley is divided and sometimes partially excised. A local tenosynovialectomy is performed, and any tissue that is densely adherent to the tendons is excised. When local anaesthesia is used the patient can flex and extend the finger on request and thereby can demonstrate whether the locking or catching has been relieved.

Figure 5 shows thickening of the tendon just proximal to the A1 pulley. In Fig. 6 positions of the A1 pulleys of the fingers and thumb and proposed skin incision can be seen. Figure 7 is an operative view illustrating the A1 pulley, thickening of the tendon, neurovascular bundles, and proposed incision of the pulley.

Figure 5

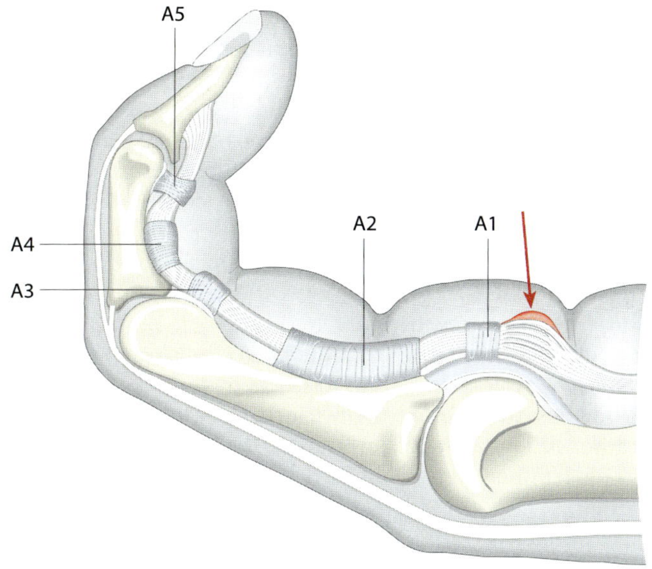


Figure 6

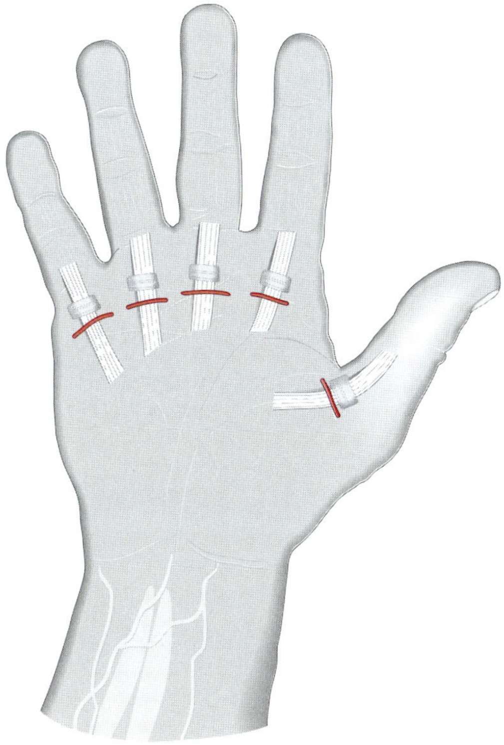

Figure 7

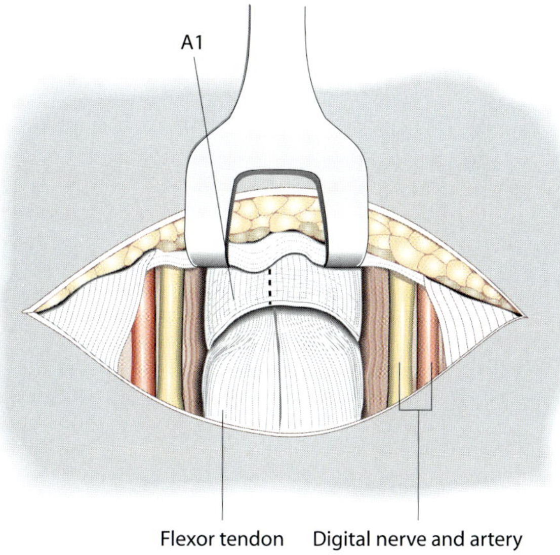

## Figure 8: Dupuytren's Contracture



Dupuytren's contracture is a progressive disease which involves the palmar fascia and the digital extensions of the palmar fascia. The disease begins usually with a small nodular thickening in the palm along the 4th or 5th ray. In its most advanced form, the disease causes a severe and crippling contracture of the palm and some fingers.

Baron Guillaume Dupuytren was born on 5 October, 1777, became chief surgeon at the Hôtel Dieu, Paris, and died in 1835. His descriptions (1831, 1832) of the gross pathological changes have been improved upon only slightly in the past 170 years, but more detail of the anatomy of the hand fascia system has changed the operative treatment. The lesions do not occur in a random pattern but rather follow certain well-defined anatomical pathways determined by the longitudinal lines of tension.

■ **Technique.** It is generally agreed that the only consistently efficacious treatment for Dupuytren's contracture is excision of the diseased palmar aponeurosis and the contracted bands in the fingers. One must carefully consider four aspects of the surgical plan: management of the skin, management of the fascia, management of the joints, and preservation or neurolysis of the nerves. John Hueston stated that "fasciectomy is little more than a dissection of the digital nerves".

Skin incisions such as multiple Y-to-V advancement flaps, Bruner zigzag incision, and midline longitudinal incision closed with Z-plasties, are the most popular and have the advantages of progressive flexible exposure and addressing the skin shortage secondary to the contracture. These incisions should not cross joint creases unless broken up by Z-plasties.

Digital nerves may be found in abnormal positions in patients with advanced Dupuytren's contractures.

General approaches to the management of the diseased fascia include fasciotomy and varying degrees of fasciectomy. The most commonly performed operation is the regional fasciectomy. Because all involved fascia and the neighbouring parts of uninvolved fascia have to be removed to prevent disease progression or recurrence, the best procedure is the "radical regional fasciectomy".

The contracture of metacarpophalangeal joints can almost always be released by fasciectomy alone. Conversely, the proximal interphalangeal joint can present a difficult problem.

In Fig. 8 the basic skin incisions are shown: middle finger: multiple Y-to-V advancement flaps, ring finger Bruner zigzag incision, and little finger: midline longitudinal incision closed with multiple Z-plasties.

Figure 8

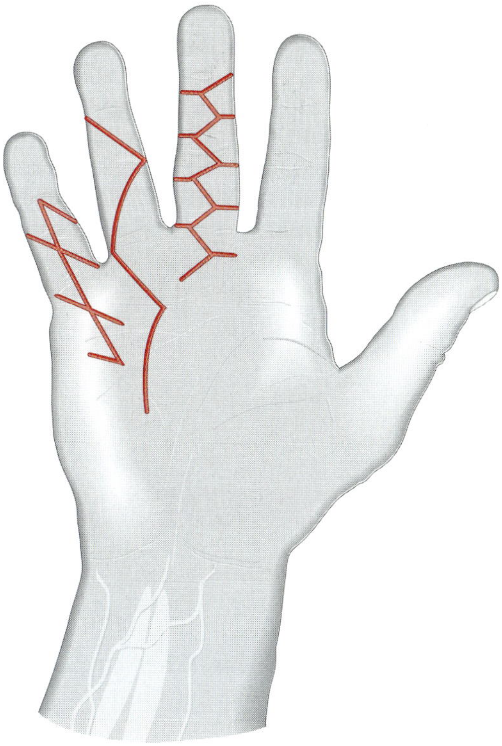

## MANAGEMENT OF FINGERTIP INJURIES

The fingertip is the part of the hand most frequently injured. Nail bed and fingertip injuries often result in time lost from work and, if improperly repaired, can be permanently disabling.

The fingertip is the end organ for touch and is richly supplied with special sensory receptors that enable the hand to "see", relaying the shape, texture, and temperature of the manipulated object. Fingertip injuries can destroy this special sensory function. The choice of surgical management after injury and successful repair of fingertip injuries requires knowledge of anatomy, the techniques of reconstruction, and sound surgical judgement.

■ **Conservative Treatment.** Wound healing by secondary intention is caused by the granulation, epithelialization, and contraction of the scar tissue and surrounding dermis that effectively reduces the subsequent size of the wound. Many different methods of conservative treatment (occlusive, semiocclusive) have been described. All of them have in common a regimen of serial dressing changes on a two to three times a week basis. Usually 3–4 weeks are needed to obtain the wound healing. This method is indicated in distal, superficial, clean defects of the tip.

## Figure 9A–D

Three types of amputation of the distal extremities: A, normal; B, oblique palmar amputation; C, transverse amputation with exposed bone; D, transverse amputation through the nail with dislocation of the nail plate.

■ **Full Thickness Skin Graft.** The indication for the full thickness skin grafts is limited exclusively to some transverse or lateral, longitudinal fingertip injuries in the distal zone. The author is not in favour of this method, because the sensitivity is far superior by using advancement or transposition flaps.

■ **Local Flaps.** When treatment by simple means is not indicated, flaps from the injured digit are useful techniques. To perform any of these flaps, adequate perfusion of the skin proximal to the damaged area is mandatory. The general indications for these flaps are the necessity to preserve finger length, to preserve the nail, and bone or tendon exposure.

## Figure 10: V-Y Flaps

These are random pattern flaps and are designed to draw a vascularized and sensate section of skin and subcutaneous tissue over the traumatic fingertip loss and allow primary healing with simultaneous closure of the donor site. Each technique uses a triangular incision through the donor site, creating a V flap. This island of tissue is advanced distally, with conversion of the V defect proximally to a Y-suture after closure. This technique was first described in the fingertip by Tranquilli-Leali (1935) and later with special reference to the neurovascular bundles by Atasoy (1970).

In Fig. 10 is seen a palmar V-Y flap with preservation of the neurovascular bundles.

The figure shows a homodigital island flap after Venkataswami (1980). Preservation of optimal function and sensation and a one-stage procedure are all features that make homodigital island transfers an attractive option. From the vascular point of view, all these flaps are based on the collateral digital artery system. The homodigital island pulp flap allows the advancement and rotation of the proximal pulp to gain the distal pulp defect. A dorsal skin segment can also be included, so a greater area of skin loss can be covered. The second advantage point is the 15 mm of distal advancement which is the maximum that can be obtained with this flap.

Figure 9A–D

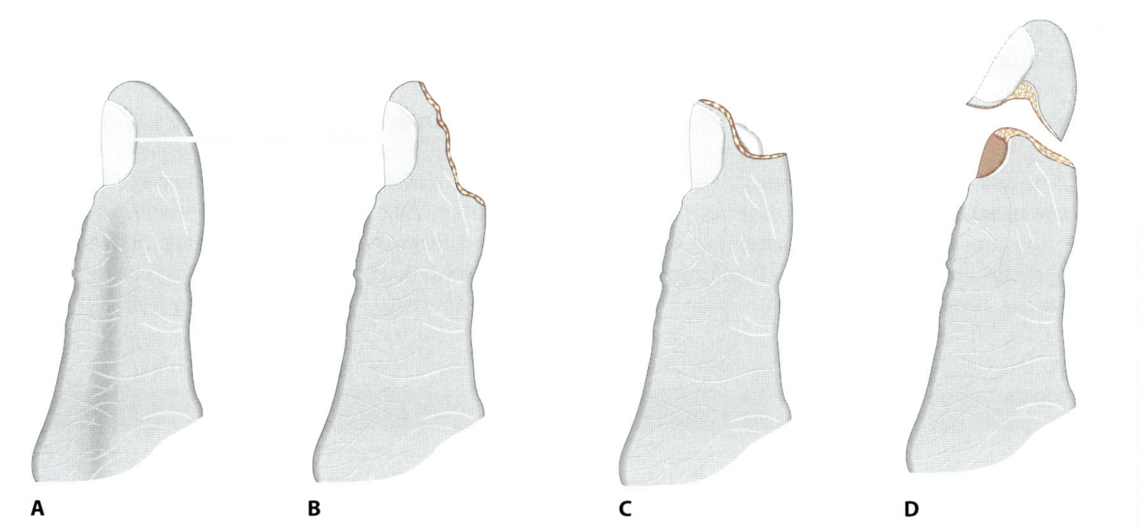


Figure 10

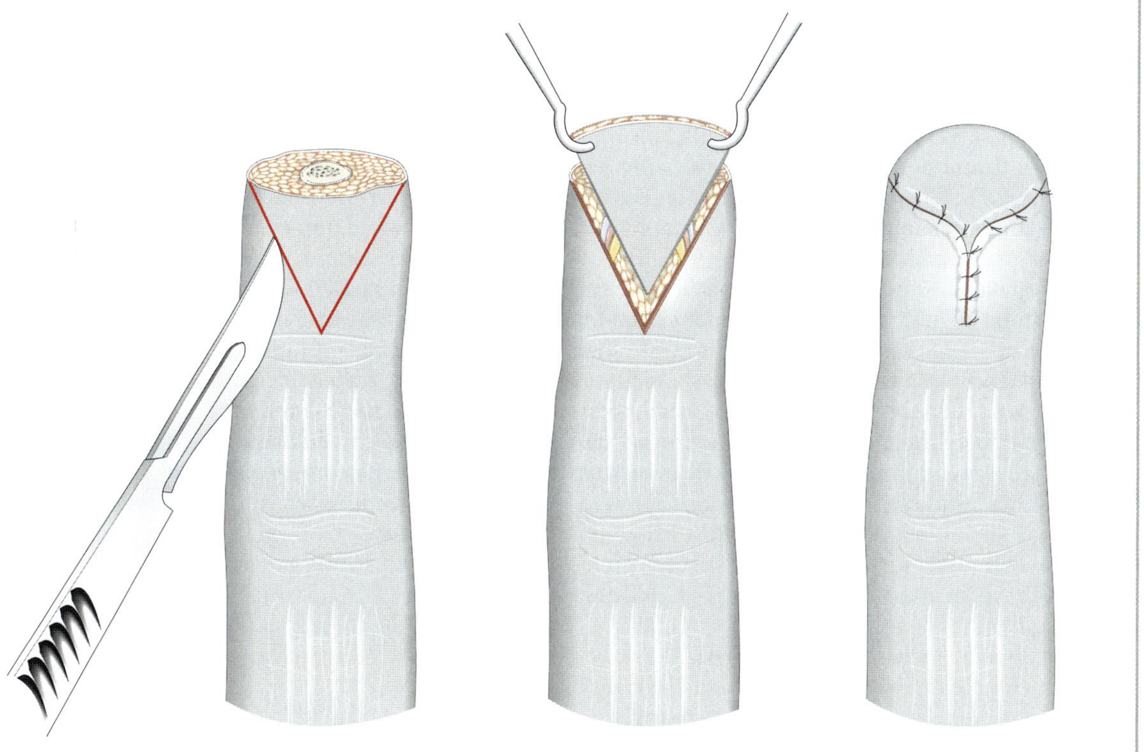

4

## Figure 11: Homodigital Island Flaps

**Partial Injury of the Nail.** If the nail is only partially injured, an attempt must be made to preserve it. The nail is an important structure cosmetically and functionally and provides efficient support of the pulp in precision handling. Normal regeneration is only possible if the matrix is intact, if the nail bed is largely undamaged, if the normal adhesion between the nail and is bed is preserved, and if the phalangeal remnant is long enough. If not, the nail will become curved and hooked.

If the nail bed has been sectioned, but each fragment is still adherent to the wound, these can be approximated and sutured. These sutures must be absorbable; otherwise their presence under the nail will be unsightly and painful.

If the nail is detached, the edges are trimmed and the nail is replaced in its bed. The nail should be perforated to allow the release of serous fluid. If the original nail is destroyed a Silastic sheath or a part of a syringe must be inserted in order to preserve the nail bed.

## INFECTIONS OF THE FINGERTIP

The hand is a common site for infection because it is so frequently injured. Sixty per cent of all hand infections are the result of trauma. The spectrum of acute bacterial hand infections is broad. The management principles are similar in type and can be summarized as follows:

A. Rest – elevation – immobilization in a functional position
B. Early and aggressive therapy, including adequate drainage of all loculations of pus and debridement of necrotic tissue

## Figure 12

**Paronychia.** Paronychia is an infection of those structures surrounding the proximal and lateral nail. Extension of a paronychia ventrally can damage the matrix of the germinal matrix, causing permanently disfiguring nail abnormalities. Paronychia is initiated by the introduction of bacteria between the nail and its surrounding structures. This is usually caused by minor trauma, such as that associated with nail biting, manicures, or hangnails.

The paronychia initially begins as erythema and discomfort in the nail fold at its proximal lateral extent. If the infection has been present for more than 24 h or if there is any fluctuance under the nail, the nail fold must be drained. The initial method of drainage can be simple elevation of the dorsal nail fold. A small amount of pus can usually be evacuated in this fashion. If this initial attempt at drainage is inadequate, if the infection extends significantly proximal to the nail fold, or if the infection fails to resolve with the above treatment, more aggressive drainage is indicated.

This is done by incising the dorsal nail fold and elevating it completely from the surface of the nail. A small strip of gauze is used as a wick for 24–48 h.

A felon is an acute subcutaneous abscess of the distal pulp of the thumb or a finger. In most cases there is a penetrating injury preceding a felon. Because of the multiple vertical fibrous septa that divide the pulp into several small compartments, it differs from other types of subcutaneous abscesses and so the pain and swelling usually develop rapidly.

By adequate early treatment an abscess can be prevented. If there is a draining sinus, incision of the sinus longitudinally with excision of the necrotic skin edges is effective. If no sinus is present, a unilateral longitudinal (J or hockey-stick incision) approach over the area of maximal tenderness is used. The scalpel blade is gently advanced in search of an abscess. If pus is encountered, the incision is enlarged to the proximal and distal limits of the abscess. The wound is irrigated and carefully explored for the presence of a retained foreign body, and then is packed with sterile gauze. The digit is splinted and elevated for 48 h, at which time the dressing is removed and the wound is inspected. Usually, a 10- to 14-day course of a first-generation cephalosporin is sufficient.

Figure 11

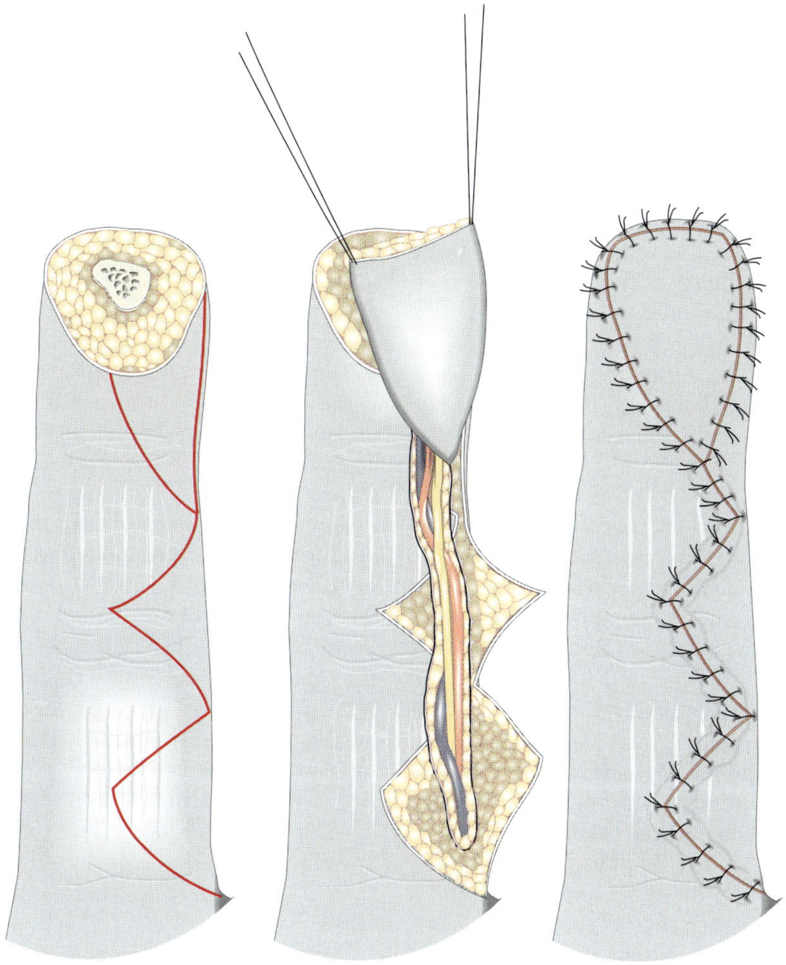

Figure 12

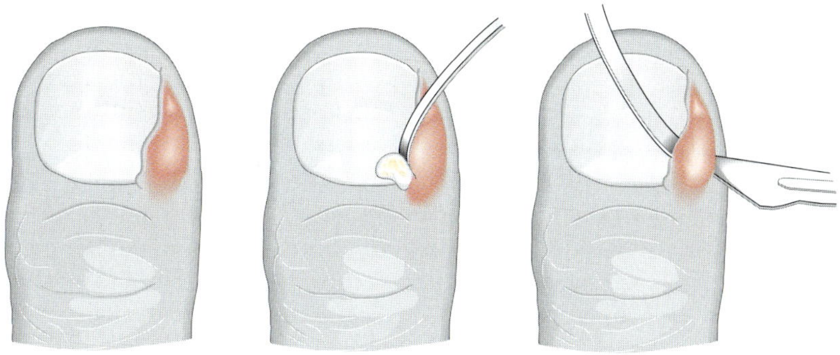

## GANGLION

A ganglion is the most common swelling found in the hand. They can arise anywhere in the hand, but the most common site (60–70%) is directly over the scapholunate ligament. The second most common ganglion of the hand and wrist is the palmar wrist ganglion (18–20%), followed by the flexor tendon sheath ganglion and the mucous cysts.

The aetiology of these cystic lesions is said to be unknown, although extensive research has shown that these ganglia are composed of a main cyst with a pedicle going from the deep part of the cyst to the underlying joint capsule. In dorsal ganglia the pedicle most often can be followed to the scapholunate ligament, in radial palmar ganglia often to the trapezio-scaphoidal joint.

■ **Operative Technique.** Most dorsal ganglia may be approached through a transverse incision over the ganglion. The main cyst and its pedicle are mobilized down to the underlying joint capsule. The joint capsule is opened along the border of the radius, and the proximal pole of the scaphoid and the ganglion and its attachment to the joint capsule is then excised off the scapholunate ligament.

Large dorsal ganglia may be excised more simply by evacuating their contents, opening the sac, and then tracing the sac down to the carpus from the inside. This is generally much simpler than attempting to preserve a large ganglion intact and to mobilise it from the outside.

The excision of a radiopalmar wrist ganglion is more difficult because of its exposure and requires precise identification of the capsular attachments. Particular care is taken to identify and protect the radial artery, which is often intimately attached to the wall of the ganglion and may even be completely encircled by the ganglion.

Flexor tendon sheath ganglia arise from the A2 pulley in the crease of the proximal phalanxes and are characteristically small (3–8 mm), tense, and on occasion painful. The cysts are attached to the tendon sheath and do not move with the tendon. A needle rupture of these ganglions is quite quick, effective and painless. At times, there are some recurrences, but the treatment can be repeated.

Mucous cysts are ganglia of the DIP joint and usually occur between the 5th and 7th decades. The cyst is approached through an "L"-shaped incision. If the skin is involved with the cyst wall, an elliptical skin-ganglion conglomerate is excised. Care is taken not to disturb the insertion of the nail matrix or the insertion of the extensor tendon.

## DE QUERVAIN'S DISEASE

In 1895, the Swiss surgeon Fritz De Quervain described a form of tenosynovitis involving the abductor pollicis longus and the extensor pollicis brevis tendons in the region of the radial styloid. Repetitive occupational trauma seems to be the most logical and most frequent aetiological agent. It is widely accepted that De Quervain's disease occurs about 8 to 10 times more often in women than in men.

De Quervain's disease has often been misdiagnosed as arthritis, periostitis neuralgia, causalgia, or a psychosomatic disorder. Pain is the predominant symptom and may be acute or gradual in onset. On examination there is often a slight thickening and swelling over the radial styloid. A test, described by Finkelstein in 1930, is almost always positive; an intense stabbing pain is elicited along the course of the long abductor of the thumb when the patient clasps the fingers tightly over the thumb and then flexes the wrist sharply into ulnar deviation. This manoeuvre, which places an unusual amount of stretch on the long abductor muscle, will produce some pain in normal persons, but in a patient with De Quervain's disease it will produce severe pain.

When treatment with steroid injections is not successful, De Quervain's disease requires surgical release.

Many published series stress the complications of surgery including incomplete liberation, neuroma of the radial nerve, tendon adhesions, keloid scars, and dislocation of the abductor pollicis longus tendon. All of these complications are easily avoided by a meticulous technique. Anatomical studies have demonstrated several relevant points. The cutaneous branch of the radial nerve crosses the area with two or more branches in about two-thirds of all cases. The abductor pollicis longus frequently presents as many (two to five) strips in about 80% of patients. The extensor pollicis brevis may be either double (5%) or absent (5%) and about 60% of the patients present with a separate compartment for the abductor pollicis longus and the extensor pollicis brevis. Therefore the observation of two tendons after the opening of one compartment should not be accepted as the complete picture, and a second compartment needs to be checked for systematically.

# Part III Breast, Head and Neck

CHAPTER 5

# Breast Surgery

Dick Rainsbury, Siobhan Laws

## INTRODUCTION

Breast surgery is evolving into a specialised area of surgical practice. Preoperative investigations are becoming increasingly sophisticated, as a result of multidisciplinary input from the surgeon, the radiologist, the pathologist, the oncologist, the nurse specialist and nuclear medicine. Better techniques are leading to more targeted procedures, and merging of the roles of clinicians is taking place. As a result, the majority of short stay surgery is for planned therapeutic procedures for benign or malignant breast disease, and diagnostic open breast biopsy is rarely indicated. Today, at least 50% of breast surgery can be carried out in short stay facilities and this figure is likely to rise with the use of targeted axillary procedures. Reconstructive surgery and mastectomy require hospitalisation, but a number of secondary procedures such as implant exchange, capsulotomy, nipple reconstruction and even breast reduction can be carried out effectively on a short stay unit.

The outcomes of short stay breast surgery can be optimised by adhering to certain principles. Indelible ink should be used to mark both the breast and the operation site in every patient.

## Figure 1A, B

Skin incisions which follow the resting skin tension lines (Langer's lines, Fig. 1) minimise scarring and optimise the cosmetic result avoiding the site of the incusion to prevent tattooning of the scar (Fig. 1B: scar placement for best cosmetic results). A monopolar diathermy pencil is a helpful adjunct to dissection, but should be operated with caution when used with non-insulated retractors, in order to avoid cutaneous diathermy damage. A high-quality headlight is indispensable when operating in narrow optical cavities, and dissection may be enhanced by the use of lighted retractors. Closure of resection defects can lead to ugly distortion of the breast and is generally unnecessary. Large resection defects require the development of parenchymal advancement flaps to reconstruct the defect, or volume replacement with autologous tissue. Skin closure may be layered with absorbable subcutaneous and subcuticular sutures, or using a single subcuticular layer. Drains are unnecessary following uncomplicated biopsy but a 'no drain' policy demands meticulous haemostasis. Discharge with a drain in situ is safe, provided there is adequate domiciliary back-up [2].

**Figure 1A, B**

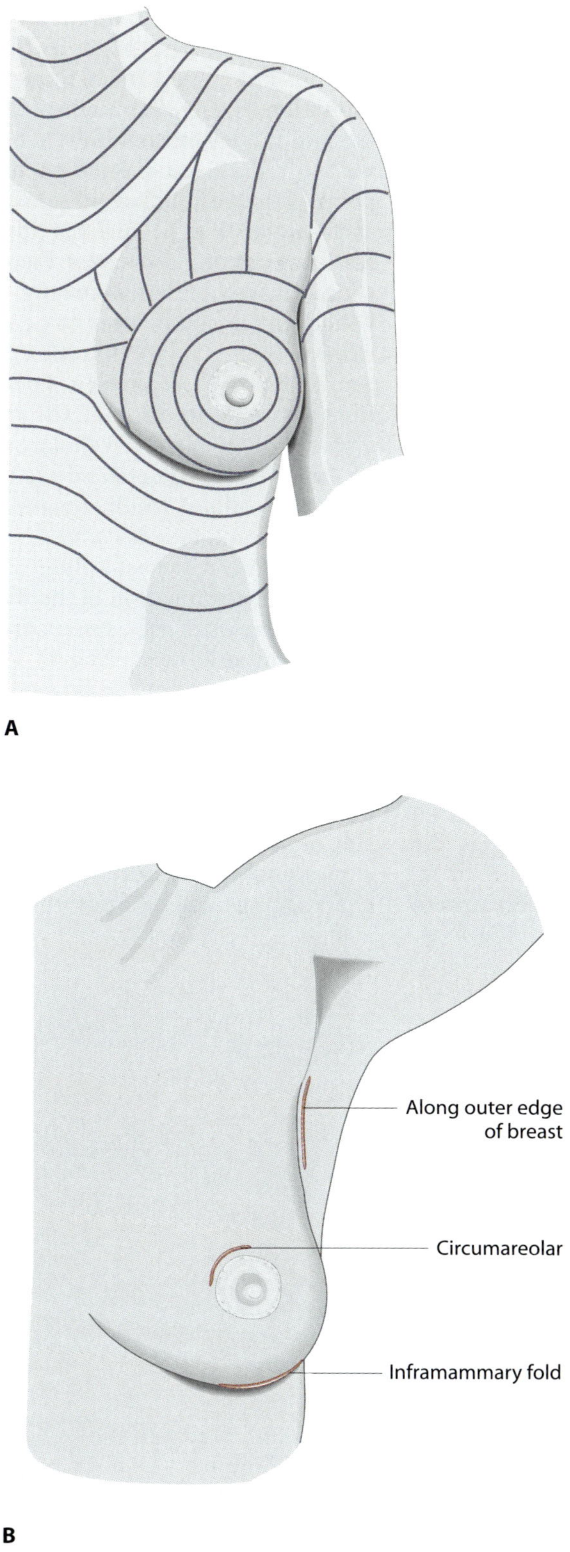
A
B
Along outer edge
of breast
Circumareolar
Inframammary fold

## Figures 2–4: Fine Needle Aspiration Biopsy

■ **Indications.** Fine needle aspiration biopsy (FNAB) is a key diagnostic component of the triple assessment of breast abnormalities, which includes FNAB, mammography and clinical examination. Its use as a diagnostic technique is gradually being superseded by core biopsy (CB), as FNAB cannot differentiate between invasive and in situ disease. False-positive results occur in <1% of cases, as a result of the severe cellular atypia found in some fibroadenomas, following radiotherapy and in patients taking HRT, and therefore CB may be a more appropriate primary investigation in these cases. The false-negative rate is higher (5–10%) and it is operator dependent. FNAB is also used therapeutically for the aspiration of cysts and abscesses. A significant but rare complication of FNAB is pneumothorax, which occurs most commonly when sampling a lesion in the axillary tail region of a slim patient. A pneumothorax caused in this way is usually small and of no clinical consequence. It resolves spontaneously and is unlikely to require aspiration or formal drainage. FNAB produces variable discomfort, which can be limited by the use of a small (23-gauge) needle.

■ **Procedure.** FNAB should be performed with the patient in the recumbent position, preferably with the assistance of a nurse. The procedure is carried out using a 20-ml syringe and a 21-g or 23-g needle, usually without local anaesthetic. The barrel of the syringe is freed, leaving 2 ml of air to enable expression of the contents of the needle onto a slide, following aspiration. The mass is identified and fixed between thumb and index finger in preparation for aspiration (Fig. 2). The angle of insertion of the needle into the lesion should be tangential to the chest wall to reduce the risk of pneumothorax, and the point of entry should avoid sensitive structures such as the areola (Fig. 3). Once the tip of the needle enters the lesion, strong negative pressure is applied to the syringe barrel, either manually or using a syringe holder, which can be used to generate high levels of vacuum (Fig. 4: aid to aspiration). Maintaining a tangential approach, aspiration is performed using multiple passes (8–10) through the lump at different angles in order to obtain a cellular sample. Cysts should be aspirated to dryness and the lesion should be no longer palpable. A residual mass following cyst aspiration, or frank blood-staining of the cystic fluid, indicate the need for aspiration of the cyst wall and cytological examination of the fluid and aspirate.

Thin smears of the aspirate are prepared on glass slides, and fixed according to local protocols. The needle and barrel of the syringe may be rinsed out with a liquid suspension medium and the contents are collected after centrifugation, to maximise cellular harvest. The amount of local pressure required for haemostasis will vary from patient to patient. One-stop reporting of cytology is carried out in many clinics, and will reassure the patient if benign. Inadequate samples can be repeated immediately.

Figure 2

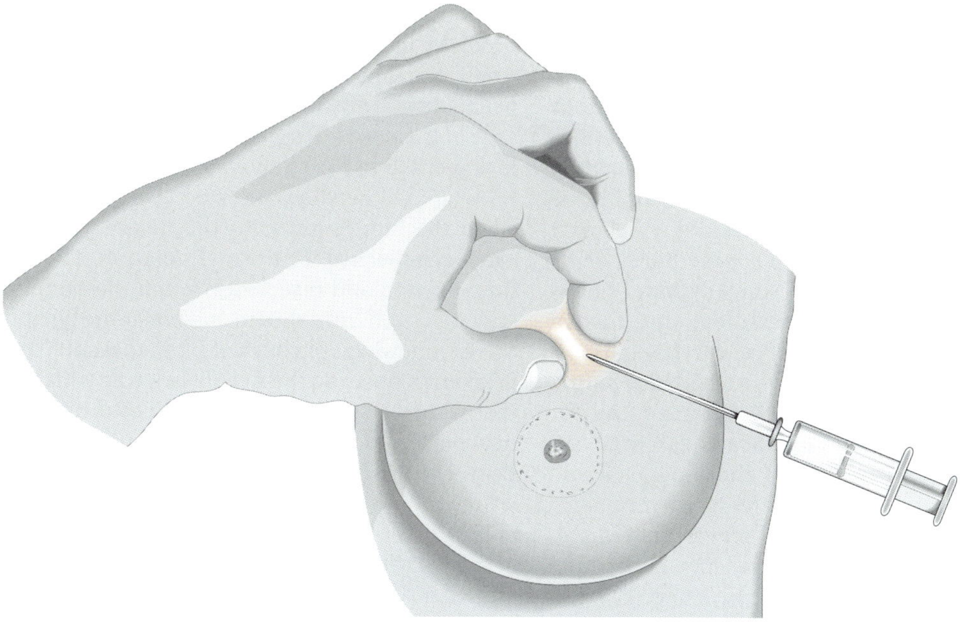

Figure 3

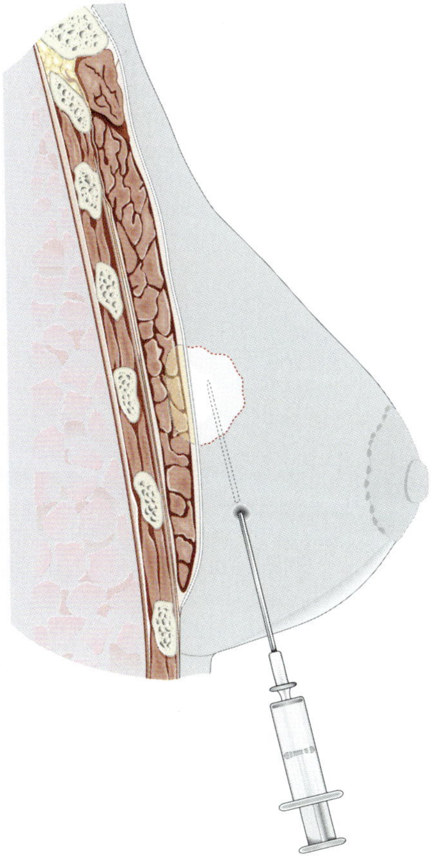

Figure 4

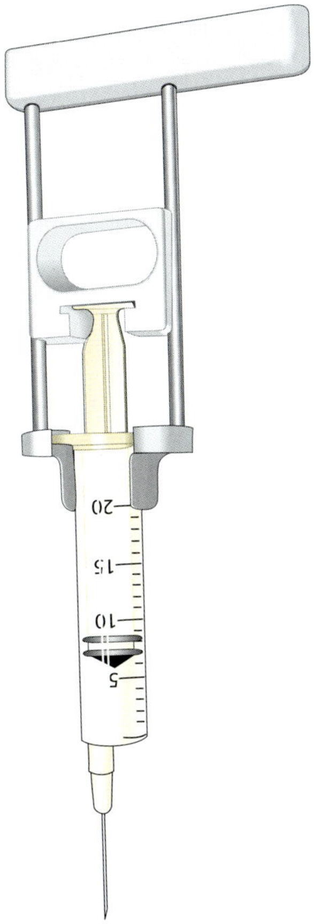

## Figure 5A, B: Core Biopsy



■ **Indications.** Core biopsy (CB) is replacing FNAB as the method of choice for the diagnosis of solid breast lesions, as it can differentiate between in situ and invasive carcinoma and will often enable tumour grade and oestrogen receptor status to be established. Sampling error with CB may be higher than with FNAB when image guidance is omitted. This is particularly true of hard, sclerotic lesions which may be more difficult to sample with a wide-bore needle than with a fine needle. Only a small cylinder of tissue sample is available for assessment, and formal histological analysis of the entire specimen is required before a final diagnosis is reached. For palpable lesions, CB can be performed freehand, but for impalpable lesions, image guidance is essential. CB provides useful confirmation of the diagnosis and oestrogen receptor status in patients deemed suitable for neoadjuvant therapy. Written consent is preferred but not essential, and patients should be warned that the main side effect is bruising. The risk of pneumothorax is similar to FNAB, and patients should be warned about the sampling error inherent in the technique, which may indicate the need for further diagnostic procedures.

■ **Procedure.** The patient is made comfortable in a recumbent position with an assistant to provide reassurance, and to apply pressure over the biopsy site during and after the procedure. Depending on the position of the tumour, the patient may need to be rolled towards the operator, and the shoulder may need to be abducted to 90°. The skin is prepared using an antiseptic solution, and the breast is draped using adhesive towels.

Lidocaine 1% is infiltrated intradermally and subdermally in the region of the selected puncture site. A small incision is made in the skin with a pointed scalpel blade in a position which will ensure that the passage of the needle from the puncture site to the lesion is tangential to the chest wall.

A 14-g CB needle is selected (Fig. 5A) and mounted in the biopsy gun and the device and its safety catch are checked for normal function. The needle is then primed and inserted through the puncture site and advanced until the tip is lying at the periphery of the lesion, which is checked by palpation. Great care is taken to position the needle in a way which ensures that when the gun is fired, the tip of the needle does not perforate the underlying pleura or overlying skin. The use of a hand-held ultrasound probe to position the tip of the needle reduces sampling error and is essential when sampling impalpable lesions (Fig. 5B). After each passage, the needle is withdrawn and firm pressure is applied over the tumour and needle track by the assistant. The cylinder of tissue is expelled into a formal-saline solution and four to six specimens are usually sufficient for diagnosis. Cores containing fatty tissue tend to float in this solution, while those containing glandular tissue and tumour tend to sink. Pressure is applied to the needle track and lesion for 5–10 min before a small dressing is applied. Postbiopsy bruising is common, but a haematoma requiring surgical drainage is rare. Patients should be provided with a contact number and return to the clinic for results, usually within 48 h.

Figure 5A, B

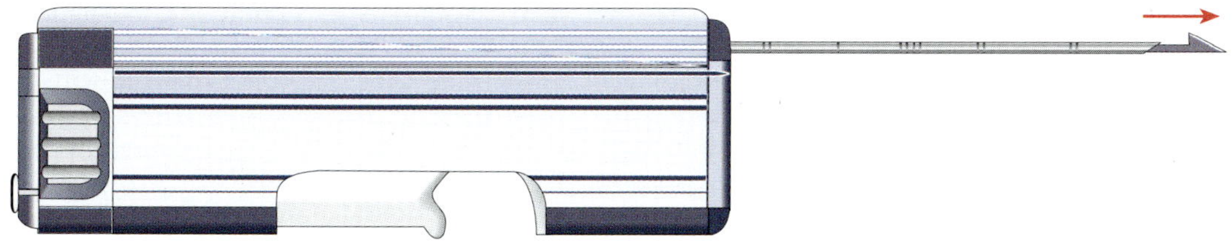

A

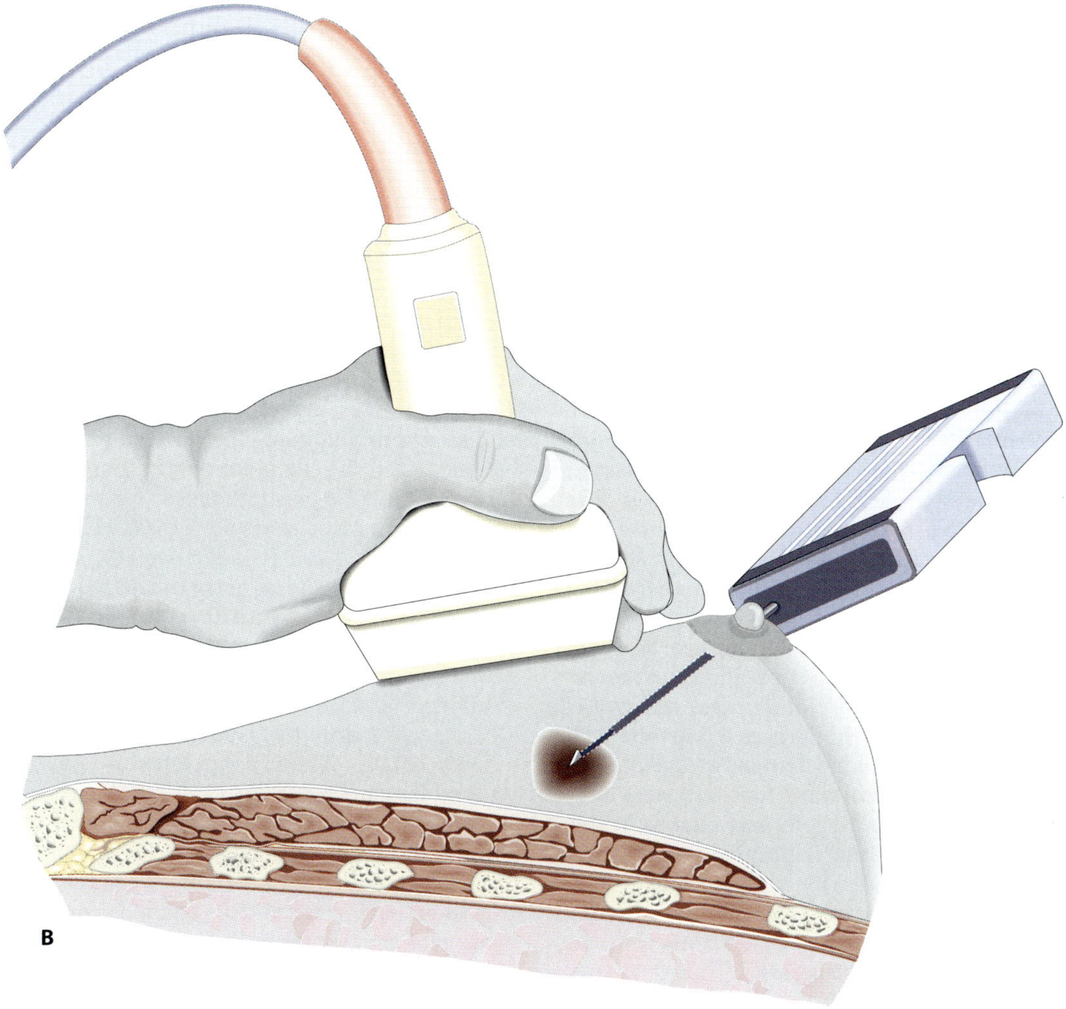

B

5

## Figures 6–8: Radiologically Guided Biopsy

■ **Indications.** Radiologically guided biopsy may be used as a diagnostic or therapeutic procedure for impalpable lesions of the breast. If the nature of an impalpable lesion cannot be diagnosed with certainty by the use of stereotactic-guided FNAB or CB, radiologically guided excision of the lesion with a narrow margin is carried out. Wide-margin therapeutic excision of lesions should only be carried out when the diagnosis has been confirmed by image-guided FNAB or CB. The surgeon should plan the skin incision to facilitate subsequent definitive surgery, and for a diagnostic biopsy the volume of breast tissue excised should be minimised (target weight <20 g) [3]. Adequate excision of the lesion should be confirmed by peroperative specimen radiology.

■ **Procedure.** A wide variety of guidewires are available for the procedure, but it is important that both the radiologist and surgeon are familiar with the type selected. The tip of the guidewire is inserted through the lesion using stereotactic guidance. This may require an oblique or tangential approach from a remote site, depending on the position of the lesion. In the ideal situation, the shaft of the guidewire is passed through the centre of the lesion, and its position is confirmed by craniocaudal and mediolateral oblique mammograms. When transfixion of the lesion with the guidewire has not been achieved, the distance between the tip of the wire and the lesion should be clearly indicated by the radiologist on both radiological views. The wire is then secured firmly to the skin with adhesive tape to prevent displacement before the patient leaves the radiology department for the operating theatre.

Under a general anaesthetic, the adhesive tape is removed and the operative site is prepared taking care not to displace the guidewire, and drapes are applied. The position of the lesion in the breast is estimated by a combination of three manoeuvres. First, gentle traction on the wire while observing for movement of the tip. Second, tapping over the reference quadrant, identifying the position resulting in the greatest movement or 'nodding' of the guidewire, a point which corresponds to the tip of the wire. Third, using both mammographic images to estimate the direction and length of the wire inside the breast.

The incision may be made to include the site of entry of the guidewire, or remotely over the estimated position of the lesion (Fig. 6; reproduced with permission from *Surgery*). When the tip of the wire lies several centimetres away from the point of entry, the procedure is facilitated by placing the incision over the lesion itself using the methods outlined above. If an incision around the site of entry is likely to produce unsightly scarring (for example, in the upper inner quadrant), a remote circumareolar incision may be preferable. When the incision is made around the site of entry it is deepened to the point of entry of the wire into the underlying glandular breast tissue. The guidewire is secured at this point by grasping it gently with Allis' forceps, including a small sleeve of breast tissue around the wire (Fig. 7; reproduced with permission from *Surgery*). Good lighting and retraction are essential, and the dissection is facilitated by the use of a hand-operated monopolar diathermy pencil, to maintain meticulous haemostasis. The area around the distal part of the wire including the hook and 2 cm of breast tissue is widely dissected. The dissection proceeds deeply, preserving a thin envelope of glandular tissue around the wire. Further Allis' forceps are applied sequentially as the dissection proceeds beyond the tip of the guidewire. At this point, the lesion is often palpable and the palpating finger can be used to guide the final part of the dissection before removal of the specimen (Fig. 8; reproduced with permission from *Surgery*).

On removal, the specimen is orientated by the use of surgical clips to mark the superior and lateral edges. The specimen is then placed in a plastic bag and sent for intraoperative specimen radiography to confirm that it contains the lesion. The patient is kept anaesthetised and if specimen radiography does not confirm the lesion, a further excision is carried out. Palpation of the wall of the resection cavity will often identify a mass lesion at this stage. Further inspection of the localisation mammograms will guide the excision of an appropriate segment of the cavity margin in those cases where the procedure is being performed for microcalcification and is not associated with a mass lesion.

When the incision is made over the lesion, some distance from the site of entry of the guidewire, tunnelling under the skin with dissecting scissors enables the identification and retrieval of the guidewire. This is drawn back through the skin into the operation field or divided just deep to the skin and is grasped with Allis' forceps before the excision is carried out as described above. When a therapeutic operation is planned for carcinoma, the same principles apply, but the procedure entails removal of the abnormality with a macroscopic 1-cm radial margin. This should be confirmed by radiography of the specimen, which is orientated with surgical clips enabling immediate re-excision of any narrow margins to be carried out.

■ **Postoperative Management.** Postoperative bruising is commonplace, particularly after removal of deep-sited lesions. Complications include wound infection, electrocautery burn and haematoma formation. Subsequent analysis of biopsy material and multidisciplinary discussion may fail to confirm removal of the mammographic abnormality. In this situation, a decision is made about the need for further excision or subsequent mammography. Guidewire complications include displacement, transection and pneumothorax. Inappropriately sited scars, postoperative haematoma formation, infection and overzealous excisions may result in a poor cosmetic outcome.

Figures 6

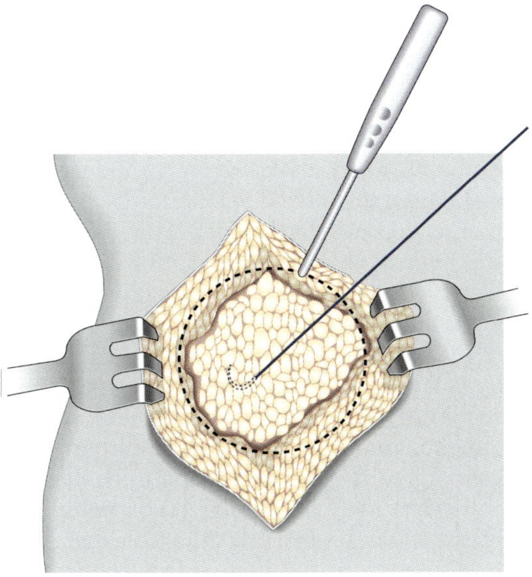

Figures 7

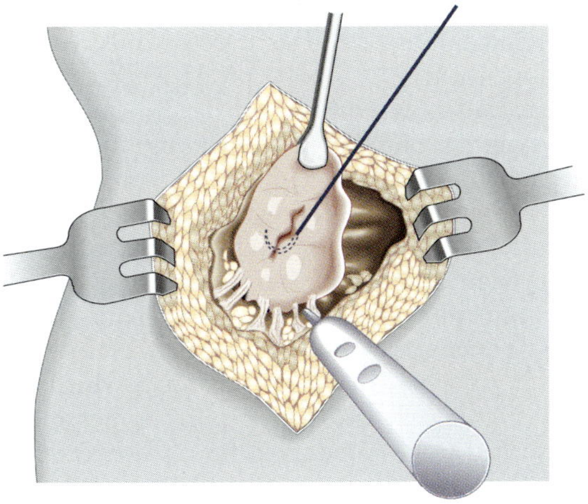

Figures 8

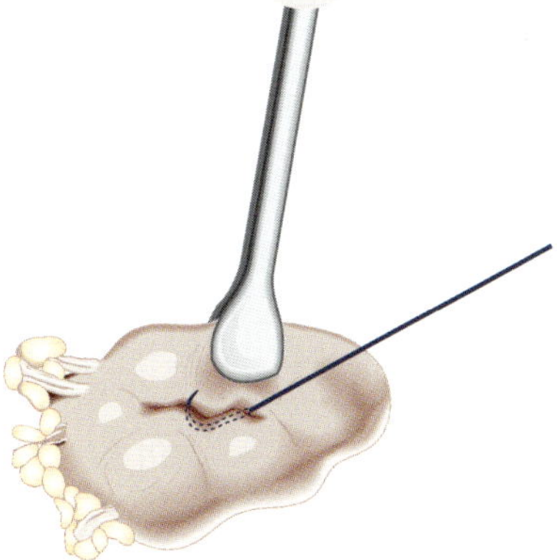

## Figures 9 and 10: Microdochectomy

■ **Indications.** Microdochectomy is the operation of choice for patients who develop a spontaneous, unilateral, persistent single duct discharge which causes staining of the clothes. The discharge is usually caused by duct ectasia, an intraduct papilloma, and occasionally in situ or invasive carcinoma. Microdochectomy is both diagnostic and therapeutic. Preoperative cytological examination of the discharge will usually demonstrate the presence of macrophages and inflammatory cells, and is generally unhelpful. Rarely, the cytological appearances will indicate an underlying papilloma or epithelial malignancy. Solitary duct discharge is often treated by major duct excision (Hadfield's procedure) in postmenopausal women as duct ectasia is the commonest cause in this age group, and major duct excision provides the most definitive cure in a group where breast feeding is no longer anticipated.

Patients should be warned that microdochectomy can lead to altered nipple shape, sensation and pigmentation, and may also affect the ability to breast feed. The risks of infection, haematoma and a poor cosmetic result arising from local distortion and ugly scar formation should be explained. Loss of part of the areola and nipple skin is rare, and may lead to delayed healing. Those at risk include smokers, the obese and patients who have undergone previous nipple surgery. Nipple discharge may recur in patients suffering from duct ectasia, but careful examination and expression of a discharge from more than one duct should alert the clinician to the underlying cause and the need to consider major duct excision.

■ **Procedure.** The patient should be advised to desist from expressing the discharge for at least a week prior to surgery. The patient is asked to confirm that the discharge has continued and to identify the site, which is marked. The patient is placed in the supine position with both arms at the side. The skin is prepared and the breast is draped in the normal way. The nipple is gently grasped between forefinger and thumb and the discharging duct is identified by gentle digital pressure. A small lachrymal probe is passed gently into the lactiferous sinus of the discharging duct and advanced with care to avoid the creation of a false passage. Ideally, the probe is passed up to its hilt, although this may not always be possible when there is an obstruction (Fig. 9: microdochectomy probe insertion). The probe is then fixed in position by passing a suture through the rim of the duct orifice, and securing this to the probe.

Careful infiltration of the subareolar tissues and the core of the nipple with lidocaine 1% with or without adrenaline aids dissection and reduces postoperative discomfort. The incision may be either radial, extending from an incision around the duct orifice to the adjacent areola border, or hemicircumferential over the areola margin, in a location which is in closest proximity to the duct. Using either approach, the subareolar fascia and veins are divided, and by retracting the areola margin with skin hooks, a mixture of blunt and sharp dissection is used to identify the duct containing the probe within the confluence of the lactiferous ducts (Fig. 10). If a radial incision is used, the probe is dissected away from the surrounding nipple, together with a small rim of skin lining the lactiferous sinus.

The probe is grasped with an Allis' forceps and dissected deeply into the reference segment of the breast. Most significant epithelial pathology is detected within 2 cm of the lactiferous sinus, and dissection beyond 4–5 cm is unhelpful in the majority of cases. When a circumareolar incision is used, the resection is carried out deep to the fascia and associated subareolar venous plexus to avoid ischaemia. This enables the further identification and dissection of the diseased duct, which is divided as close to the tip of the nipple as possible. The resection cavity is checked for a palpable mass, and the duct is incised and inspected for visible pathology, such as a duct papilloma. Care is taken with haemostasis and the wound is closed with absorbable subcutaneous and subcuticular sutures, without a drain. A small square of paraffin gauze with an overlying eye pad modified with a central aperture for the nipple provides a comfortable dressing. The patient is asked to report any undue discomfort or swelling, and the wound is inspected at 1 week.

Figure 9

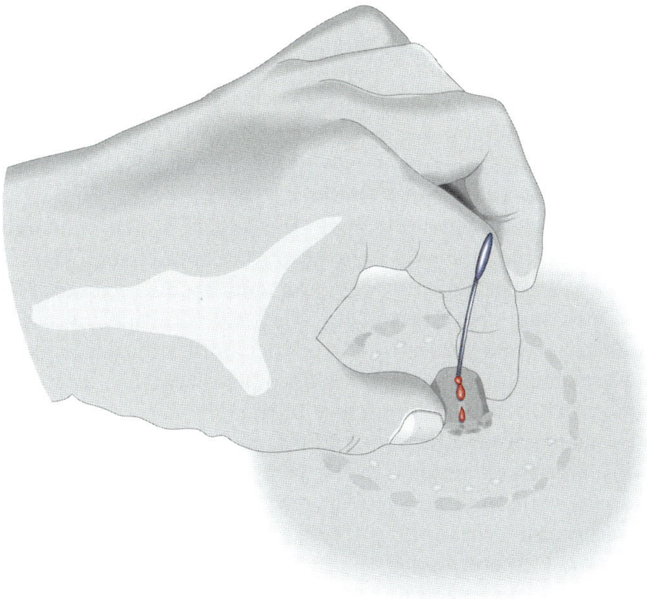

Figure 10

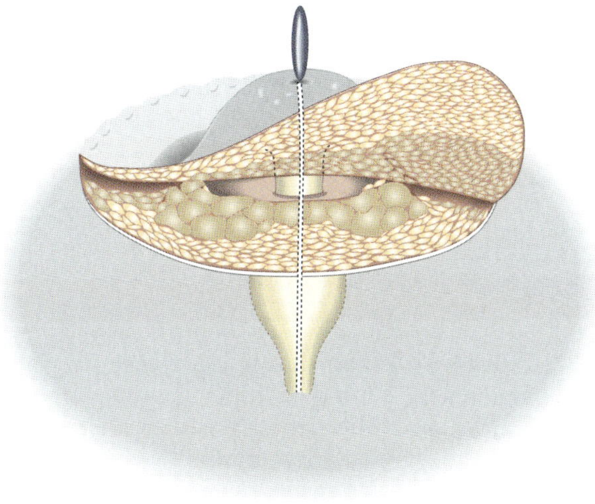

## Figure 11–13: Major Duct Excision: Hadfield's Procedure

**Indications.** Hadfield's procedure aims to divide all the major lactiferous ducts at the level of the lactiferous sinuses. Ducts comprising the core of the nipple as well as any opening widely onto the surface of the areola need to be identified and divided in order to achieve complete excision, and avoid a recurrent discharge. Major duct excision is the procedure of choice for recurrent periductal mastitis and for its complications, including recurrent subareolar sepsis and mamillary fistula. The procedure is also indicated for the management of the solitary duct discharge in postmenopausal women. The retroareolar dissection in Hadfield's procedure is extensive, and it is important to perform this dissection in the subfascial plane, deep to the subareolar venous plexus, in order to minimise the risk of nipple and areola ischaemia.

Risks of the procedure include necrosis, infection, haematoma formation and altered nipple sensation, shape, size and colour. These risks are higher following Hadfield's procedure than in patients undergoing microdochectomy. A number of patients are smokers who are overweight and who have had previous unsuccessful nipple surgery for recurrent sepsis. Peroperative antibiotic prophylaxis is advisable in any patient with a history of recurrent subareolar sepsis, using a broad spectrum preparation with anti-anaerobic activity (e.g. co-amoxiclav). Patients should be warned of the risk of recurrence and the inability to breast feed following this type of surgery.

**Procedure.** The patient is prepared as for microdochectomy and the subareolar region is infiltrated with lidocaine 1% deep to the venous plexus. A circumareolar incision is made passing from 3 o'clock to 9 o'clock and deepened through the fascia, dividing and ligating any subareolar veins. A plane is developed between the deep surface of the fascia and the underlying fat, freeing the areola from the underlying breast tissue. This manoeuvre divides any aberrant lactiferous ducts opening more peripherally onto the surface of the areola, and identifies the core of lactiferous ducts which converge behind the tip of the nipple. A curved haemostat is passed through the incision and around the core of lactiferous ducts (Fig. 11). Gentle traction inverts the nipple and places the ducts under tension, ready for division with a small scalpel blade. The ducts should be divided as close to the dermis as possible, and this manoeuvre can be facilitated by placing the fingertip in the inverted nipple to guide the level of duct division (Fig. 12).

Once divided, any remaining lactiferous duct remnants lying on the under surface of the inverted nipple can be trimmed away using a sharp pair of dissecting scissors. The proximal divided core of lactiferous ducts is grasped with Allis' forceps, and a 2–3 cm cone of tissue is excised from the central part of the breast, which includes the terminal portion of these ducts (Fig. 13). After careful haemostasis, the resulting defect is closed with interrupted absorbable sutures. The nipple is everted without using sutures, as these may jeopardise an already compromised nipple blood supply and are not necessary to maintain eversion. The wound is closed with subcutaneous and subcuticular absorbable sutures, and the dressings and postoperative instructions are as for microdochectomy.

## EXCISION BIOPSY

**Indications.** Open removal of an entire breast lump is carried out with decreasing frequency, with the increasing accuracy of non-invasive investigations. Excision biopsy may be carried out for diagnostic reasons, when the results of triple assessment are discordant or inconclusive. Biopsy has a therapeutic role to play in the removal of unsightly or painful benign lesions, at the patient's request.

**Procedure.** Excision biopsy may be carried out using general or local anaesthetic, but excision of deep-sited lesions or lesions within the confluence of lactiferous ducts may be difficult to carry out under local anaesthetic. The patient is placed in the supine position, with the shoulder abducted to 90° if the lesion lies in the outer half of the breast or axillary tail. The skin incision may be placed directly over the lump or in the circumareolar position, according to the patient's wishes. Remotely sited circumareolar incisions minimise visible scarring, but they entail extensive subcutaneous tunnelling, excellent retraction and high intensity illumination to localise the lesion and carry out its removal.

The lesion should be excised with a narrow intact margin using a diathermy pencil or a scalpel blade for sharp dissection. The specimen is then orientated according to the Unit's protocol and sent for histopathology. Meticulous haemostasis is carried out and the superficial layers are closed with absorbable sutures. No attempt is made to obliterate the resection defect, and drains are not recommended.

Figure 11

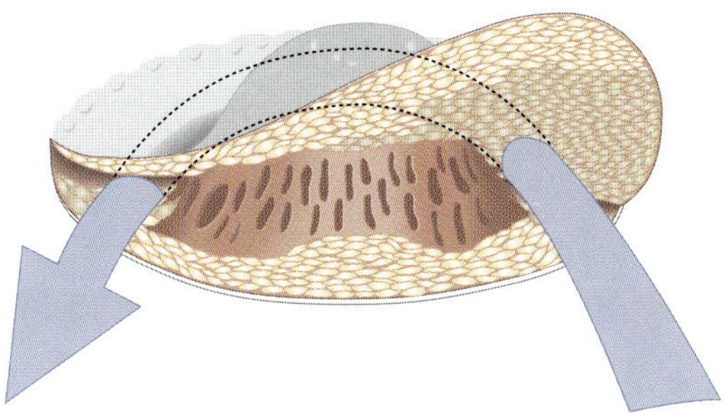

Figure 12

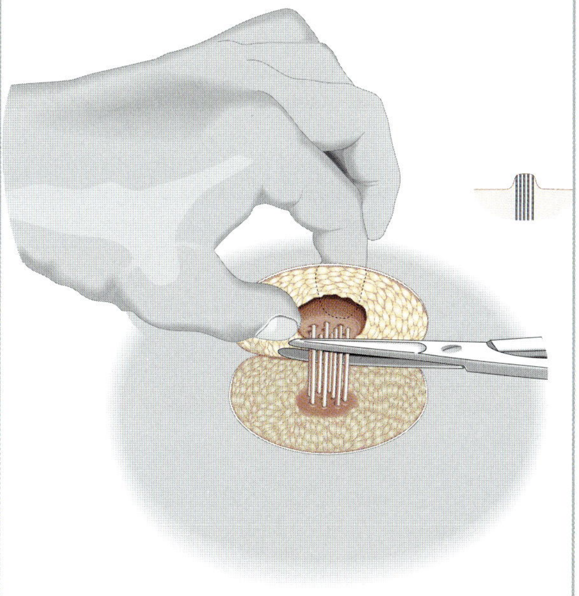

Figure 13

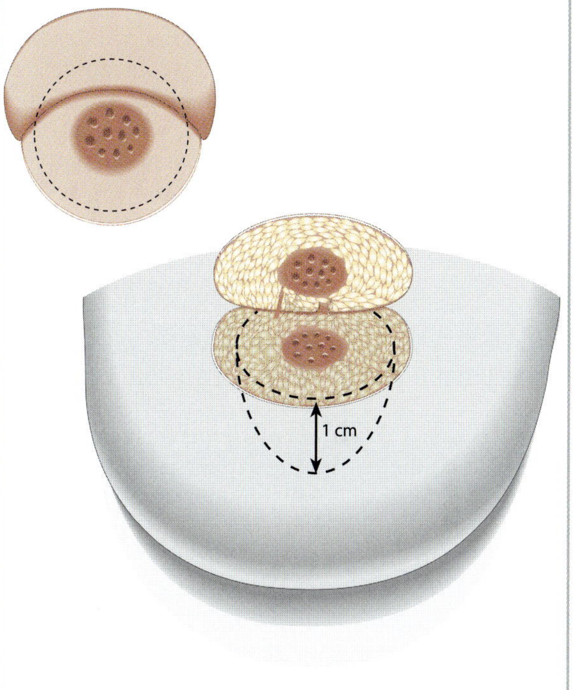

**Postoperative Management.** The main complication of breast biopsy is haematoma formation. This is usually contained, and requires no active intervention. An expanding haematoma requires formal evacuation under general anaesthetic. Most breast biopsies heal with minimal scarring, although hypertrophic and keloid scars are occasionally encountered, particularly in the upper inner quadrant of the breast. Other complications include infection, failure to excise the clinically identified lesion, and recurrence (typically following the excision of phyllodes tumours and fibroadenomata).

## Figures 14, 15: Wide Local Excision



**Indications.** Wide local excision (WLE) of breast carcinoma aims to excise at least 1 cm of macroscopically normal breast tissue with a minimum 2 mm microscopic margin [4].

If a WLE meeting these criteria results in loss of >20% of breast volume, the cosmetic results are likely to be poor, and a mastectomy may be indicated. Similar cosmetic penalties may arise from excision of upper inner quadrant lesions associated with as little as 10% volume loss. WLE is generally contraindicated for central, subareolar tumours (within 2 cm of nipple-areola complex) and in patients with multifocal disease. Extensive in situ disease, extensive lymphatic invasion and young age (<30 years) are relative contraindications to WLE. New methods of volume replacement and volume displacement, using autologous tissues to reconstruct wider resection defects, are extending the role of breast-conserving surgery to include patients who would otherwise require mastectomy as a result of extensive volume loss.

**Procedure.** WLE is normally performed under a general anaesthetic with the patient in the supine position with the ipsilateral shoulder abducted to 90° on an armboard. The skin, axilla and upper arm are prepared with an antiseptic solution, and towels are placed to enable access to the breast and axilla. Most patients undergoing WLE have an axillary procedure (see below). An incision is made over the tumour using Kreissl's lines, bearing in mind that a subsequent mastectomy may be necessary. Alternatively, the tumour may be excised through a circumareolar incision when it is sited in the upper pole of the breast to avoid unsightly scarring, but this approach requires extensive undermining of the skin to gain access to the reference quadrant. The excision of skin overlying a carcinoma is unnecessary unless there is frank invasion and may lead to poor cosmesis.

A cylinder of breast tissue is excised from subcutaneous fat down to and including pectoralis fascia, orientated to remove the lesion with a minimum 1 cm macroscopic radial margin (Fig. 14: specimen once excised). In Fig. 15 the skin is undermined and then cut down vertically at the margin beyond the tumour down to the pectoral fascia. The specimen is marked and specimen radiography may be carried out according to the Unit protocol and sent for histology. Meticulous haemostasis is vital and no attempt is made to close the resection defect. Routine skin closure is performed without placing a drain.

**Postoperative Management.** Early complications include wound haematoma, wound infection and wound breakdown. If a positive margin is reported, the wound is reopened and re-excision of the adjacent cavity wall is carried out.

**Late Complications.** Localised volume loss combines with the effects of radiotherapy to produce localised deformity as a result of scarring, contraction and parenchymal fibrosis. These effects are minimal in the majority of patients, but become more common with extensive volume depletion (>20% breast volume), and in patients who have experienced postoperative infection, haematoma formation and wound breakdown. Other late complications include local recurrence (<1% per annum) and lymphoedema of the breast.

Figure 14

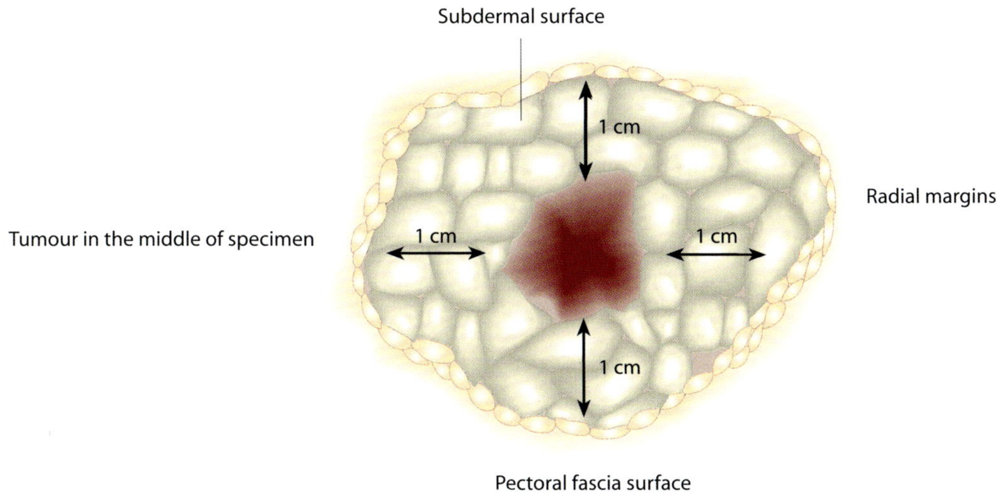


Figure 15

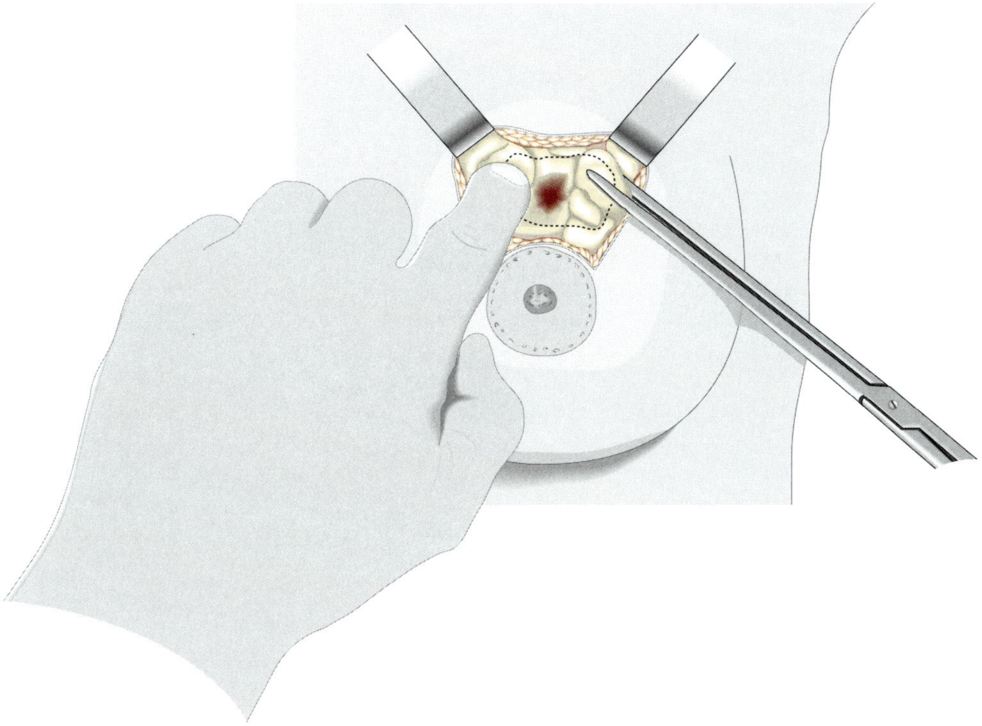

## Figure 16: Axillary Surgery

Axillary surgery is currently undergoing a critical review with the advent of sentinel node biopsy as a diagnostic procedure (Fig. 16: schematic plan of axilla). Axillary sampling and level 1, 2 or 3 axillary dissection appear to have equivalent prognostic value, but each approach is associated with morbidity. Patients undergoing axillary sampling followed by radiotherapy have a higher incidence of shoulder stiffening when compared with patients having level 3 axillary dissection, who have a higher incidence of arm lymphoedema.

Figure 16

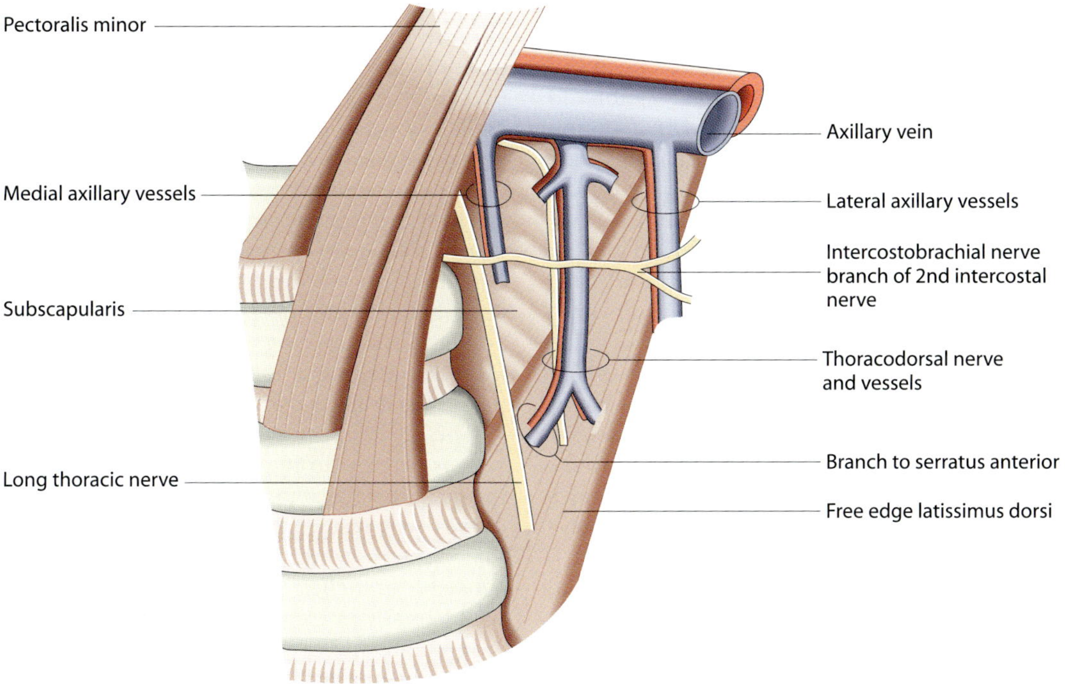
Pectoralis minor
Medial axillary vessels
Subscapularis
Long thoracic nerve
Axillary vein
Lateral axillary vessels
Intercostobrachial nerve branch of 2nd intercostal nerve
Thoracodorsal nerve and vessels
Branch to serratus anterior
Free edge latissimus dorsi

## Figures 17–20: Axillary Dissection



■ **Indications.** The axilla is divided into three levels, namely level 1, level 2 and level 3, which correspond to dissections below, behind and above pectoralis minor, respectively [5]. The current indications for axillary clearance include patients with a tumour >1 cm in diameter, those with positive sentinel nodes and those with operable malignant lymph nodes in level 1, 2 or 3. Axillary clearance is excellent treatment for nodal metastases and is the preferred axillary surgery in many centres, as it provides accurate staging, excellent regional control and optimum prognostication. Patients should be warned of a 5–10% risk of lymphoedema, which increases with the use of adjuvant axillary irradiation. Intercostobrachial neuralgia is a relatively uncommon but troublesome complication of division or entrapment of the nerve at the time of surgery, and may be prevented by preservation of the dominant branches of this nerve.

■ **Procedure.** The patient is draped as described for WLE. The arm may be draped separately to allow movement of the shoulder during surgery and to aid retraction of pectoralis minor if dissection is continued to level 3. A lateral tilt away from the surgeon and the use of a headlight simplify the procedure. The surgeon may prefer to be seated. A vertical 8–10 cm excision is made just behind the lateral border of pectoralis major running down from the apex of the axilla towards the axillary tail. Alternatively, a transverse incision is made within the skin crease from the anterior axillary fold across the hollow of the axilla to the posterior axillary fold (Fig. 17). The incision is deepened by sharp dissection to expose the lateral edge of pectoralis major, and a space is developed between the deep surface of pectoralis major and the underlying clavipectoral fascia (CPF) (Fig. 18). Medial retraction of the lateral border of pectoralis major by the assistant facilitates this step.

The lateral pectoral nerves and thoracoacromial vessels emerge through the CPF as they pass towards the deep surface of pectoralis major. Damage to these nerves will result in atrophy of most of pectoralis major and loss of the anterior axillary fold. Small but constant branches of the thoracoacromial vessels pass laterally into the axillary fat and require careful coagulation and division to avoid avulsion and damage of this important neurovascular bundle.

Figure 17

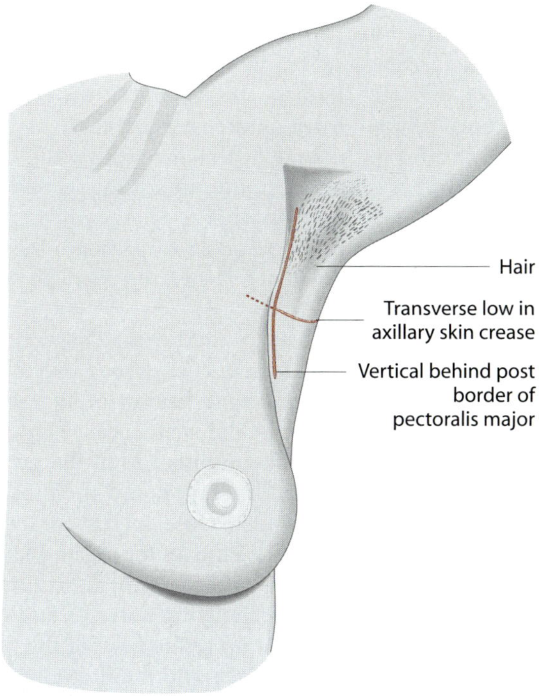


Figure 18

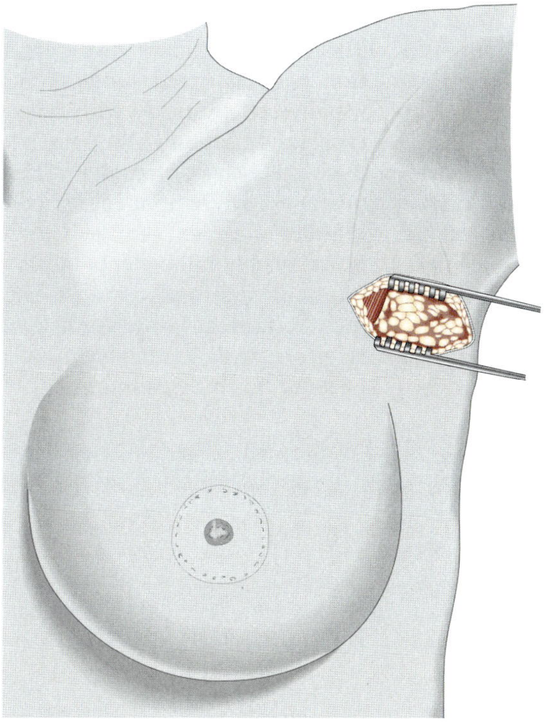

Both layers of the CPF are incised along the path of the free edge of pectoralis minor, sweeping laterally towards the arm. This opens the roof of the axilla and enables access to its contents, and exposure of the anterior wall of the axillary vein running across the upper border of the axilla (Fig. 19. A: superficial dissection; b deep dissection). Loose areola tissue overlying the anterior and inferior surface of the axillary vein, together with any nodes, are dissected in a caudal direction. This dissection is best carried out using a combination of diathermy forceps dissection and bipolar diathermy scissors. Clearance of the fatty and lymphatic tissue lying inferior to the vein exposes two or three lateral thoracic veins draining into the inferior border of the axillary vein and, more laterally, a larger subscapular vein draining into the posterior border of the axillary vein. Occasionally, a lateral axillary vein drains directly into the subscapular vein. Each tributary must be carefully identified and the lateral tributaries divided between surgical clips.

Continuing the dissection in a caudal direction along the subscapular vein reveals the subscapular artery lying just behind the vein, which is joined by the thoracodorsal nerve, emerging from under the axillary vein and running obliquely over subscapularis to join the vascular bundle about 2 cm below the axillary vein (Fig. 20. A: dissection from above; B: dissection from below). The long thoracic nerve is plastered to the surface of the serratus anterior by the overlying serratus fascia and must be identified by clearing the fatty tissue which lies in the inverted triangular space between the thoracodorsal nerve and the chest wall. For a level 1 dissection, the tongue of fibrofatty tissue which encases the anterior and inferior borders of the axillary vein is divided as it passes behind the lateral border of pectoralis minor up towards the first rib.

The last key structure to identify is the intercostobrachial branch of the second intercostal nerve, which typically emerges from the second intercostal space some 2 cm anterior to the long thoracic nerve. Gentle downward traction of the partially mobilised axillary content puts the nerve under tension, which feels like a 'bowstring'. The nerve is dissected away from its surrounding fatty envelope, and is dissected free from the already divided lateral thoracic veins which cross the nerve and often branch around it. The dissection is completed by clearing the axillary contents away from the latissimus dorsi, thoracodorsal trunk and long thoracic nerve, taking care not to damage these structures. The lateral branch of the third intercostal nerve is usually sacrificed in the course of this procedure; the lateral thoracic vessels are encountered for the second time and require further division to allow removal of the specimen. Care must be taken to preserve the caudal, more vulnerable part of the long thoracic nerve.

■ **Level 2 and Level 3 Dissection.** The pectoralis minor muscle is exposed, and this is facilitated by adduction and flexion of the shoulder. A window is made in the costocoracoid membrane, which is the medial continuation of the pectoral fascia medial to pectoralis minor, and the muscle is either retracted or divided close to the coracoid process. This manoeuvre exposes level 2 and level 3 nodes, which are excised by diathermy dissection of all lymphatic and fatty tissue lying anterior and inferior to the wall of the vein up to the level of the first rib, the first intercostal space, and the first digitation of serratus anterior para. The axilla is checked for any residual lymphatic tissue and thorough haemostasis is carried out. The wound is closed in layers with non-absorbable sutures over a suction or siphon drain, which is brought out through the dependent aspect of the dissection cavity.

■ **Postoperative Management.** The main early complications of axillary dissection are seroma formation and restricted shoulder movements. Seromas usually settle quickly with repeated aspiration, and early mobilisation of the arm is recommended to reduce the risk of shoulder stiffness. Transient early postoperative lymphoedema is observed in a small number of patients and usually settles spontaneously. Delayed lymphoedema (after 1–2 years) is a more ominous sign and requires early aggressive treatment to prevent progression. Intercostobrachial neuralgia resolves gradually in most patients, but may become chronic in a minority.

Figure 19A

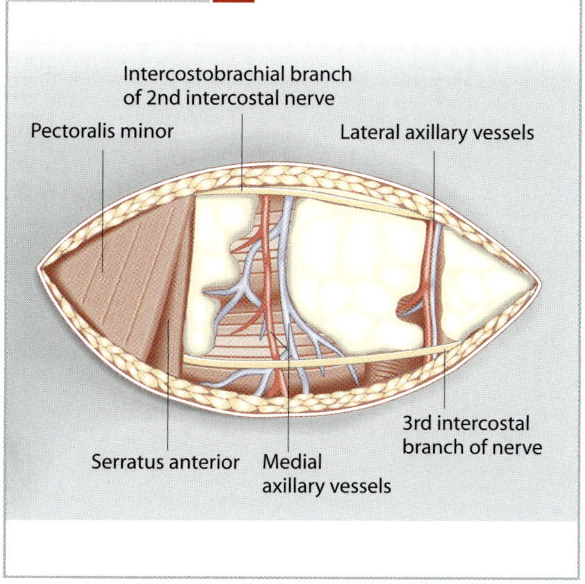


Figure 19B

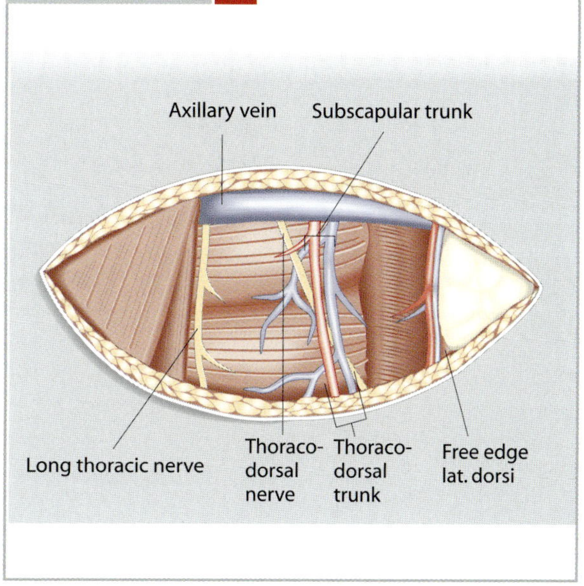


Figure 20A

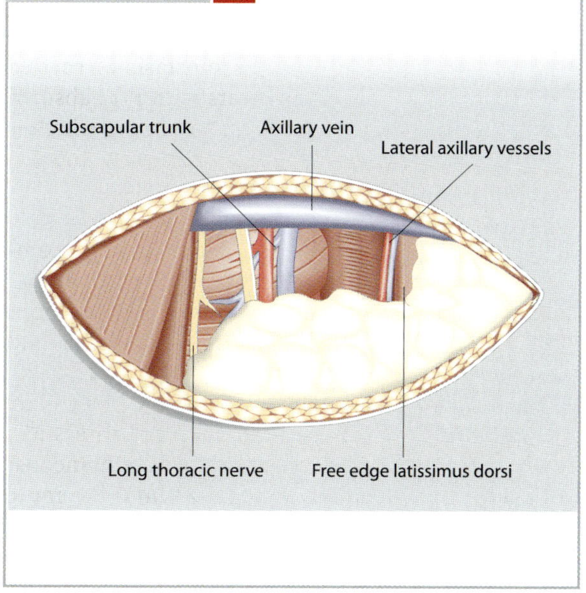


Figure 20B

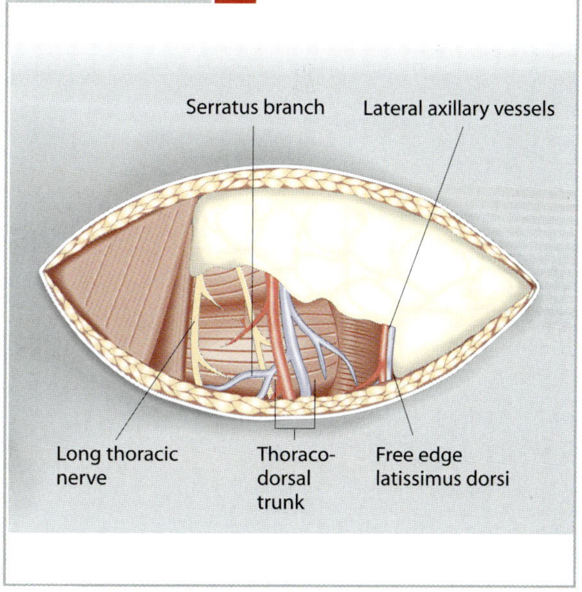

## Figure 21: Breast Abscess

Figure 21

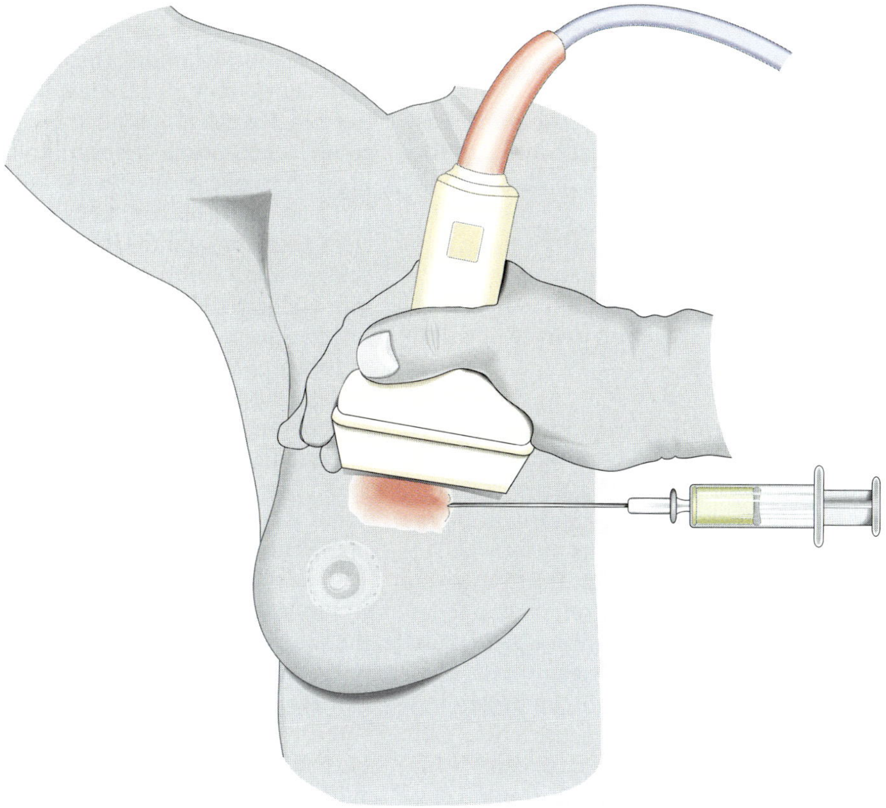

## AXILLARY SAMPLING

**Indications.** Axillary sampling involves removal of a minimum of four lymph nodes from the lower part of the axilla, inferior to the intercostobrachial nerve. The indications for axillary sampling vary from Unit to Unit, but there is general consensus that this approach is appropriate for the management of small invasive carcinomas (<1 cm) and patients with extensive DCIS lesions (>5 cm) in whom the risk of invasive disease is significant. The patient should be informed that further surgery or radiotherapy is recommended in those who are found to have nodal involvement.

**Procedure.** The patient is placed in the position used for axillary dissection, although separate towelling and movement of the arm is not required. Through a longitudinal or transverse incision the clavipectoral fascia is identified and a window of sufficient size is made to enable identification of the intercostobrachial nerve running from medial to lateral in the upper aspect of the operation field. Fatty axillary tissue is gently dissected away from the chest wall from medial to lateral, using a combination of blunt and sharp diathermy-assisted dissection. Care is taken to avoid dividing the intercostobrachial nerve and the lateral branch of the third intercostal nerve, and the dissection proceeds between these two nerves. A minimum of four nodes are identified by a combination of sharp and blunt dissection and finger exploration. It is unusual to encounter the long thoracic nerve or the thoracodorsal trunk during this procedure, but sometimes the dissection has to be extended above the intercostobrachial nerve or below the third nerve in order to harvest all four nodes. Meticulous haemostasis is achieved, and the wound is closed in layers without a drain.

**Postoperative Management.** Recovery is rapid and any seroma formation usually settles with one or two aspirations. Shoulder stiffness and arm lymphoedema are rare sequelae.

## SENTINEL NODE BIOPSY

Sentinel lymph node dissection (SLND) is likely to replace more invasive axillary procedures in the majority of patients with breast cancer. The sentinel lymph node is defined as the first node in the lymphatic basin to which the primary tumour drains. SLND is used to stage the clinically node negative axilla in patients with operable invasive breast cancer. It may also be used in patients with extensive DCIS, where the surgeon would normally perform nodal sampling. SLND is a staging examination and not a treatment per se. Local protocols will determine the subsequent axillary management in patients with a positive sentinel node, which will include further axillary surgery or irradiation. The overall false-negative rate for a sentinel node biopsy is 5%, which may result in suboptimal adjuvant treatment and distressing axillary recurrence in a small number of patients.

Local protocols for SLND are agreed with the Nuclear Medicine and the Pathology Departments. Most centres use a combination of Tc 99m colloidal albumin and patent blue dye. The radiolabelled colloid is injected intradermally or into the subareolar tissue or just cephalad to the site of a recent biopsy the day before surgery. The lymphoscintigraphy is performed at a minimum of 2 h after injection of the tracer, and static anterior, lateral and anterior oblique views are obtained. A sentinel node is found in the axilla in >95% of cases, and occasionally in intramammary and internal mammary sites.

**Procedure.** Surgery is performed within 24 h of the tracer injection. The patient is anaesthetised and prepared and draped as for a wide local excision and axillary dissection. Patent blue V dye (Laboratoire Guerbet, Aulmay-sous-bis, France) is injected intradermally in the skin overlying the tumour, or into the subareolar region or cephalad to a recent biopsy scar. The breast is gently compressed to augment the action of the lymphatic pump and promote passage of blue dye to the axilla. Some 5 min later, a transverse incision is made just inferior to the hair-bearing region of the axilla and deepened by blunt dissection to identify a blue-stained lymphatic running just deep to the clavipectoral fascia. This blue channel is traced proximally and distally until the first blue node or sentinel node is identified. The gamma probe is calibrated according to the manufacturer's recommendations, and is used to confirm that the blue node also contains a high radioactive count which should be approximately 10% of the count in the primary tumour.

If the sentinel node is not identified with the blue dye, the gamma probe is used to identify any hot or non-staining sentinel nodes. Following removal of the first sentinel node, the axillary basin should be searched for the presence of other sentinel nodes, which should be numbered in the order in which they are removed. Background count is recorded for 10 s over the ipsilateral arm, and a node is identified as a sentinel node if it meets any of the following criteria: first, a hot node with radioactive counts 10 times greater than background; second, a blue-stained node; third, a blue lymphatic leading to a non-stained node.

■ **Postoperative Management.** The rates of lymphoedema, intercostobrachial neuralgia and seroma formation are similar to axillary sampling. The radiolabelled colloid and patent blue dye can cause anaphylactic reactions, and the blue dye may colour the urine and stools during excretion. Discolouration may persist in the skin for many months.

## BREAST ABSCESS

■ **Indications for Intervention.** An abscess may occur in the lactating or non-lactating breast and result from different bacterial infections. Streptococcal and staphylococcal organisms predominate in the lactational abscesses, and in addition anaerobic bacteria are found in the non-lactational abscess. Prompt identification and treatment of breast infections with appropriate antibiotics can prevent the subsequent development of an abscess in many cases. The treatment of choice for an abscess is by repeated ultrasound-guided needle aspiration and antibiotics. The puncture site is prepared with aseptic solution and a 19-g needle is advanced into the pocket or pockets of pus. Aspiration is performed to dryness and the procedure is repeated until the infection has settled. Appropriate antibiotic therapy for lactational abscesses includes flucloxacillin or erythromycin, adding metronidazole for non-lactational abscesses. Co-amoxiclav is a useful alternative.

In the lactating patient, repeated aspiration with ultrasound-guidance using a 19-g needle and concurrent appropriate antibiotics may abort infection and prevent the need for formal incision and drainage. Self or mechanical expression of the milk may hasten resolution, but suppression of lactation with bromocryptine may be indicated in cases of painful progressive breast engorgement. Incision and drainage is indicated if the mass is fluctuant, if there is associated superficial skin necrosis or the abscess fails to resolve after repeated aspirations. Underlying pathology such as carcinoma, tuberculosis and factitious causes must be considered in those cases which fail to respond to aggressive surgical management.

■ **Procedure.** Incision and drainage is best carried out with the patient under a general anaesthetic in the supine position and the breast prepared and towelled to allow free access. A radial incision is made over the site of maximum fluctuance to minimise damage to the underlying duct system. Pus is evacuated, and collected for microbiological examination, checking that an appropriate culture medium is available when atypical organisms are suspected. The abscess loculations are gently broken down with the finger and the abscess cavity is washed out thoroughly with an antiseptic solution. Generous biopsies are taken from the wall of the abscess and sent for histological examination to exclude malignancy. The cavity may be packed with saline soaked gauze or other suitable dressing, or alternatively closed gently over a large corrugated drain.

■ **Postoperative Management.** The cavity normally heals within 4–6 weeks, providing no atypical infection or underlying malignancy has been identified.

## CONCLUSION

The popularity of short-stay surgery for the management of a wide range of benign and malignant breast conditions is increasing, to the benefit of patients and healthcare providers. This development is linked to the earlier detection, more precise preoperative diagnosis, and better peroperative localization of small breast lesions and their associated lymph nodes through the use of modern imaging and sampling techniques. Results can be optimised by a clear understanding of anatomy, the judicious use of local anaesthesia and haemostasis, and by a meticulous surgical technique.

## SELECTED REFERENCES


1. Kriessl CJ (1951) The selection of appropriate lines for elective surgical incisions. Plast Reconstr Surg 8:1–27
2. Holcombe C, West N, Mansel RE, Horgan K (1995) The satisfaction and savings of early discharge with drain *in situ* following axillary lymphadenectomy in the treatment of breast cancer. Eur J Surg Oncol 21:604–609
3. National Co-ordinator Group of Surgeons Working in Breast Cancer Screening. Quality Assurance Guidelines for Surgeons in Breast Cancer Screening. NHS BSP Publication No 20, 1994. NHS BSP Publications, Sheffield
4. Guidance on Cancer Services (2002) Improving outcomes in breast cancer: Manual update, 2002. National Institute of Clinical Excellence, London
5. O'Dwyer (1991) Axillary dissection in primary breast cancer. BMJ 302:360–361

CHAPTER 6

# Head and Neck Surgery

**Mario Colombo-Benkmann, Norbert Senninger**

## THYROID SURGERY

Indications for thyroid surgery can be divided into three groups: functional indications comprising all forms of hyperthyroidism, morphological indications, i.e. large benign goitres, and oncological indications, if cancer is suspected or evident. However, regardless of the indication, the surgical approach is uniform except for the extent of removal of tissue. The amount of thyroid tissue to be removed has been a matter of constant debate. In the case of hyperthyroidism, unilateral lobectomy is considered to be adequate for an autonomous adenoma. In Graves' disease more radical concepts such as total thyroidectomy have recently been propagated (Barakate et al. 2002), especially for the control of extrathyroidal symptoms. By contrast a thyroid remnant of about 4 g was considered to be an adequate operative goal in the past. In multinodular euthyroid goitre more radical concepts have also been applied recently because clinical experience has shown that despite subtotal resection, recurrent goitre may develop with a latency of several decades (Gibelin et al. 2004).

In incidental papillary thyroid cancers of up to 1 cm, unilateral lobectomy has been regarded as being oncologically sufficient and not requiring remnant thyroidectomy. More recently, even for incidentally diagnosed sporadic medullary thyroid cancer, this type of less than radical surgery has been claimed to be acceptable (Raffel et al. 2004). However, in all other types of thyroid cancer total thyroidectomy is the procedure of choice. Eliminating all thyroid tissue reduces the risk of recurrence, allows successful adjuvant radioiodine treatment (Kim et el. 2004), as well as the utilization of thyroglobulin levels for follow-up.

In unilateral surgery both lobes should be explored digitally or if available by a fingertip ultrasound probe. The use of magnifying loops nowadays is recommended.

Operative procedures in thyroid surgery follow a uniform sequence of operative steps: (1) collar Kocher's incision followed by creation of the upper and lower skin flaps; (2) dissection of the lower part of the sternocleidomastoid muscle from the strap muscles; (3) median separation of the strap muscle midline raphe with transsection of the strap muscles only if needed; (4) preparation of the upper pole and ligation of the superior thyroid vessels; (5) identification of the parathyroid glands and the recurrent laryngeal nerves; (6) ligation of the lower inferior thyroid artery during thyroid subtotal resection or transection in total thyroidectomy; (7) ligation of lower pole veins; (8) undermining of the thyroid isthmus and transsection in unilateral lobectomy or bilateral thyroid resection; (9) resection of pathological thyroid tissue followed by adaptive sutures or removal of the entire thyroid; (10) placing of drains if needed; (11) reconstruction and readaptation of strap muscles; (12) closure of platysma and subcutaneous layer; and (13) skin closure.

If cancer is evident, systematic dissection of the central lymph nodes (in between the internal jugular veins) is performed.

## Figure 1

Good intraoperative exposure is facilitated by the patient's position on the operating table, with extension of the neck. This should not be excessive to avoid postoperative neck pain. In general all thyroid and parathyroid operations are carried out through a collar Kocher's incision. The incision line is drawn with a marker, 2 cm above the sternal notch, ascending bilaterally. If transverse skin creases are present at a suitable position, the incision may be placed there. The lateral ends of the incision line extend according to the size of the thyroid. In small nodules of the isthmus a suprasternal incision of 2 cm length may be sufficient, while in very large goitres the length of incision may extend laterally to the medial borders of the sternocleidomastoid muscle. However, in most instances the incision ends just 1 cm lateral to the medial borders of the sternocleidomastoid muscle.



## Figure 2

The incision is started using a scalpel to transect the epidermis and dermis, while subcutaneous fat and platysma are divided with a diathermy needle. Care needs to be taken not to injure the fasciae of the strap muscles and the sternocleidomastoid muscles, since this may cause adhesions between the muscular tissue and the platysma with subsequent indentations especially visible during swallowing.

Figure 1

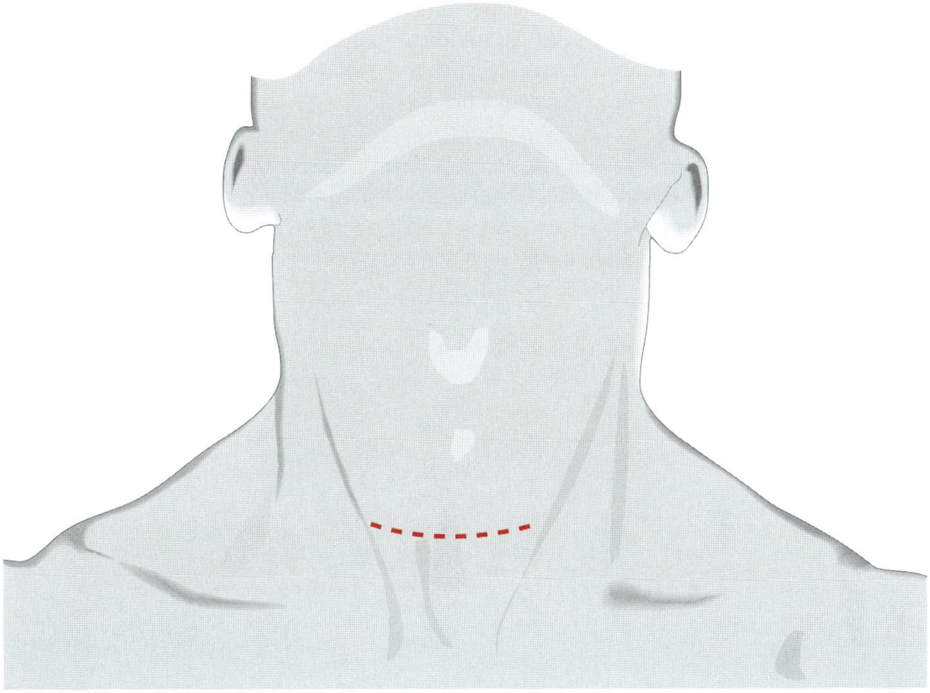

Figure 2

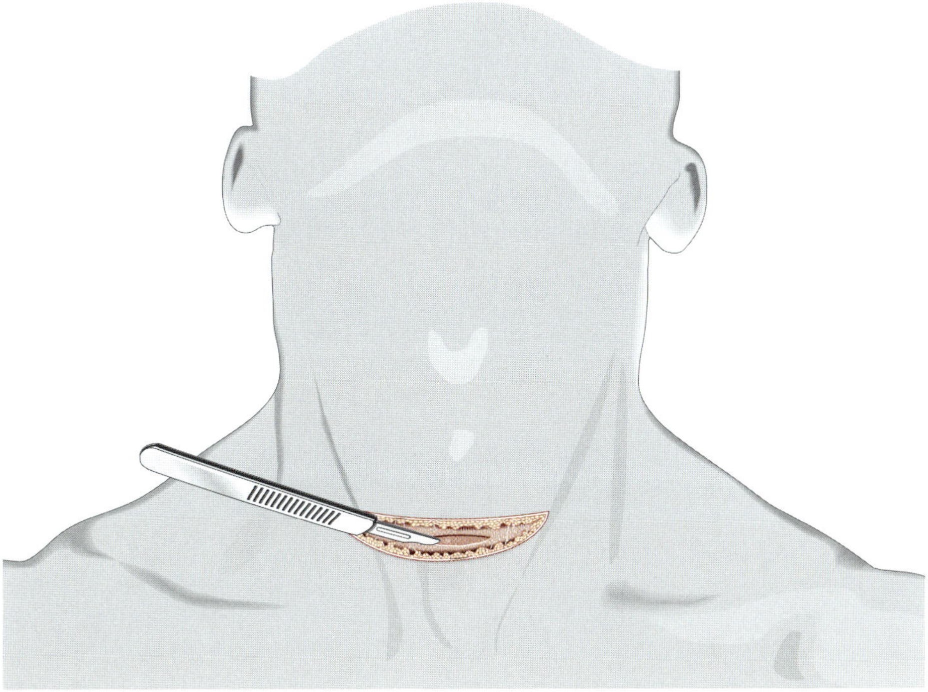

## Figure 3

Care needs to be taken not to damage the superficial veins. However, when indicated they can be divided and are ligated with 3-0 absorbable sutures. For reasons of clarity of the sketches, the retraction hooks necessary of adequate esposure are omitted in the subsequent figures. In addition, the dissected and separated strap muscles being clamped are omitted for better visibility.

## Figure 4

Mobilisation of the upper and lower flap is carried out bluntly with a gauze over the thumbs up to the notch of the thyroid cartilage and down to the sternal notch. This can be performed in the layer dorsally to the previously ligated cervical veins and this allows a bloodless exposure of the strap muscles. To facilitate separation of the strap muscles from the sternocleidomastoid muscle, the medial border of the latter is dissected thoroughly without injuring its fascia.

Figure 3

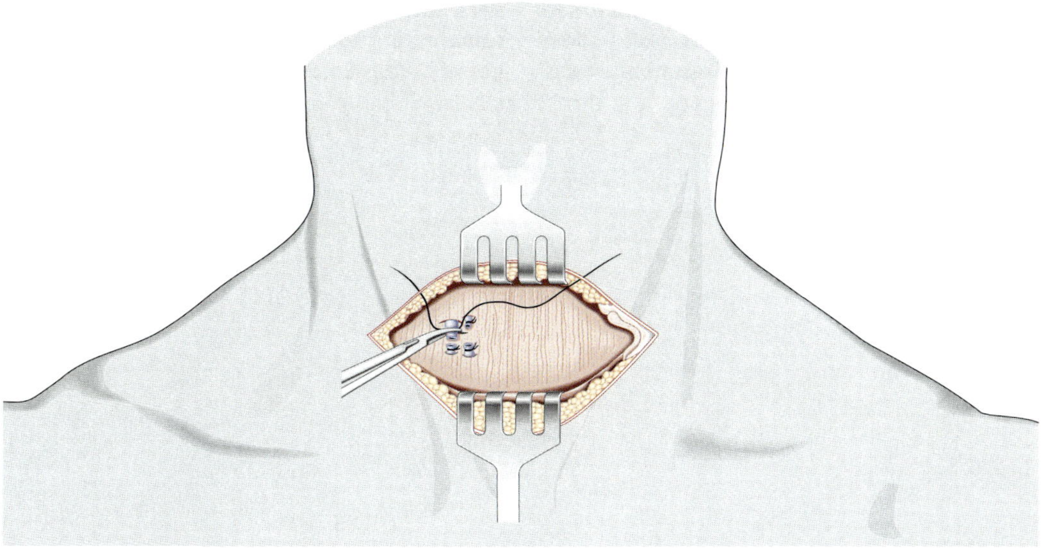

Figure 4

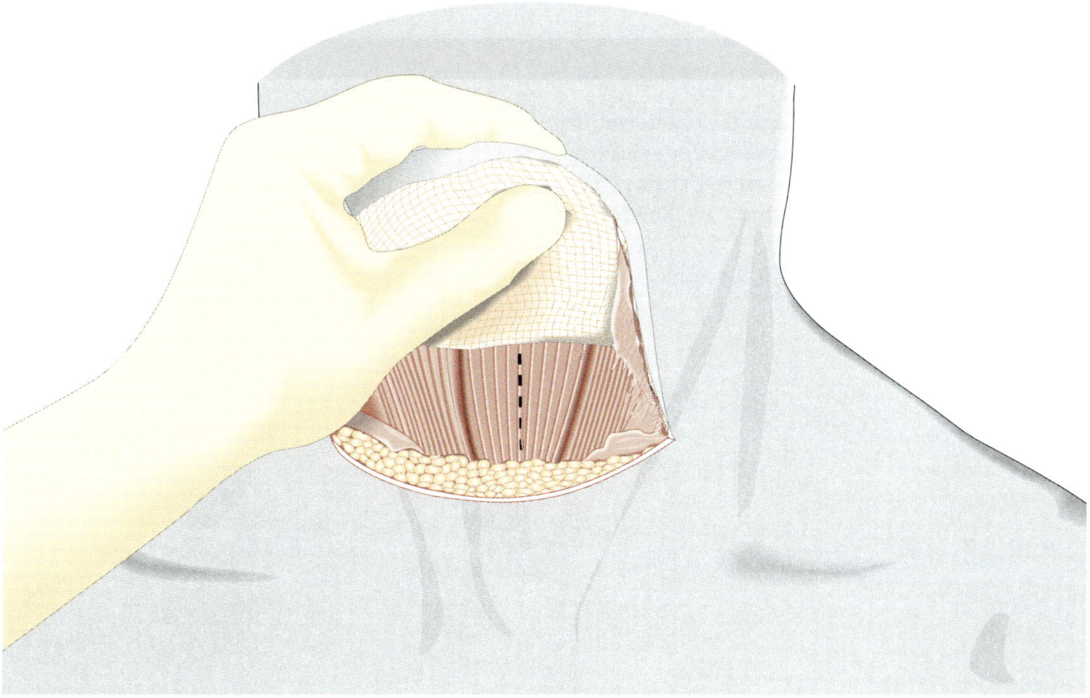

## Figure 5

Mobilisation of the strap muscles involves their separation via the midline raphe. This is best accomplished with an Allis forceps and Metzenbaum scissors. Subsequently the medial border of the strap muscles is mobilised from the underlying thyroid gland in the same way.



## Figure 6

Further separation from the thyroid is achieved by digital mobilisation using both index fingers allowing complete exposure of the target tissue. This should be done gently to avoid injury of the subcapsular thyroid veins.

Figure 5

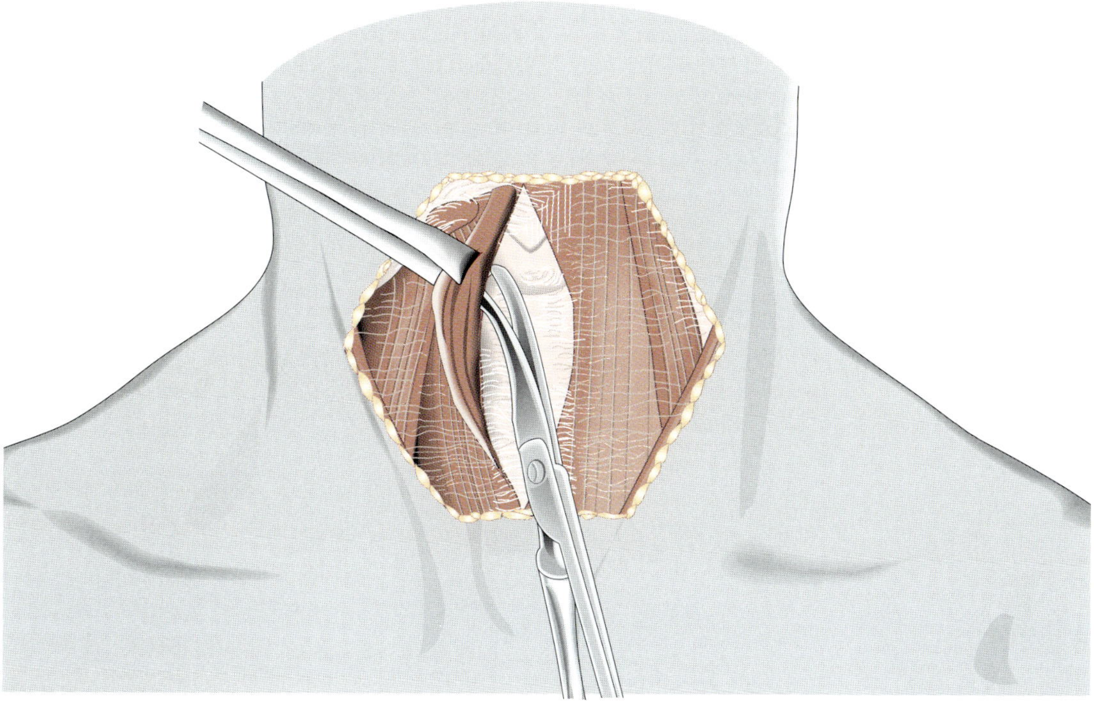

Figure 6

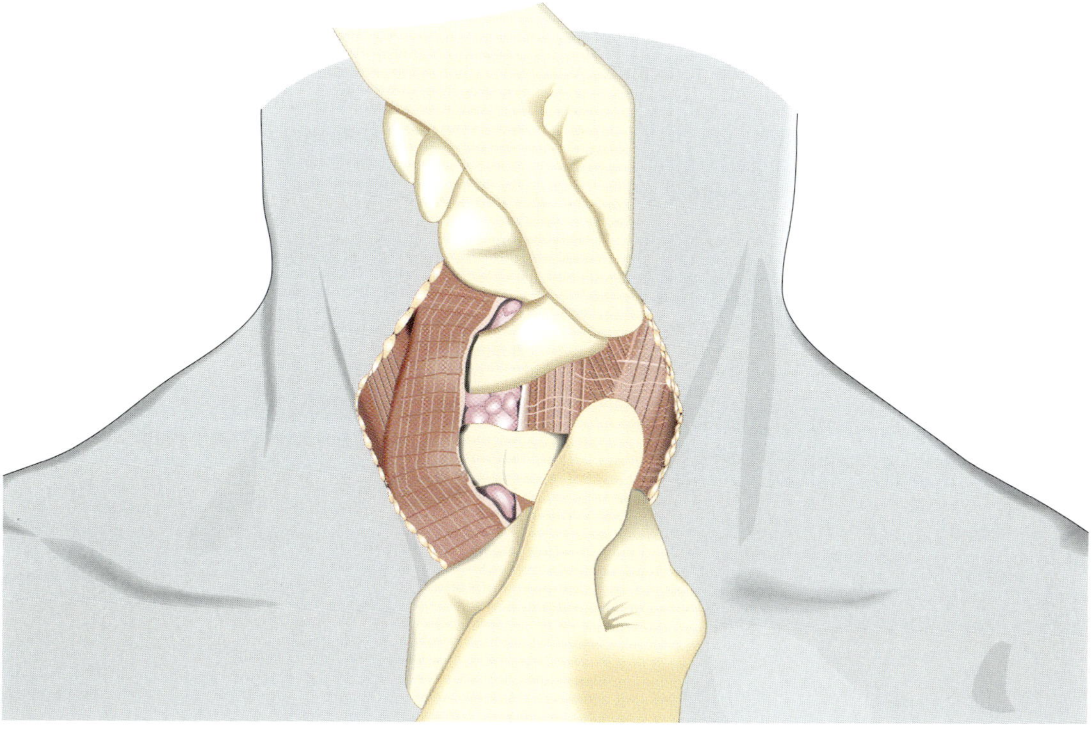

## Figure 7

Routine division of the strap muscles is controversial. It facilitates the exposure of the thyroid and parathyroids, but it is argued that in small glands this may not be necessary. Moreover, formation of scar tissue is considerably enhanced. In oncologic thyroid surgery, however, this manoeuvre is recommended to allow a thorough dissection of the central lymph node compartment.

Transection of the strap muscles should always be carried out under the protection of a spatulum. While the use of Kocher clamps is optional, they do facilitate readaptation of the strap muscles at the end of the operation. Transection can be carried out with a knife or diathermy.



## Figure 8

After exposure of the gland, dissection of the superior pole is started by entering the space between the upper pole and the cricoid cartilage which carries no blood vessels. The thyroid lobe is retracted caudally, which can be achieved by stay sutures or Allis clamps placed at the lower end of the upper pole of the thyroid lobe. The thyroid lobe is retracted laterally to allow better exposure of the superior pedicle containing the superior pole vessels and the superior laryngeal nerve lying usually posteromedial to the vessels. The lobe is carefully separated from the peritracheal fascia by gently opening the jaws of scissors or haemostats, which also allows separation of the vessels from the external branch of the superior laryngeal nerve. Care should be taken not to injure the cricothyroid muscle.

Figure 7

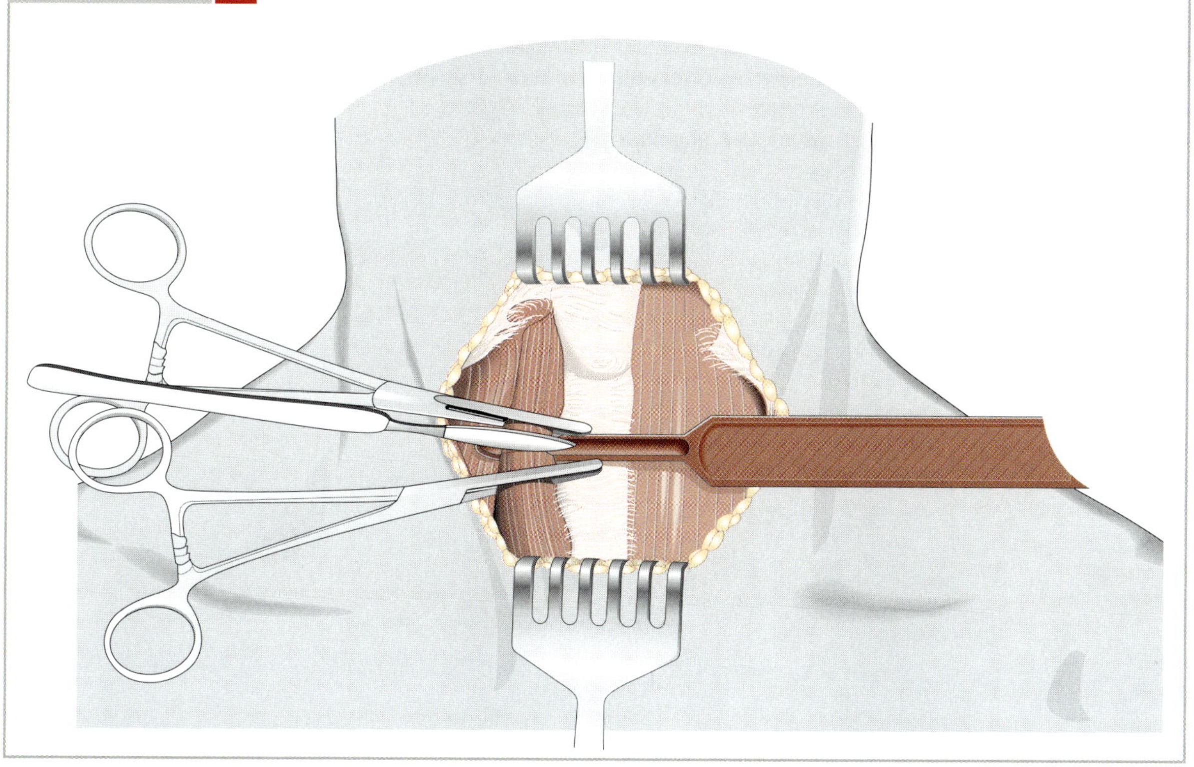

Figure 8

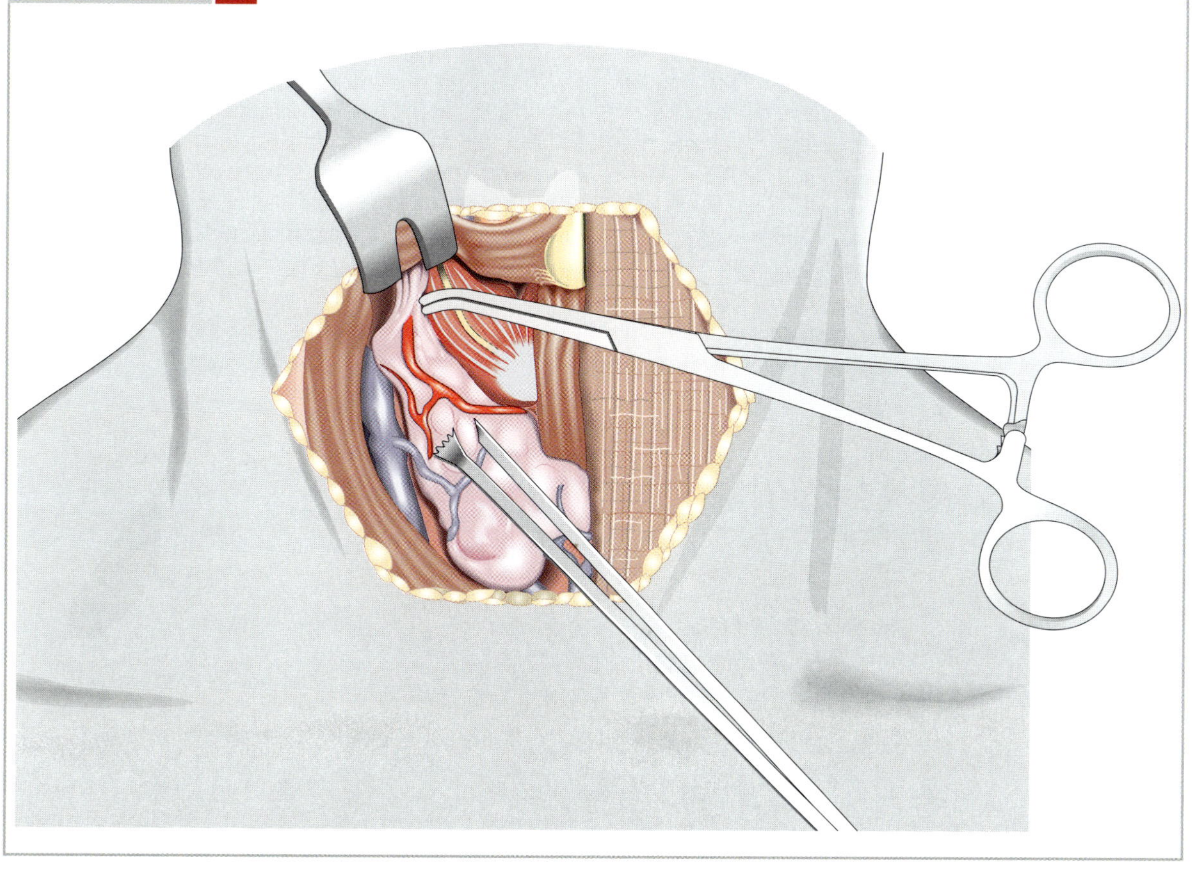

## Figure 9A, B

Once the vessels are separated from the external branch of the superior laryngeal nerve, an Overholt or Lahey clamp may be introduced posteriorly to the superior thyroid pedicle. Ligation of the superior thyroid vessels is carried out with 2-0 absorbable threads (Fig. 9B). The caudal ligature is placed and knotted first.

**Figure 9A, B**

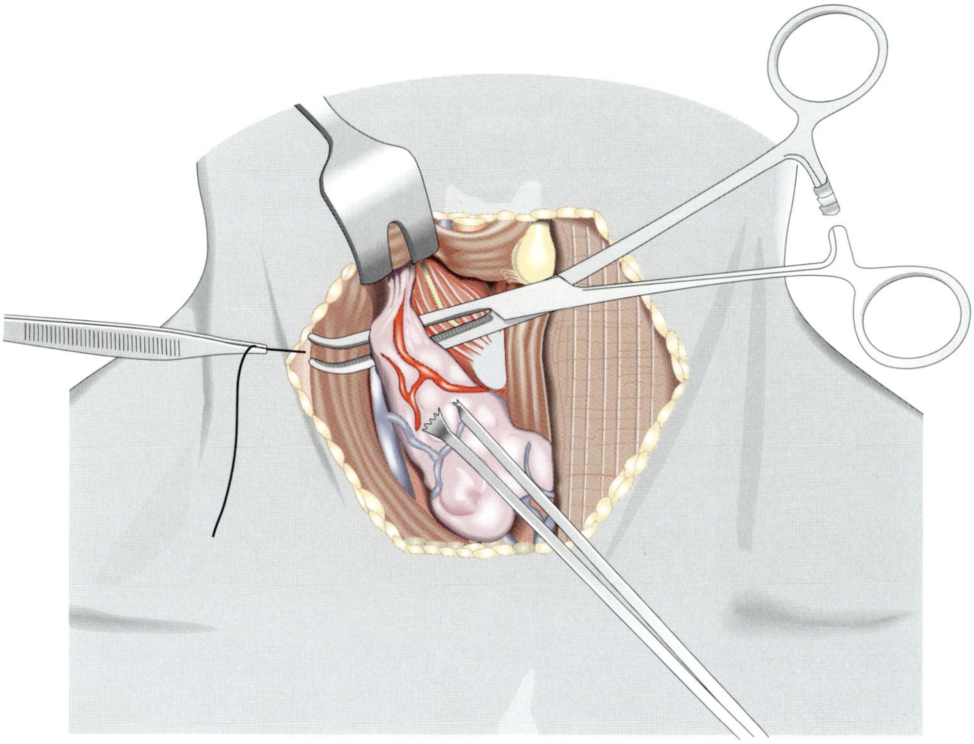

A

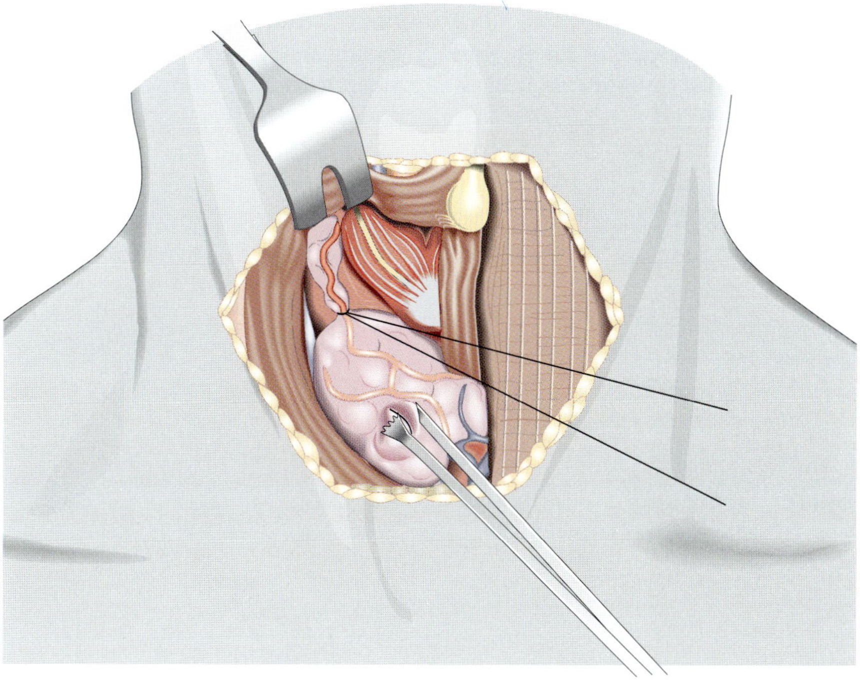

B

## Figure 10

Exerting gentle tension will facilitate placement of the cephalad ligature, which is introduced using the Overholt or Lahey clamp. This ligature is knotted with an adequate distance between it and the previous knot to allow safe transection of the vessels. As an alternative, titanium clips or a LigaSure™ clamp can be used to occlude the superior thyroid vessels before their transection.



## Figure 11

Subsequently the lobe is retracted medially to allow exposure of the lateroposterior aspect of the thyroid gland. As a first step the middle thyroid vein is ligated with 3-0 absorbable threads. This is accomplished by using an Overholt or Lahey clamp placed posteriorly to the vein.

Figure 10

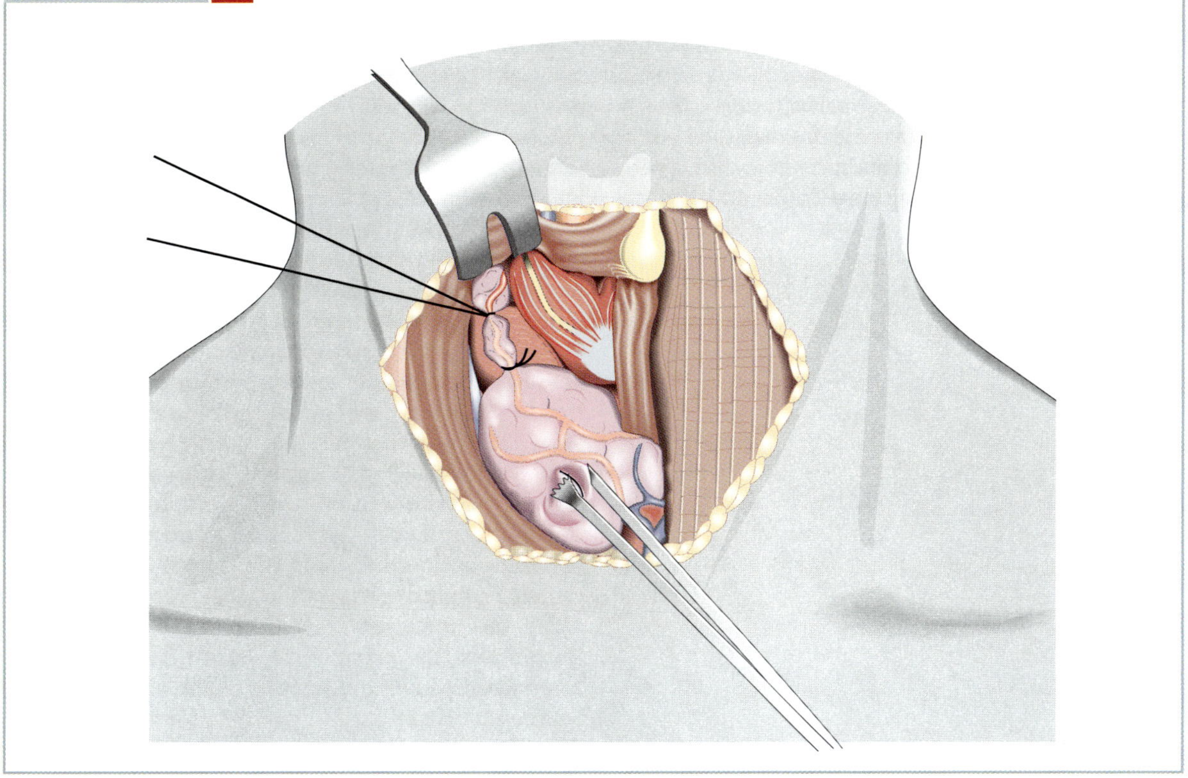

Figure 11

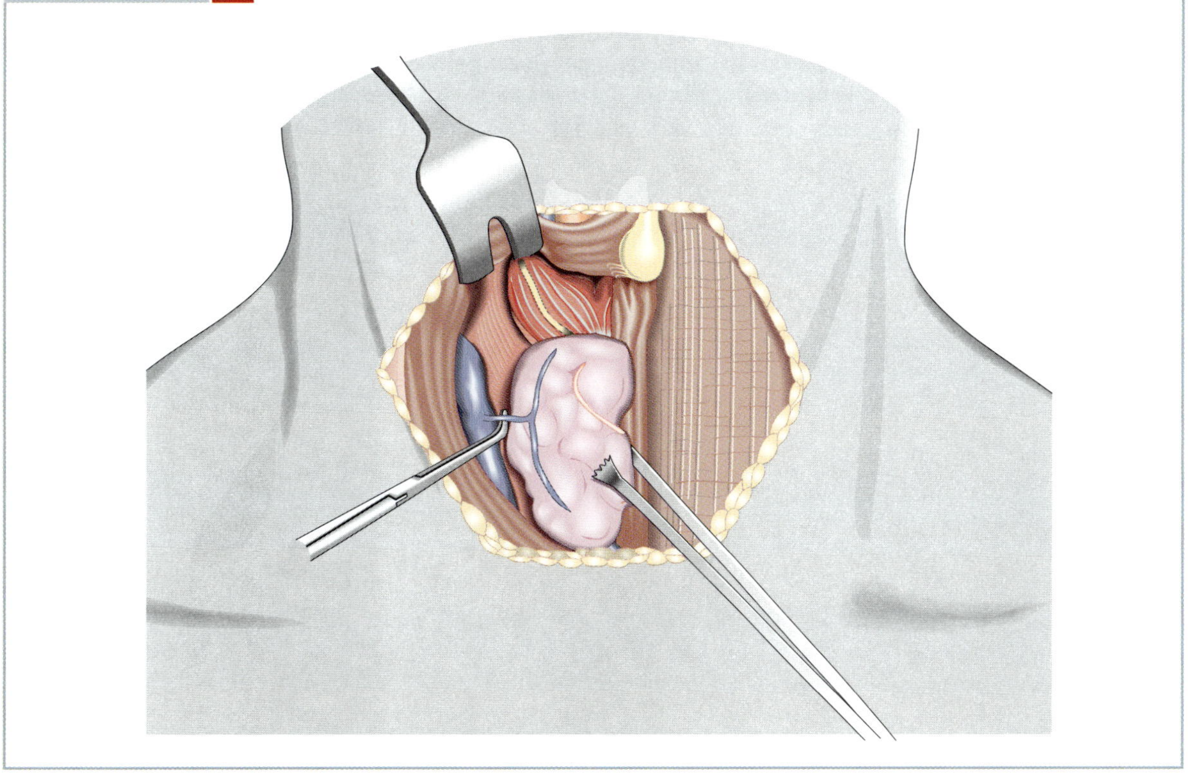

## Figure 12

As a next step the inferior thyroid artery is dissected out of the fatty tissue lying posterior to the thyroid gland. The recurrent laryngeal nerve must be clearly identified but usually the nerve is not dissected out in its entirety but allowed to remain covered with a connective tissue sheath to minimise injury to its blood supply.

## Figure 13

Care is to be taken not to damage the recurrent laryngeal nerve during dissection of the inferior thyroid artery. The most common sites where a recurrent laryngeal nerve is at risk of injury are near the inferior thyroid artery, near the ligament of Berry, and at the inferior pole of the thyroid gland.

Nearly 30 variations in the relation between the recurrent laryngeal nerve and the inferior thyroid artery have been described. At that level the most common position of the nerve is posterior to the inferior thyroid artery. This is particularly true of the left nerve, as the right nerve more commonly runs anterior to the artery or between the branches of the artery. The recurrent laryngeal nerve may also lie between the trachea and the thyroid gland or laterally or posteriorly to the tracheoesophageal groove. The nerve is also at risk of injury during division of the inferior thyroid veins if it leaves the tracheoesophageal groove within the mediastinum and runs along the posterior surface of the thyroid gland. Despite this, the nerve is consistently found in most cases within a few millimetres of the artery and the ligament of Berry.

## Figure 14

The inferior thyroid artery is then separated from the recurrent laryngeal nerve. Care must be taken while dissecting near the nerve to preserve its anterior branches, which may divide a considerable distance away from the larynx. Prior to entering the larynx, the nerve commonly divides into two branches. This may occur at variable distances from the larynx, even prior to encountering the thyroid itself.

Figure 12

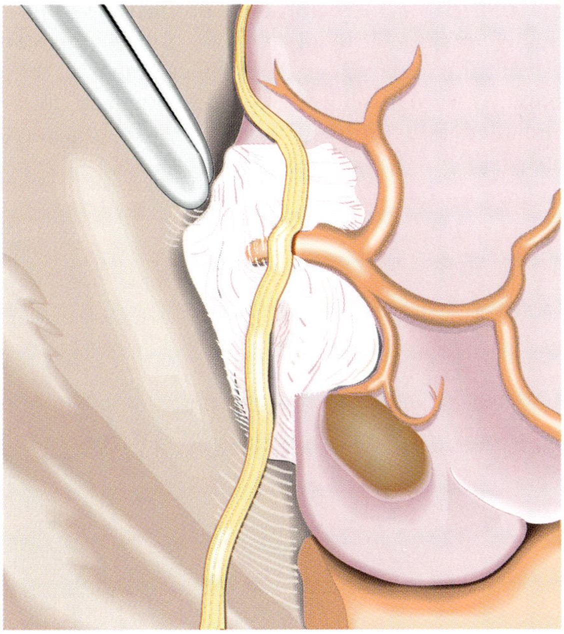

Figure 13

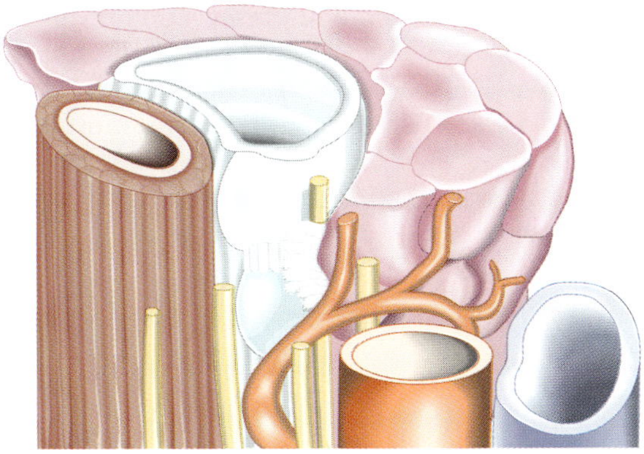

Figure 14

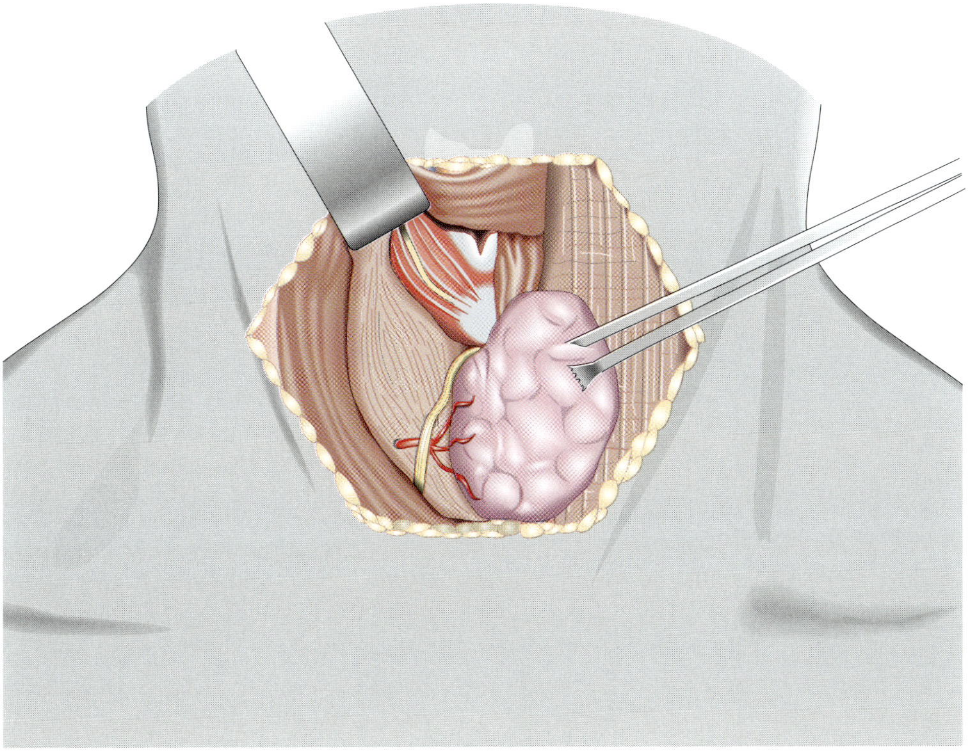

## Figure 15

After clear visualization and preservation of the recurrent laryngeal nerve the posterior surface of the upper pole is examined for the delicate brown upper parathyroid gland. The upper glands are more variable in position than the lower ones. If the gland is identified, it is carefully dissected off the thyroid capsule and left on the carotid sheath posteriorly. It is usually not possible to identify a discrete feeding vessel with the upper gland. If the gland turns dark in colour it is devascularised and may need to be implanted into the ipsilateral sternocleidomastoid muscle.



## Figure 16

Subsequently the inferior thyroid artery is ligated with 2-0 absorbable threads. In lobectomy or total thyroidectomy the artery is transected.

Figure 15

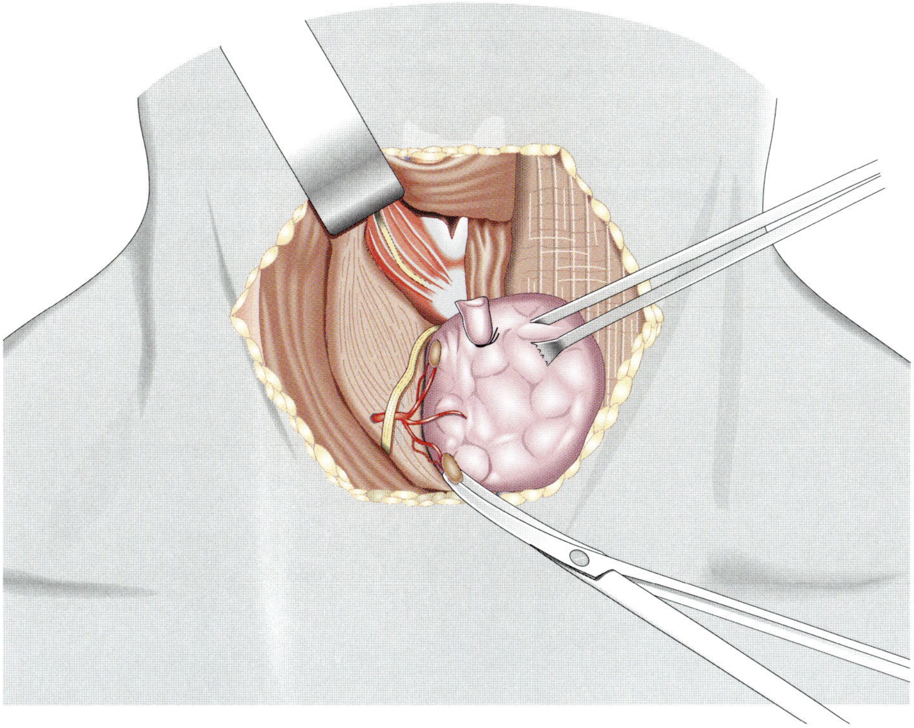

Figure 16

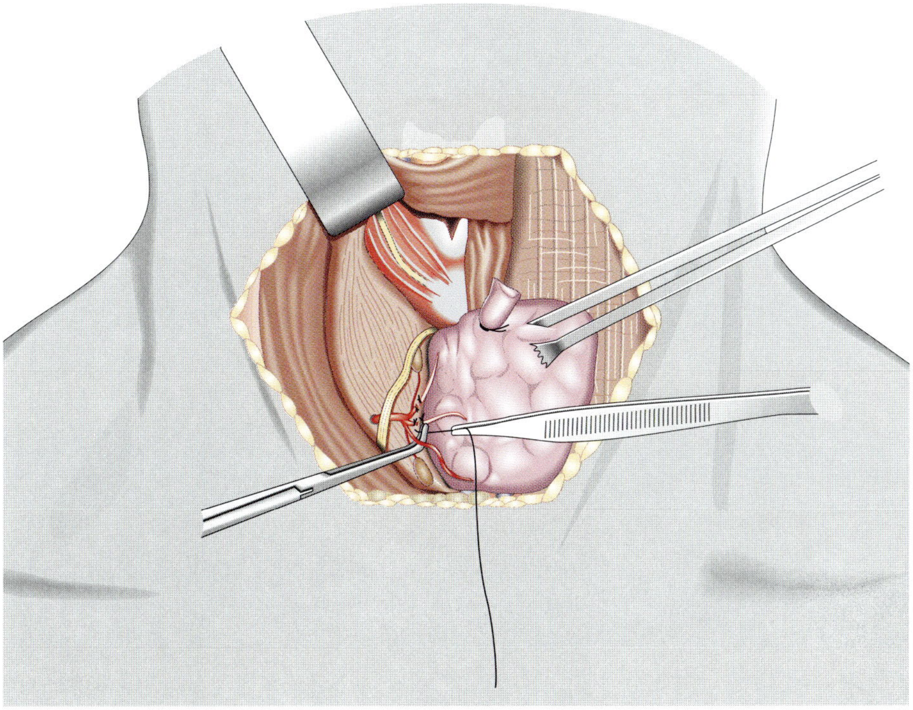

## Figure 17A, B

The lower border of the isthmus is dissected free from connective tissue taking care not to injure a thyroid ima artery, which is encountered in up to 10% of operations. If present this artery is ligated with 2-0 absorbable threads.

Subsequently the inferior thyroid veins are dissected free with Metzenbaum scissors. An Overholt or Lahey clamp is placed posteriorly and a 2-0 absorbable ligature is pulled through. Ligation is completed by a second 2-0 thread followed by transection. If total thyroidectomy is intended, the isthmus is dissected free from the trachea followed by mobilisation of the upper pole of the contralateral lobe as described above.

Figure 17A, B

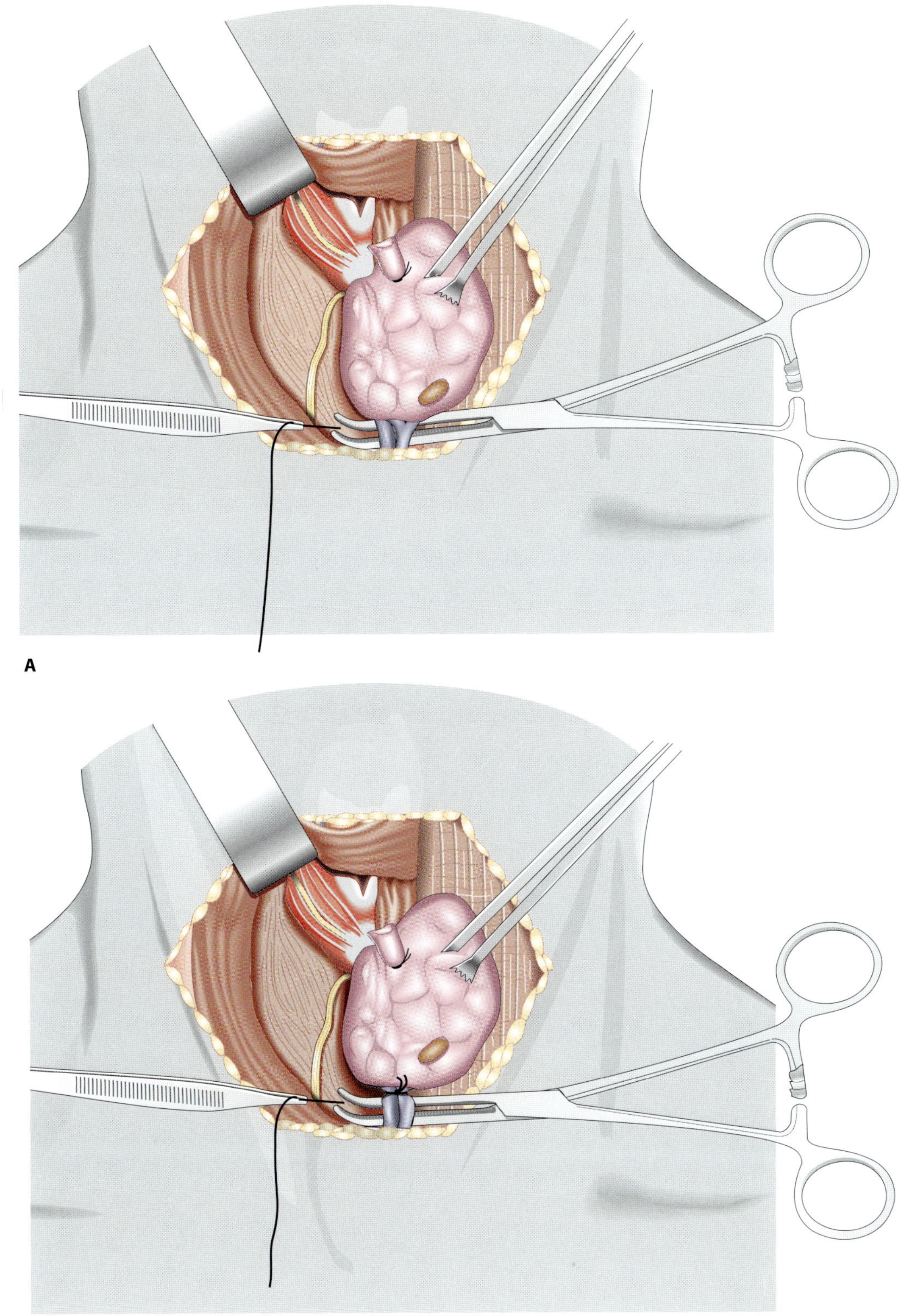

A

B

## Figure 18

If lobectomy or subtotal resection is intended, the isthmus is undermined from its superior border with an Overholt clamp, which is used as a guide for a grooved dissector. The strap muscles are omitted for better visibility.



## Figure 19

The grooved dissector is used to protect the trachea from injury while two Kocher clamps are placed on the isthmus.

Figure 18

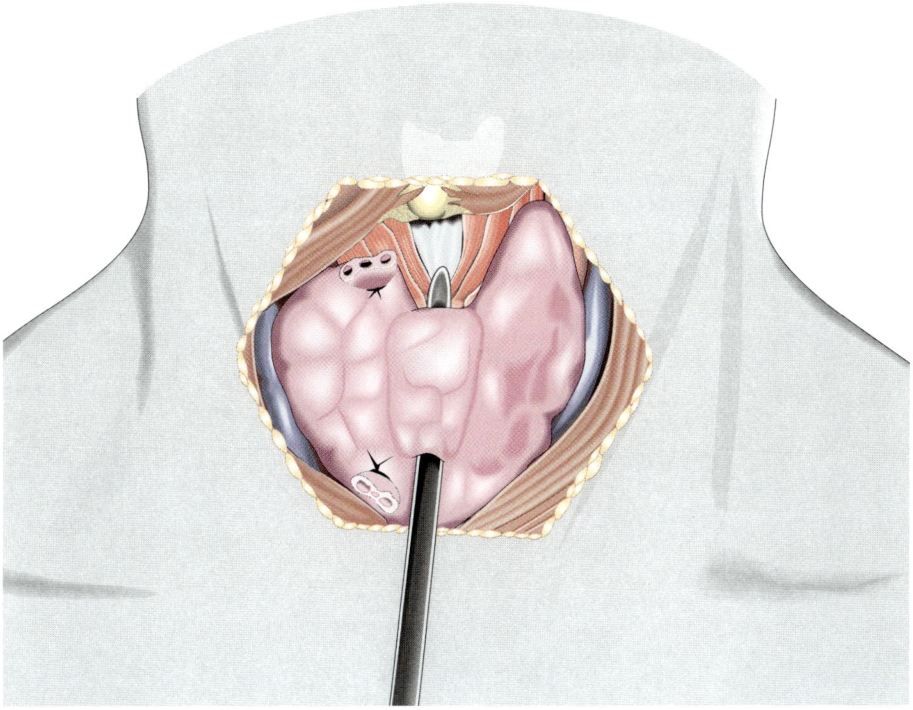

Figure 19

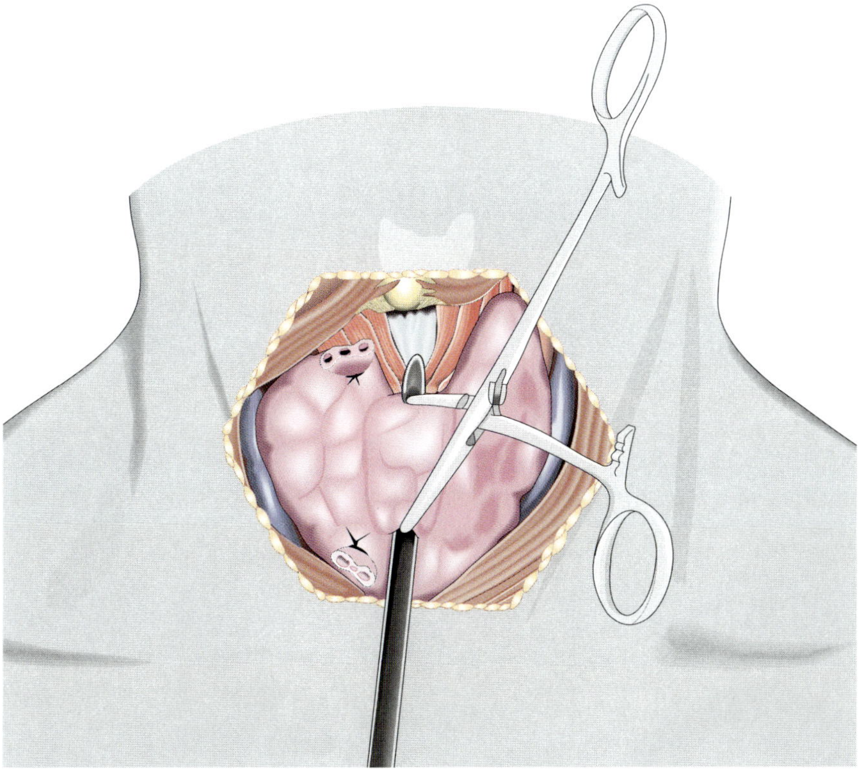

## Figure 20

Subsequently the isthmus is transected and oversewn using 2-0 absorbable suture material. The strap muscles are omitted for better visibility.

Figure 20

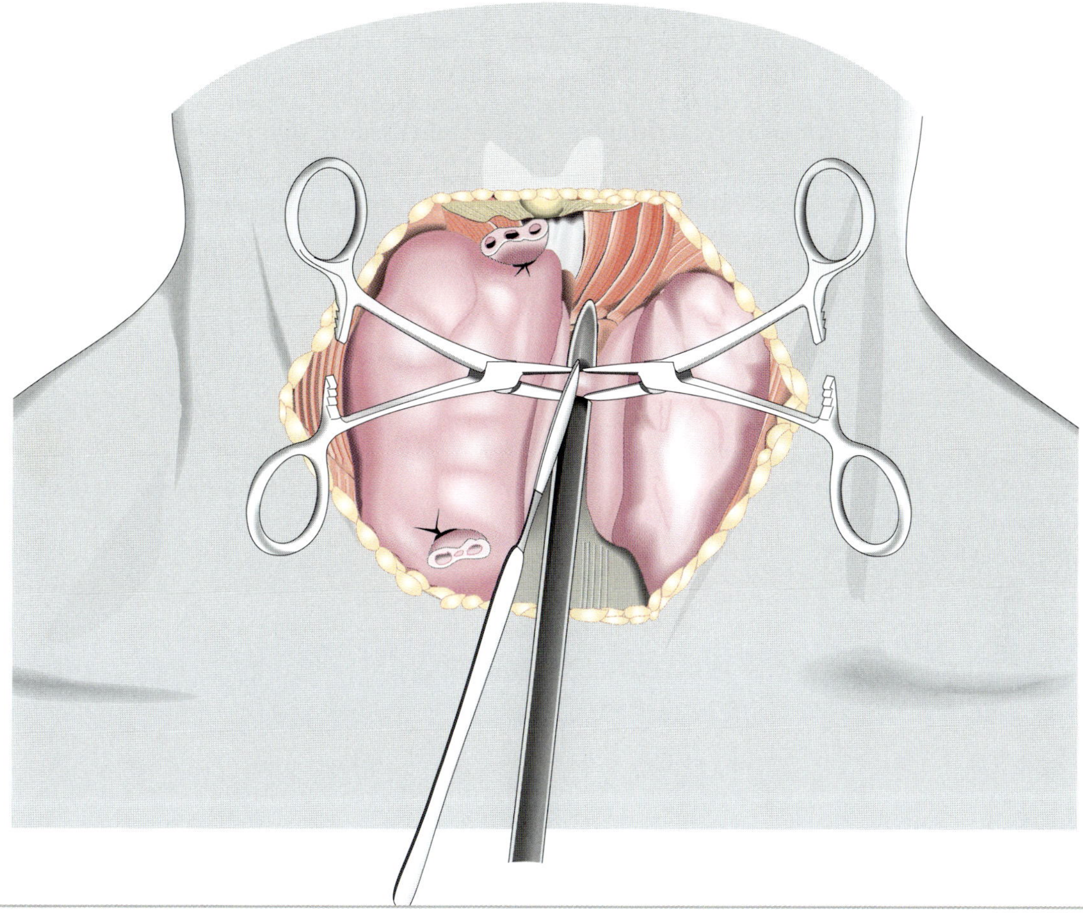

## Figure 21A, B

Subtotal resection is carried out after placing Kocher clamps around the thyroid lobe, defining the plane of resection. While incision of the thyroid capsule is performed with a knife, resection is carried out with scissors instead to avoid incidental dorsal transection of the thyroid with the risk of injury of the trachea and the recurrent laryngeal nerve.

This will result in a thyroid remnant of adequate size. Care should be taken not to leave any hyperplastic thyroid tissue in situ.

Figure 21A

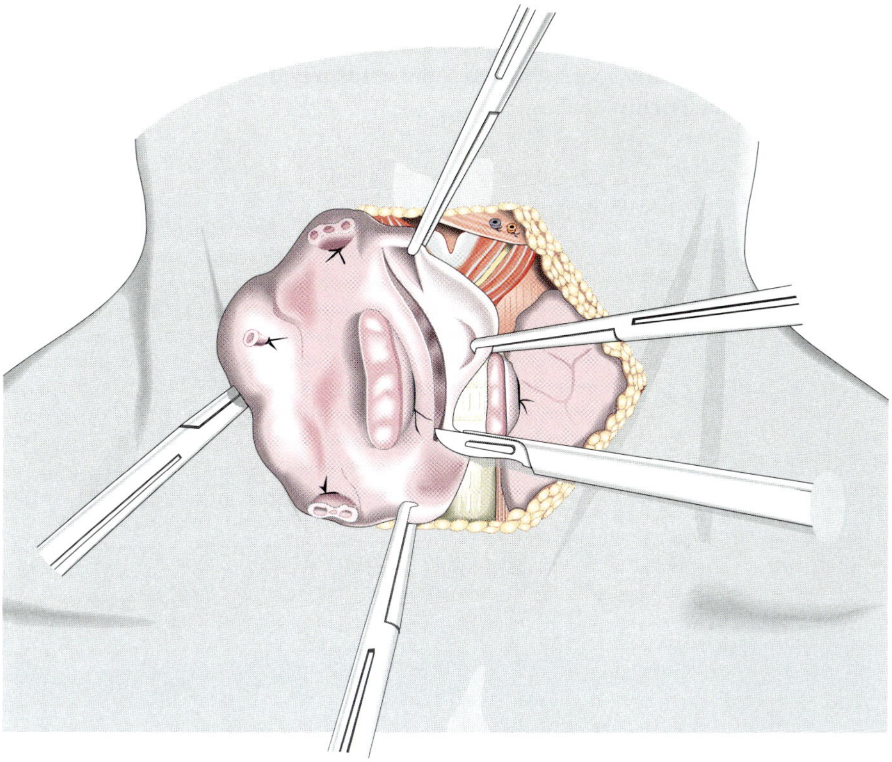

Figure 21B

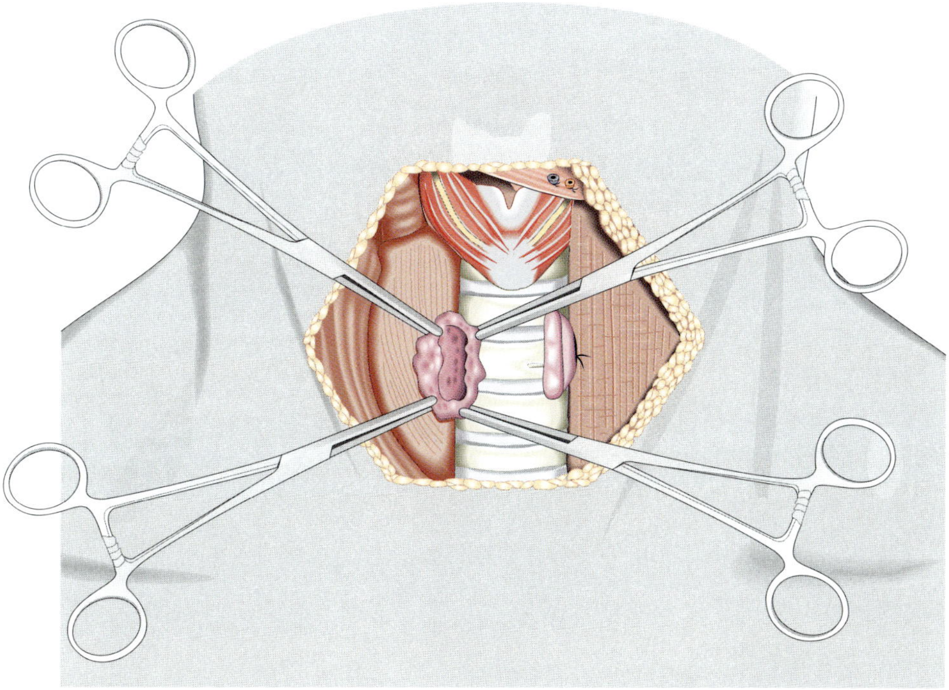

## Figure 22A, B

The thyroid remnant is sutured using a continuous 3-0 absorbable thread, which also serves to control parenchymal bleeding. Occasionally parenchymal bleeding is controlled with diathermy or single suture.

After subtotal thyroid resection a remnant of about 2–4 g, i.e. 2×1/2×2 cm, is left in place to preserve further thyroid function.

Figure 22A, B

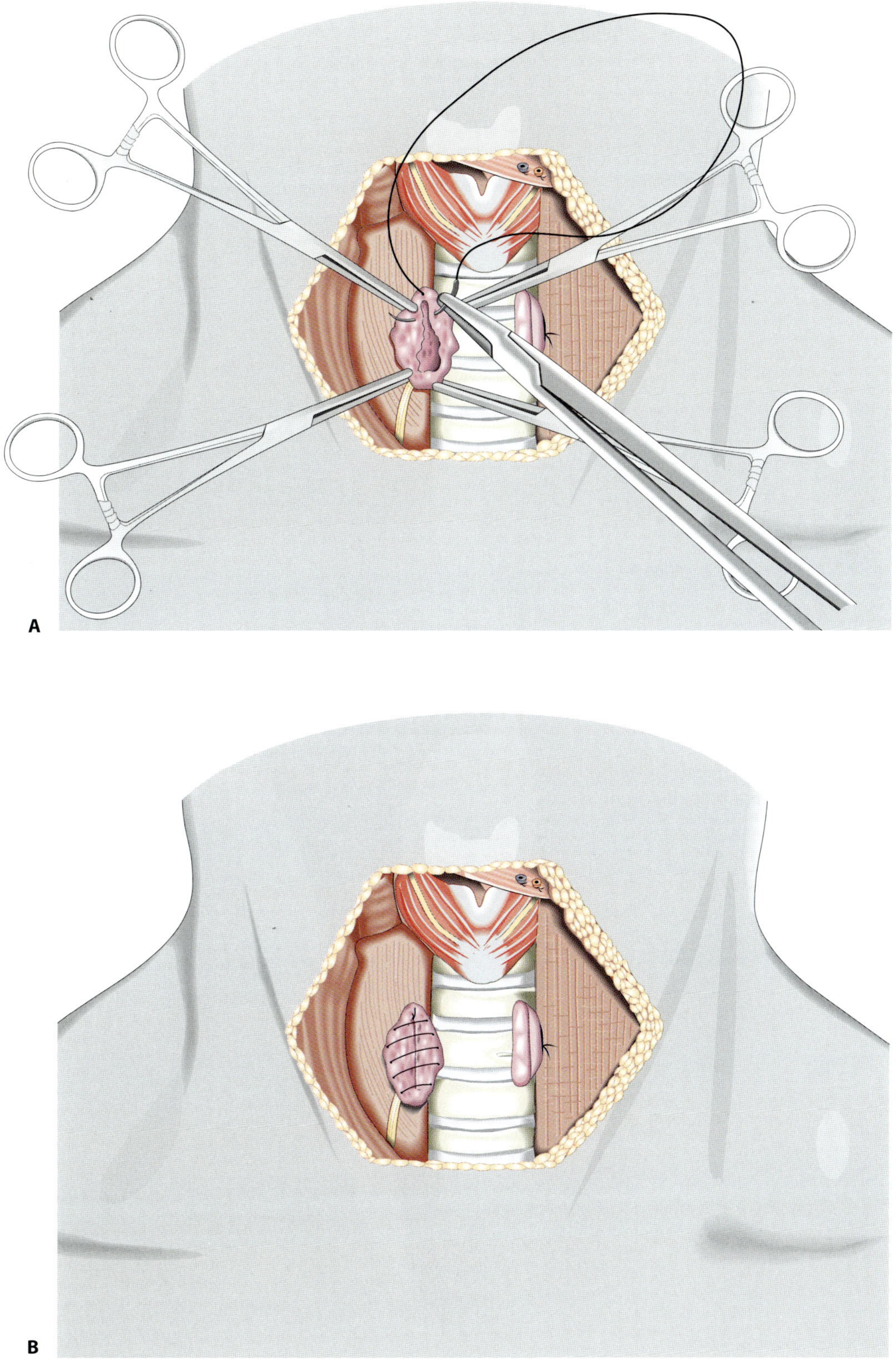

## Figure 23

If lobectomy is carried out, the thyroid is mobilised by transecting the connective adhesions to the trachea.



## Figure 24

Two suction drains may be used, one on each side of the neck, exiting the neck just above the sternal notch or laterally.

Figure 23

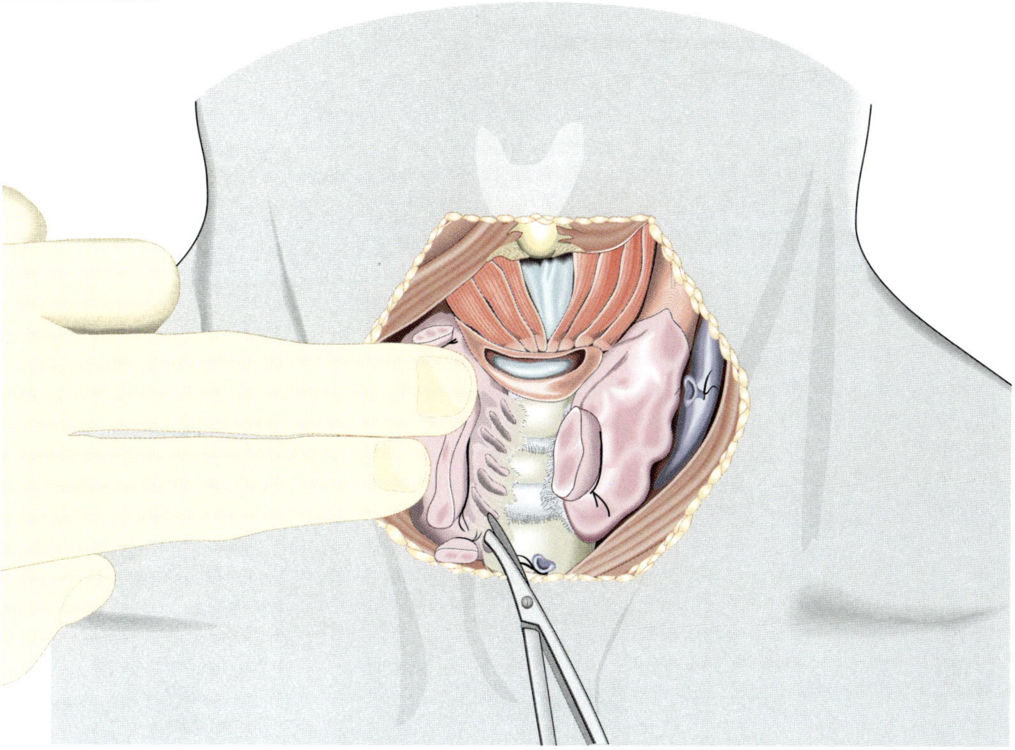

Figure 24

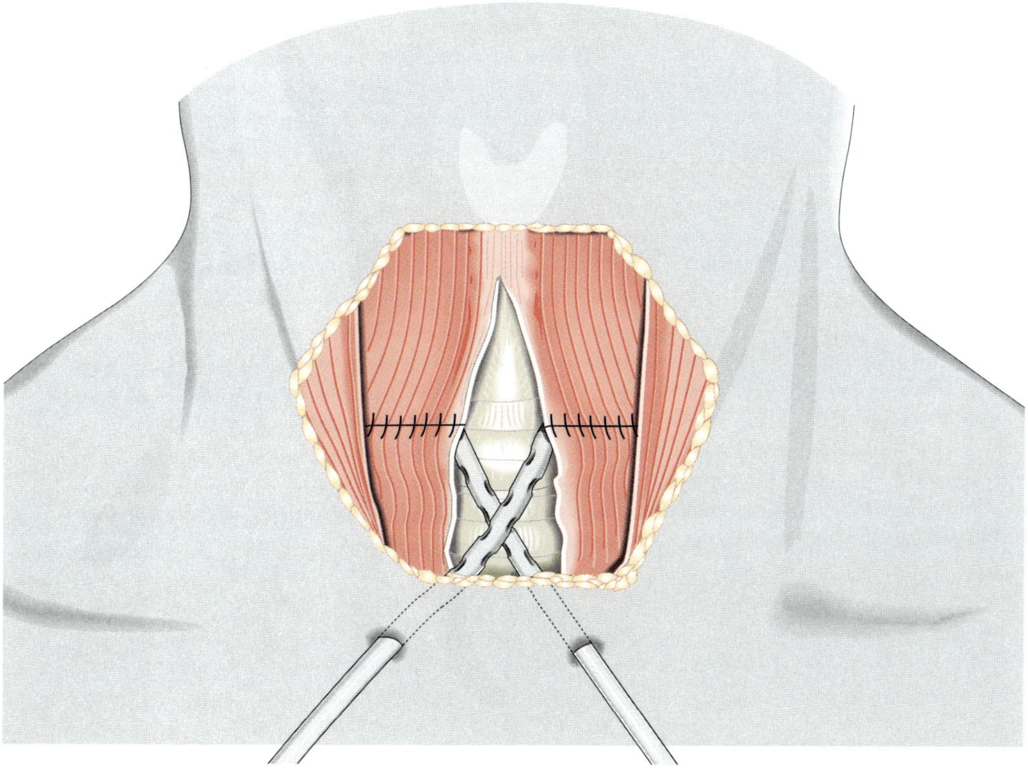

## Figure 25

The strap muscles are approximated and sutured together with an absorbable 3-0 thread.

Figure 25

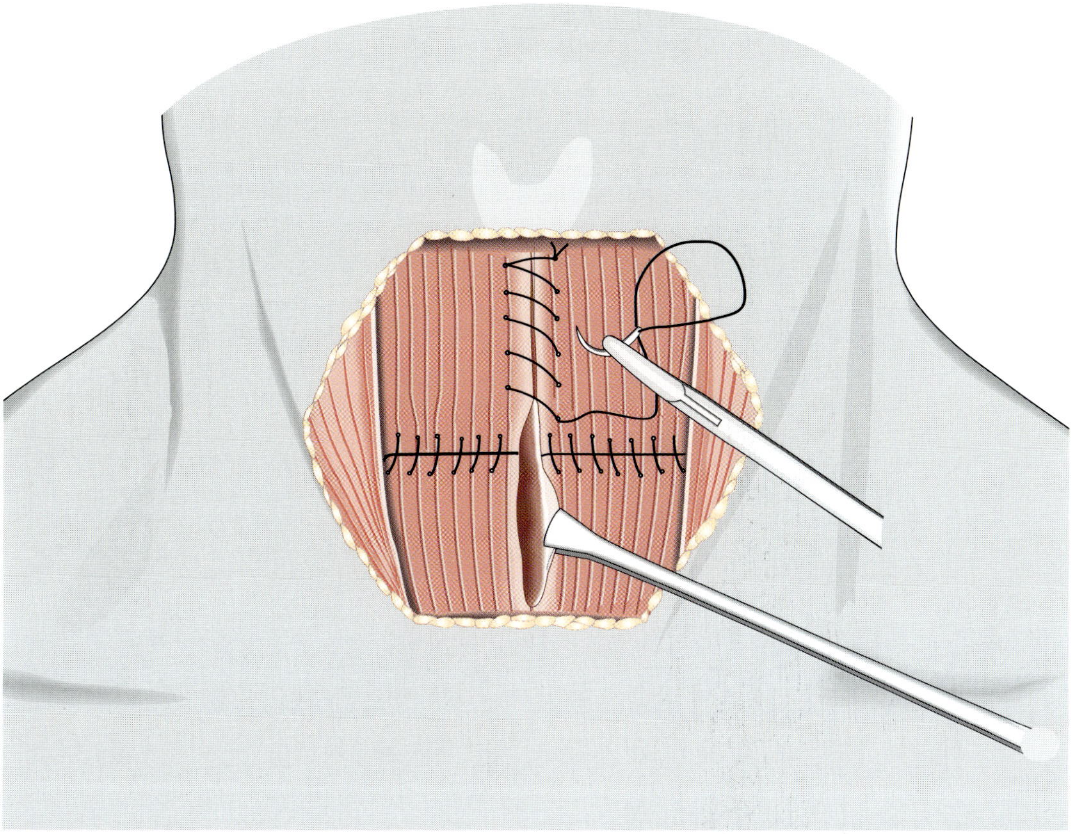

## Figure 26

Platysma and the subcutaneous layer are sutured with a single layer of 4-0 absorbable suture material.



## Figure 27

Skin closure is accomplished with a subcuticular 4-0 suture, which is either absorbable or unabsorbable.

Figure 26

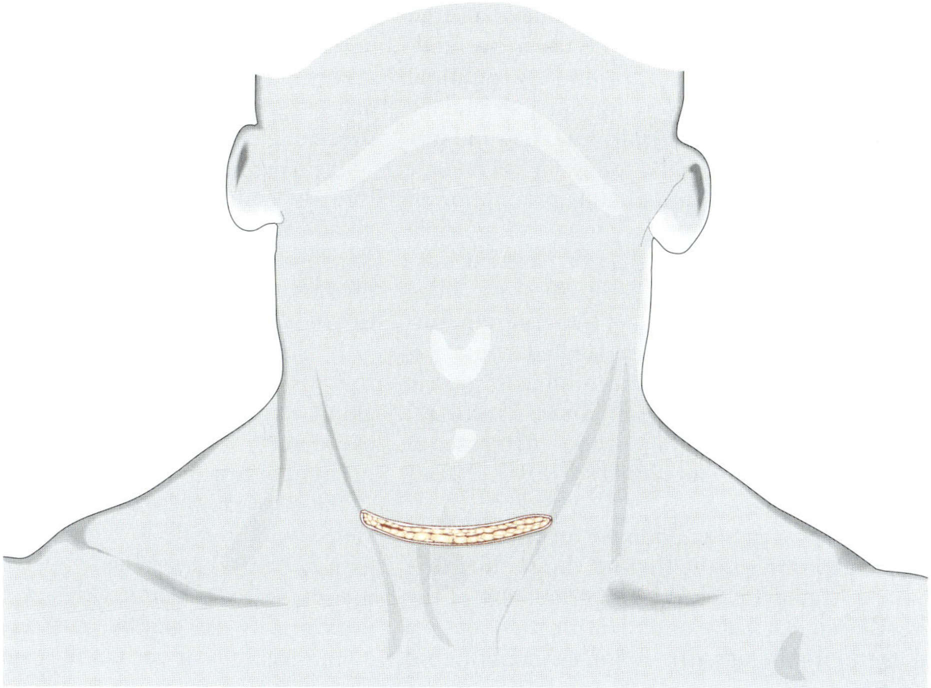

Figure 27

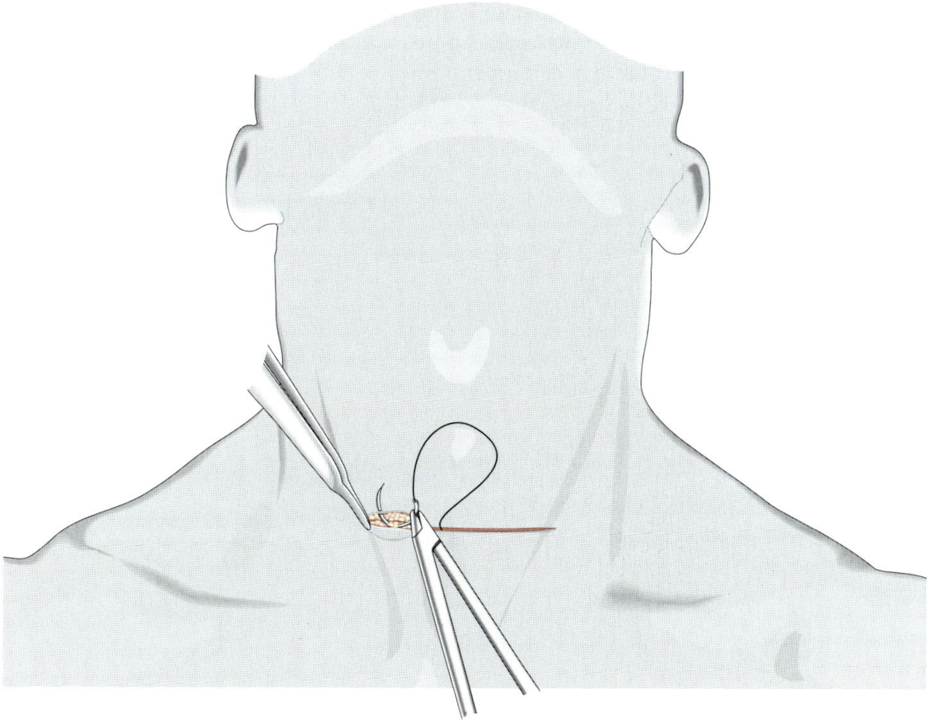

## PARATHYROID SURGERY

Indications for parathyroid surgery depend on the symptom pattern and the nature of the hyperfunction: primary (autonomous adenoma(s)), multiple gland hyperplasia (e.g. MEN syndrome), secondary (hyperplasia due to chronic hypocalcaemia) and tertiary (autonomous adenoma(s) following secondary hyperparathyroidism). If autonomous production of parathyroid hormone due to a single or multiple parathyroid adenoma is the cause of elevated hormone levels, surgery is indicated regardless of symptoms (Farnebo 2004). In secondary hyperparathyroidism asymptomatic patients are treated conservatively, while symptoms such as urolithiasis, gastric and duodenal ulcers, osseous pain and pathological fractures indicate the need for surgery (Schlosser et al. 2004). In parathyroid carcinoma surgery is the only therapeutic option.



The operation starts as outlined for thyroid surgery. After exposure of the thyroid the middle thyroid vein is ligated, followed by identification of the recurrent laryngeal nerve and identification and removal of the pathologically abnormal parathyroid gland. If intraoperative parathyroid hormone measurement is available, a drop of at least 50% below the preoperative level is regarded as sufficient to terminate surgery. Otherwise all other parathyroids are inspected to exclude a second adenoma.

If no adenoma is found in the vicinity of the thyroid, depending on whether the superior or inferior glands are missing the most common aberrant sites are the sheath of the carotid artery, the cornua of the thymus and the mediastinum. Occasionally an intrathyroidal parathyroid adenoma may be present.

In secondary hyperparathyroidism all parathyroid tissue is removed except for 25–50% of one gland, which is either left in place and marked with a clip or autotransplanted into muscle (sternocleidomastoid or brachioradialis).

Patients with primary hyperparathyroidism associated with multiple endocrine neoplasia with all glands being hyperplastic are treated in the same manner as for patients with secondary hyperparathyroidism. If all glands have evolved already into adenomas, 25% of one gland is autotransplanted.

### Figure 28

The most common location of the upper parathyroid glands is next to the upper half of each lobe of the thyroid at the dorsolateral aspect. If a superior gland is missing, the carotid sheath should be explored up to the level of the bifurcation and if no gland can be found there, the posterior mediastinum may be the site of an aberrant gland.

### Figure 29

The inferior glands show a more variable topography. Most commonly they are located in the vicinity of and below the inferior thyroid artery. If an inferior gland is missing, a thymectomy is carried out.

Figure 28

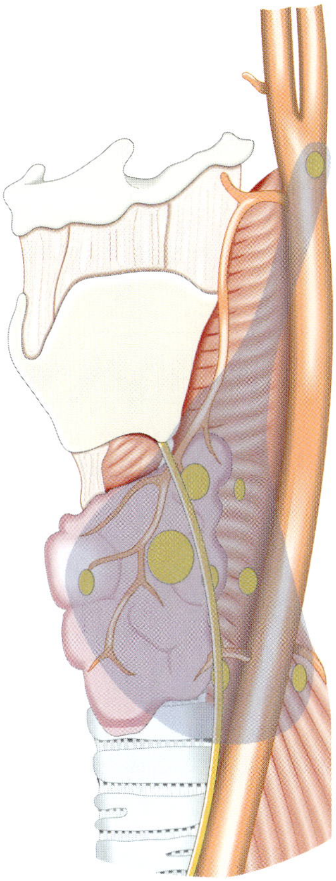

Figure 29

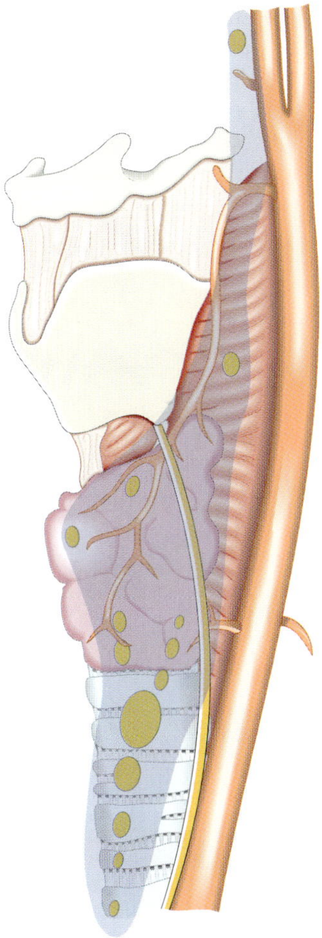

## Figure 30

As a first step the middle thyroid vein is ligated with 3-0 absorbable threads. This is accomplished by using an Overholt or Lahey clamp placed posteriorly to the vein.



## Figure 31

The thyroid lobe is mobilised with clear identification of the recurrent laryngeal nerve and the parathyroid glands are then sought.

Figure 30

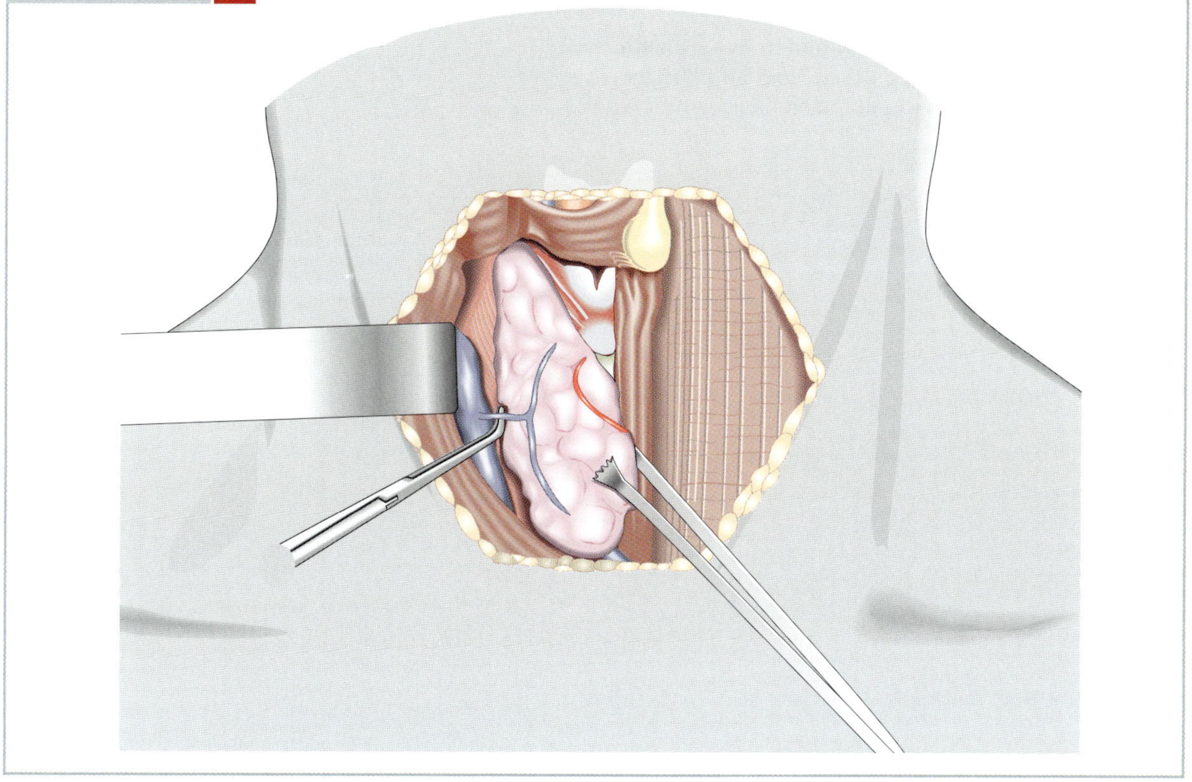

Figure 31

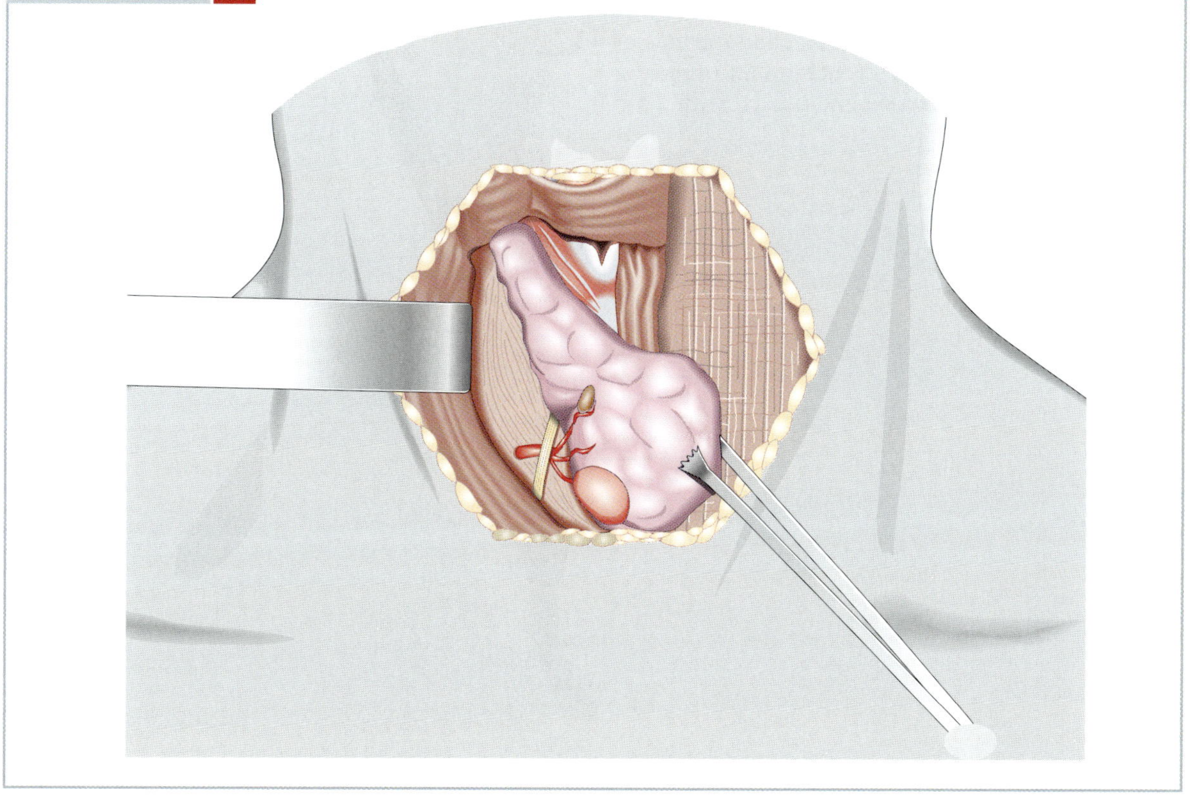

## Figure 32

If found to be enlarged, the adenoma or hyperplastic gland(s) are separated from the thyroid and dissected out of the connective tissue.



## Figure 33

After identification of the adenoma, an Overholt or Lahey clamp is placed on or behind the vascular stalk, and the stalk is divided and ligated with a 3-0 absorbable ligature.

Figure 32

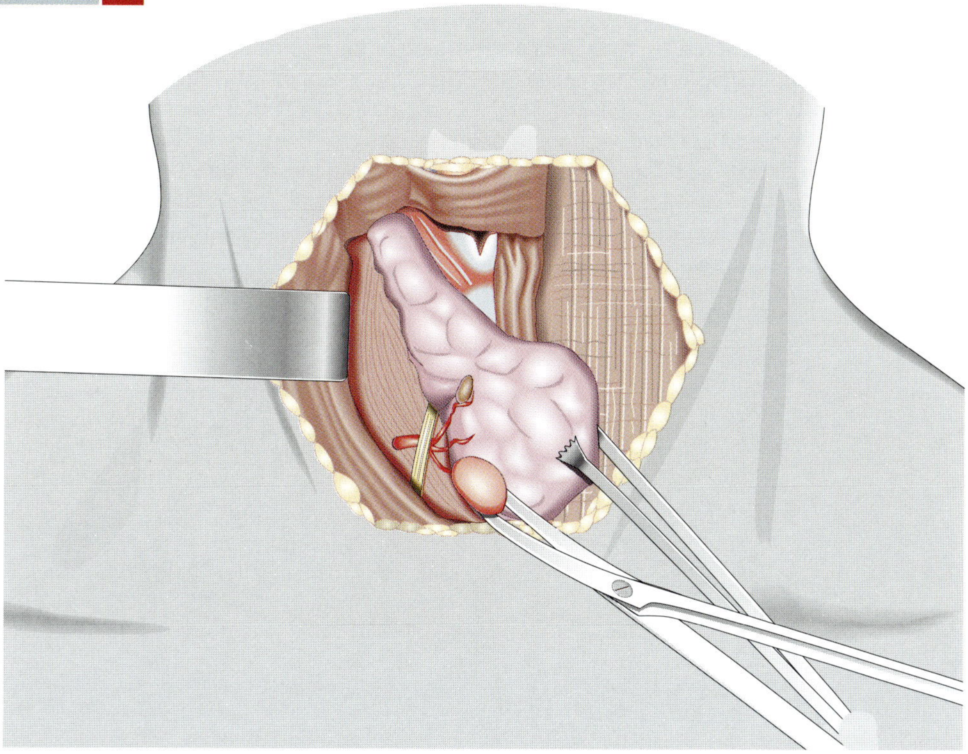

Figure 33

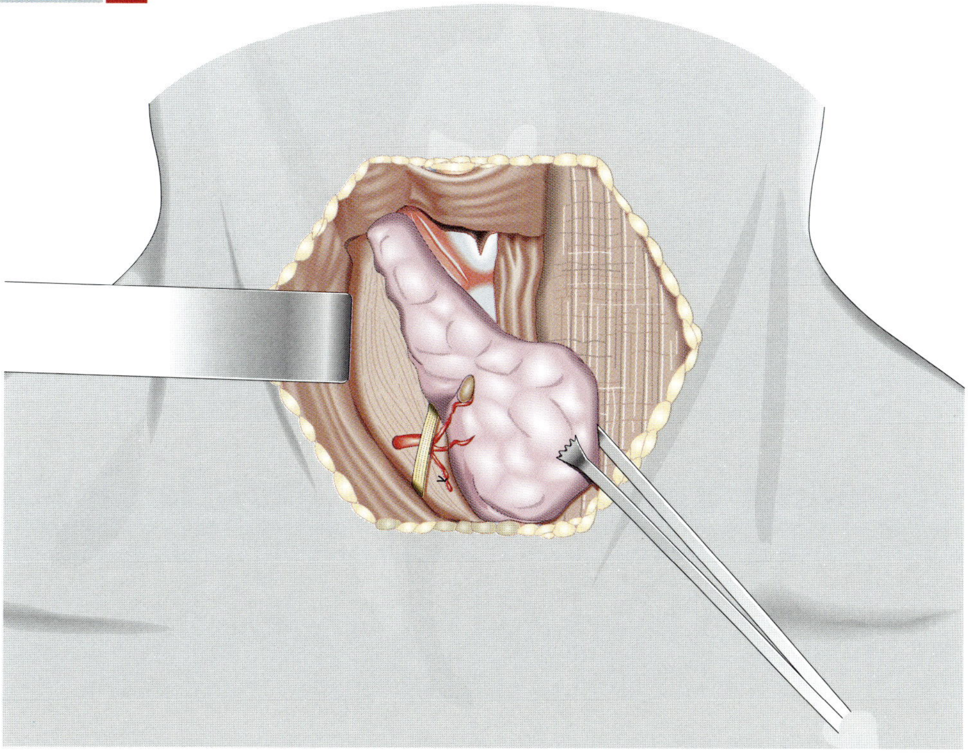

## Figure 34A, B

The strap muscles are reconstructed by running sutures (Fig. 34A). In symptomatic secondary hyperparathyroidism 3 1/2 to 3 3/4 glands are removed. The remnant can be left in place and marked with a clip provided the blood supply has not been compromised. In the case of devascularisation, a safer strategy is to cut the gland into thin slices and implant it into the adjacent sternocleidomastoid muscle. The site of implantation should be marked with a metal clip in the event of future recurrent hyperparathyroidism, especially when operating for secondary hyperparathyroidism. In the latter case, some surgeons prefer to implant the questionable gland into a forearm muscle such as brachioradialis so that it is easily accessible without reopening the neck (Fig. 34B).

Figure 34A, B

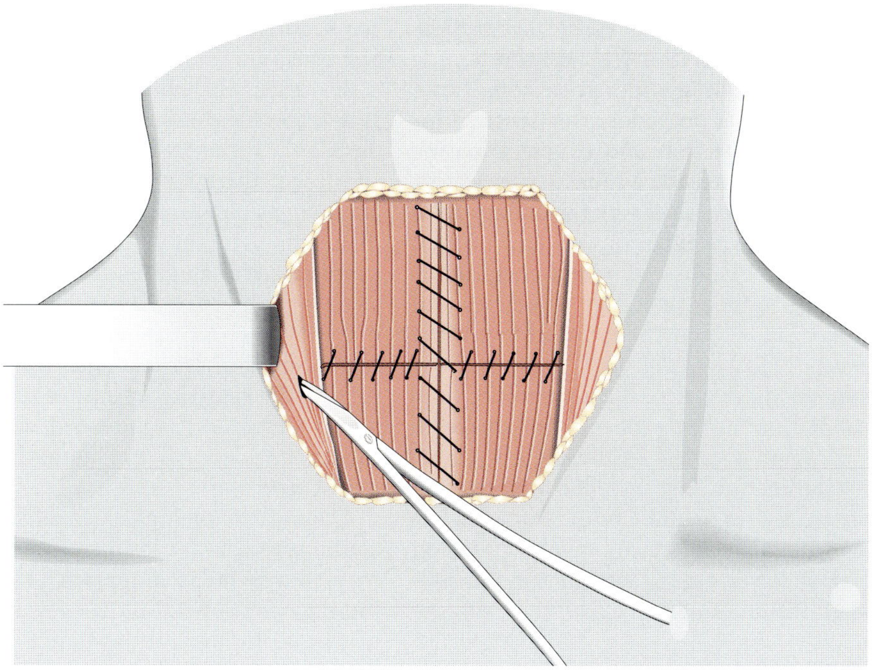


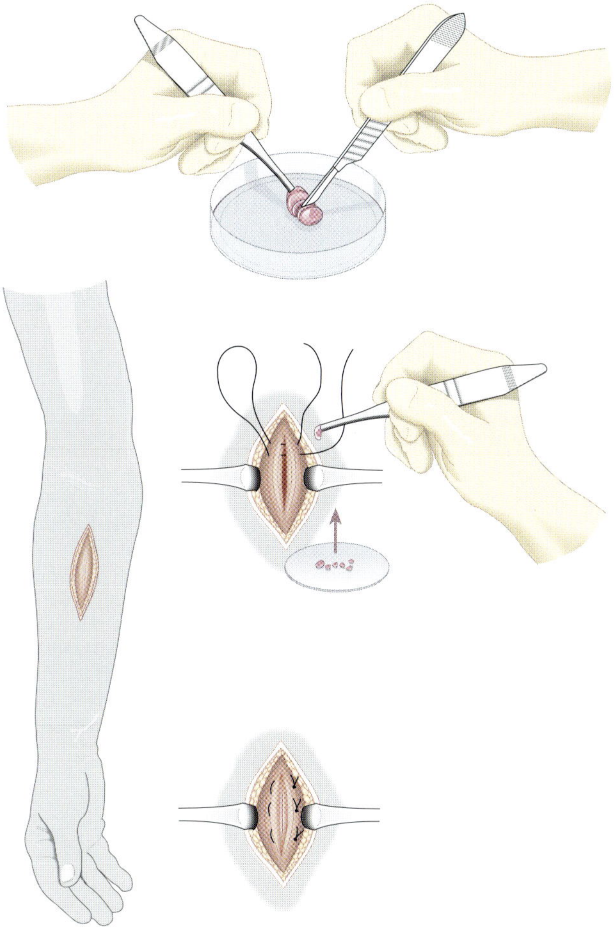

6

## CONCLUSIONS

Thyroid and parathyroid surgery both follow an essentially similar operative strategy. The objective is to eliminate diseased tissue while preserving functional integrity whenever possible. Essential steps involve meticulous preparation and exposure of the target tissue as well as structures and tissues at risk of accidental injury such as the superior laryngeal nerves, the recurrent laryngeal nerves and normal parathyroid glands. The use of magnifying loops does help to achieve these operative objectives and their use is strongly recommended to achieve these operative goals.

In unilateral nodular goitre, hemithyroidectomy should be carried out as the procedure of choice to avoid remnant thyroidectomy in those cases where histological examination has unveiled malignancy. However, if there is a single unilateral lesion which is not suspicious for cancer, resection to a lesser extent such as upper or lower pole resection may be adequate, although this approach is currently losing favour.

Bilateral nodular goitre not suspicious for cancer may be treated by bilateral subtotal thyroid resection; however, if there is any doubt about the nature of a lesion all thyroid tissue should be removed on that side. Also some authors favour total thyroidectomy in multinodular goitre to avoid recurrence, which is associated with an increased risk of complications (Gibelin et al. 2004).

To expedite decision making regarding definitive operative strategy, suspicious thyroid nodules may be examined by frozen section in selected cases to exclude malignancy (Udelsman 2001). In the presence of preoperative high quality cytological results, a frozen section in most instances is of little extra value and thus can be omitted.

If cancer is evident, total thyroidectomy and systematic central lymphadenectomy are carried out during the same procedure.

After surgery for hyperthyroidism without nodular changes only some patients will achieve euthyroidism. Thus recently total thyroidectomy has been propagated for all patients with Graves' disease (Barakate 2002), especially in the presence of ophthalmopathy to reduce the amount of antigen perpetuating an autoimmune response and specific symptoms. Also in the situation of secondary thyrotoxicosis total thyroidectomy is indicated, while for a single autonomous adenoma, unilateral thyroid lobectomy is performed.

Diagnostic imaging, such as Sestamibi and ultrasound scanning, for localising parathyroid adenomas may allow a focused approach in patients undergoing their first operation; however, the maximum use of diagnostic methods available is required for persisting or recurrent hyperparathyroidism prior to reexploration. Primary and tertiary hyperparathyroidism are a clear indication for surgical therapy, while operative treatment of secondary hyperparathyroidism is based on its symptoms (Farnebo 2004; Schlosser et al. 2004). While parathyroidectomy in most instances is a straightforward procedure, intraoperative negative findings require a systematic surgical clearance of the neck and upper mediastinum.

In the future new operative procedures such as the minimally invasive or video assisted approaches may change the surgical management of thyroid and parathyroid diseases substantially.

## SELECTED REFERENCES


Barakate MS, Agarwal G, Reeve TS, Barraclough B, Robinson B, Delbridge LW (2002) Total thyroidectomy is now the preferred option for the surgical management of Graves' disease. ANZ J Surg 72:321–324

Farnebo LO (2004) Primary hyperparathyroidism. Update on pathophysiology, clinical presentation and surgical treatment. Scand J Surg 93:282–287

Gibelin H, Sierra M, Mothes D, Ingrand P, Levillain P, Jones C, Hadjadj S, Torremocha F, Marechaud R, Barbier J, Kraimps JL (2004) Risk factors for recurrent nodular goiter after thyroidectomy for benign disease: case-control study of 244 patients. World J Surg 28:1079–1082

Kim S, Wei JP, Braveman JM, Brams DM (2004) Predicting outcome and directing therapy for papillary thyroid carcinoma. Arch Surg 139:390–394

Raffel A, Cupisti K, Krausch M, Wolf A, Schulte KM, Roher HD (2004) Incidentally found medullary thyroid cancer: treatment rationale for small tumors. World J Surg 28:397–401

Schlosser K, Zielke A, Rothmund M (2004) Medical and surgical treatment for secondary and tertiary hyperparathyroidism. Scand J Surg 93:288–297

Udelsman R (2001) The thyroid nodule. Ann Surg Oncol 8: 89–90

# Part IV Abdomen

In these next chapters on short stay abdominal surgery a description will be given of the following abdominal operations: diagnostic laparoscopy, laparoscopic and mini-cholecystectomy, and conventional and laparoscopic appendicectomy. The use of diagnostic laparoscopy was first reported by general surgeons as part of the assessment of patients with acute abdominal pain in 1978. Many studies have subsequently shown that laparoscopy significantly improves surgical decision-making in patients with acute abdominal pain, in whom the diagnosis is uncertain. Approximately 15% of female patients admitted under a general surgeon will have a gynaecological condition, thus strengthening the view that all females with suspected appendicitis should undergo laparoscopy before appendicectomy. In recent years diagnostic laparoscopy has also been used to help stage gastrointestinal cancers prior to laparotomy, and has proven especially useful in gastro-oesophageal malignancies which have a significant incidence of peritoneal metastases which preclude curative surgery.

Gallstones represent a major health problem in western Europe, with approximately 70,000 cholecystectomies being performed each year in the United Kingdom. They occur more commonly in women than men, with only 10% of males between 60 and 70 years of age having gallstones compared to 30% of women in the same age group. Approximately 25% of patients with gallstones will develop symptoms related to their gallstones, the commonest presentations being biliary colic, pancreatitis, and acute and chronic cholecystitis. Cholecystectomy is the treatment of choice for patients with symptomatic gallbladder stones who are medically fit for surgery. Operative mortality is low at approximately 0.25%, but is increased in elderly patients and those with coexisting medical problems, especially cirrhosis of the liver. There is currently no indication for undertaking cholecystectomy in patients with asymptomatic gallstones, as the increased risk of developing gallbladder cancer in these patients is less than the risk of elective cholecystectomy. The operation may be performed using one of two techniques, either laparoscopically or by open surgery using a small incision, a procedure known as mini-cholecystectomy. Several randomised controlled trials have shown no benefit for laparoscopic cholecystectomy compared to mini-cholecystectomy, in terms of postoperative analgesic requirements, time in hospital and time to return to normal activities, but others have shown that the laparoscopic approach is associated with shorter hospital stay and less time off work.

Acute appendicitis is the commonest intra-abdominal surgical emergency, occurring in approximately 10% of the population in Western countries. The peak incidence is around 30 years of age and the disease is commoner in males than in females. It is a bacterial infection secondary to blockage of the lumen, usually by a faecolith, which is often progressive eventually leading to gangrene of the appendix, perforation and peritonitis. The variable position of the appendix, which may be retrocaecal, pelvic, retroileal or supraileal, leads to appendicitis mimicking many other disease processes, but once the diagnosis is made prompt operative intervention should be undertaken.

CHAPTER 7

# Diagnostic Laparoscopy

Iain C. Cameron, William E.G. Thomas

## INTRODUCTION

Diagnostic laparoscopic examination of the abdominal cavity has become increasingly popular with general surgeons over the past 20 years. The procedure is carried out with the patient under general anaesthetic and lying supine on the operating table. The first step in the operation is to create a pneumoperitoneum, which may be done using either the open ('Hasson') technique or the closed technique.

## Figure 1

The open technique begins with a subumbilical incision of approximately 2 cm which may either be vertical or transverse. The subcutaneous fat is divided until the linea alba comes into view, which is divided over a 1-cm distance between two clips. The same two clips are then reapplied to the underlying peritoneum, which is divided and access gained to the peritoneal cavity. A finger is then placed into the abdomen to ensure that there are no adhesions beneath. The cannula is introduced under direct vision into the peritoneal cavity through the small window created in the linea alba and peritoneum and fixed in place using a purse string suture to ensure a tight seal and prevent continual leakage of gas during the procedure. Insufflation of the peritoneal cavity with carbon dioxide is commenced by connecting the gas supply to the side port of the cannula, and continued until it has been filled to a pressure of 12—15 mmHg. This technique virtually abolishes the risk of major vascular injury, although injuries to the bowel may still occur. Many surgeons prefer to use this method routinely whilst others selectively employ this technique when patients have had previous abdominal surgery.



## Figure 2

The closed technique involves creating a carbon dioxide pneumoperitoneum using a Veress needle and electronic insufflator. The Veress needle is most commonly inserted at the subumbilical site after a stab incision has been made in the skin using a pointed scalpel. A different site may be selected if subumbilical adhesions are suspected. Insertion of the Veress needle is a blind procedure with the potential for complications including perforation of a viscus and vascular injury, and must be performed under general anaesthetic with the patient fully relaxed. The safest technique involves holding the Veress needle like a pen and lifting the fascia of the abdominal wall either manually or with the help of Littlewood's forceps. The Veress needle is passed through the anterior abdominal wall towards the pelvis and a definite click is felt as the linea alba and peritoneum are breached.

Figure 1

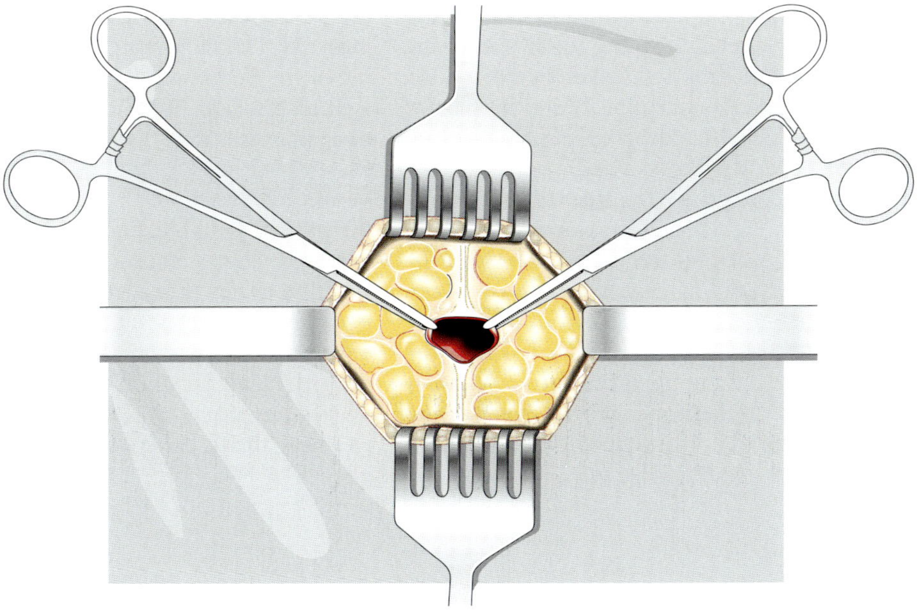

Figure 2

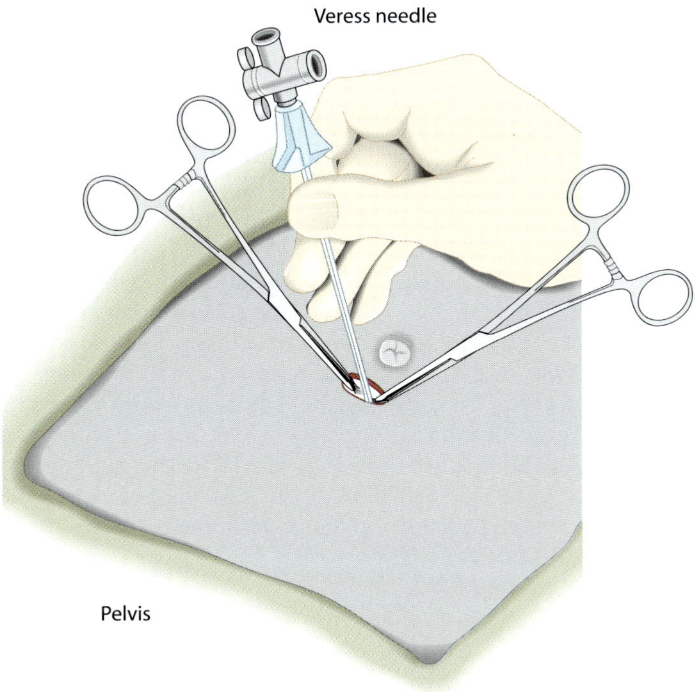

## Figure 3

Various tests can now be performed to ensure that the tip of the Veress needle is lying freely within the peritoneal cavity. The 'drop test' involves closing the tap of the Veress needle and then filling the part of the needle above this with a drop of saline. This drop will disappear down the Veress needle when the tap is opened if the needle tip is lying free within the peritoneal cavity, although sometimes abdominal wall countertraction may be required to free the tip of the needle. Alternatively, the 'syringe aspiration' test can be used to confirm the correct placement of the needle tip. Ten millilitres of saline is injected into the peritoneal cavity and if the tip of the Veress needle is lying freely within the peritoneal cavity then the saline cannot be aspirated. If the needle is not within the peritoneal cavity it should be withdrawn and reinserted. The commonest site of incorrect positioning of the Veress needle is in the anterior abdominal wall. Aspiration of yellow stained or blood stained fluid indicates that the needle tip is incorrectly positioned in either a loop of bowel or a blood vessel. The Veress needle should be withdrawn and providing the patient is stable, the needle may be repositioned correctly, the pneumoperitoneum created and inspection of any damaged structures undertaken. If it is suspected that a significant vascular injury may have occurred, a mini-laparotomy is recommended immediately after the Veress needle is withdrawn to assess the injury. (For reason of clearity, the clamps elevating the fascia are omitted.)



## Figure 4

Insufflation is commenced with carbon dioxide via the Veress needle initially at a slow flow rate of <1 l/min. A high insufflation pressure (>8 mmHg) at this low flow rate indicates malposition of the needle tip and insufflation should be stopped. If the insufflation pressure remains low and the patient appears to be tolerating the insufflation, the flow rate is increased to 3.5 l/min and the peritoneal cavity filled to a pressure of 12—15 mmHg. The Veress needle is withdrawn and the first port which will allow introduction of the laparoscope is inserted in the subumbilical region. The trocar is held in the right hand with the butt pressed firmly against the palm. The periumbilical region is tented upwards with the left hand or with the help of Littlewood's forceps applied to the fascia, and the trocar is inserted parallel to the axis of the aorta aiming at a position in the centre of the pelvis. Using a disposable sheathed cannula a click is heard, due to snapping of the sheath over the trocar point, as soon as the peritoneal cavity is breached. The trocar is withdrawn before the cannula is advanced further, and the gas supply is connected to the side port of the cannula to maintain the pneumoperitoneum.

Figure 3

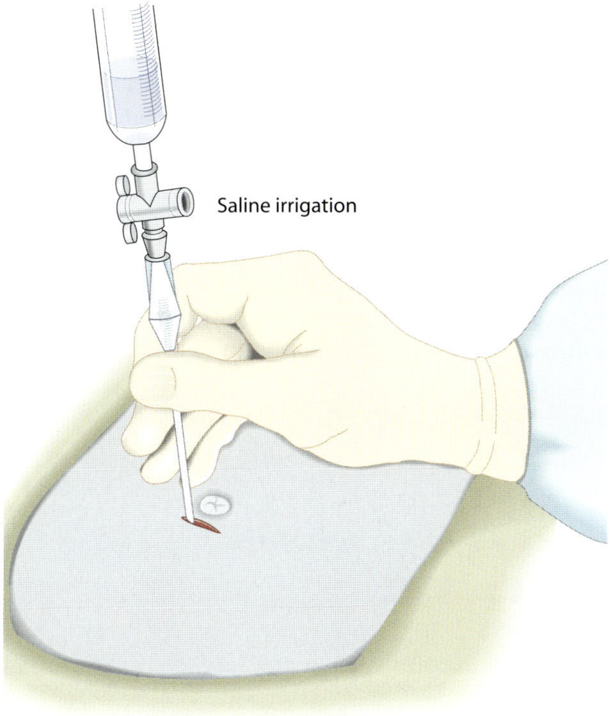


Figure 4

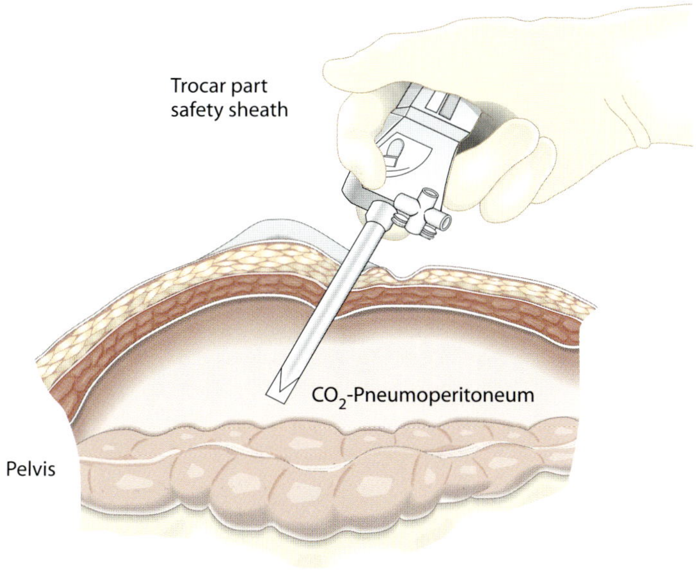

## Figure 5

A 10-mm laparoscope (0° or 30°) is inserted via the subumbilical port after the camera and light source have been attached, and the system has been 'white balanced'. The peritoneal cavity is examined and further ports (usually one or two) are inserted under direct vision. The precise placement of these ports depends on the purpose of the laparoscopic examination, which may be diagnostic, usually in patients with undiagnosed abdominal pain, or undertaken as part of the staging of an oesophagogastric or pancreatic cancer. During a laparoscopy for non-specific abdominal pain it is usual to assess the entire peritoneal cavity. The gallbladder is assessed for any signs of recurrent inflammation such as a thickened wall and omental adhesions, as are the liver and diaphragm. The left lobe of the liver is lifted to assess the stomach but views of the pancreas are not possible unless the lesser sac is opened. The small bowel is examined next with the entire length being assessed for abnormalities. The patient may then be tilted head down for assessment of the pelvic organs including the appendix and samples are taken of any free fluid for microbiology and cytology, with any suspicious areas or nodules being biopsied.

Figure 5

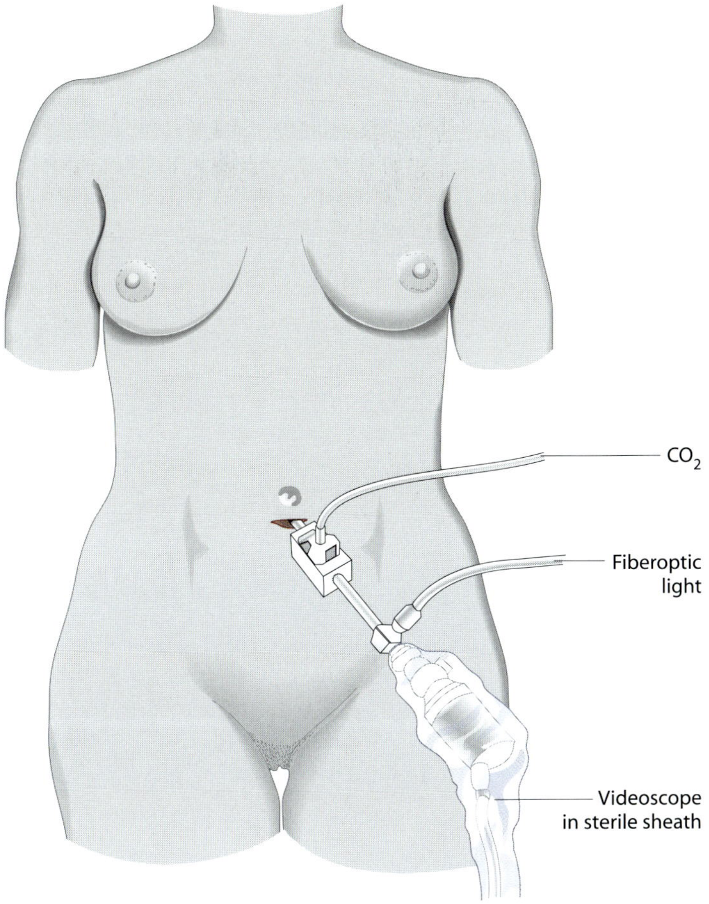

CHAPTER 8

# Laparoscopic Cholecystectomy

Iain C. Cameron, William E.G. Thomas

## INTRODUCTION

Laparoscopic techniques for the removal of the gall bladder were first described in 1989, and laparoscopic cholecystectomy has now become the operation of choice in many centres for dealing with symptomatic gallstones. Initial concerns were raised about the number of common duct injuries with this technique (rates of up to 1% were reported), but improvements in training for this procedure have seen the prevalence of these injuries reduce to the same levels as seen in the open cholecystectomy era.

The operation is undertaken with the patient under general anaesthesia with tracheal intubation, allowing monitoring of vital cardiovascular and respiratory parameters.

## Figure 1

The patient is placed supine on the operating table and the skin sterilised from above the costal margin down to a point midway between the umbilicus and the symphysis pubis. A pneumoperitoneum is then created, with initial access to the peritoneal cavity by either the open 'Hasson' technique or by using a Veress needle, as previously described. The laparoscope is introduced via the 10-mm umbilical port to allow the remaining three ports to be inserted under direct vision. The sites of placement of the remaining three ports are shown in the figure.



## Figure 2

The 10-mm epigastric port is the second to be inserted. A skin incision is made about 3 cm below the xiphisternum and the trocar is inserted so that the intra-abdominal entrance site is just to the right of the falciform ligament. Two further 5-mm ports are placed laterally, port 3 having the most variable position depending on surgeon preference and port 4 being placed laterally just above the level of the umbilicus. The patient is then placed at approximately 10° of reverse Trendelenburg and the table rotated slightly to the left. The surgeon stands on the patient's left side with the assistant next to them and the scrub nurse on the opposite side of the table.

Figure 1

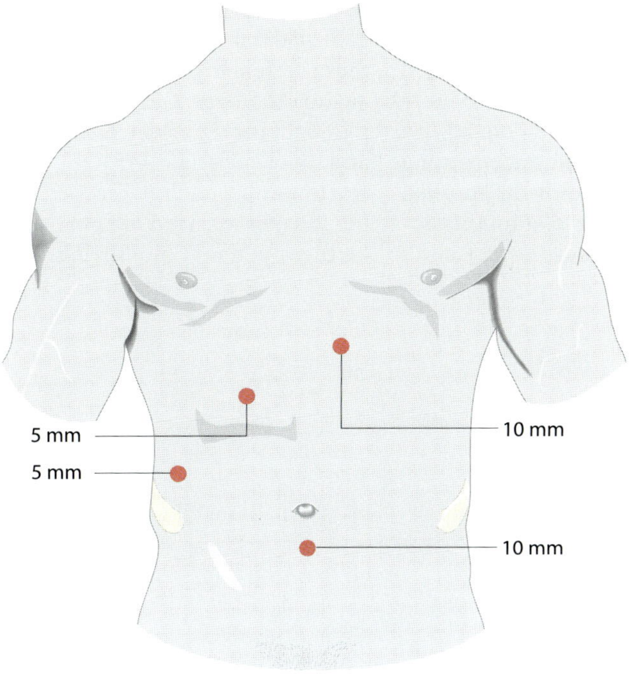


Figure 2

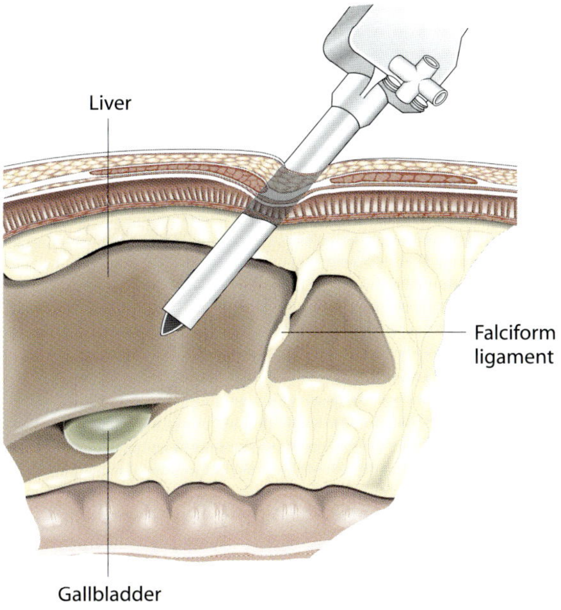

## Figure 3

A toothed grasper is placed via the most lateral port (port 4) and the fundus of the gall bladder is grasped and, with progressive traction, is retracted up and over the anterior lip of the liver. This manoeuvre pulls up the gall bladder and Hartmann's pouch, with Calot's triangle and the common bile duct coming into view as a result. The assistant holds the toothed retractor in place as it is essential to maintain this position in order to dissect out the structures in Calot's triangle. It is not always possible to push the tip of the gall bladder over the anterior hepatic edge, and in these cases the GB tip should be pushed gently against the liver, taking care not to damage the liver parenchyma, in order to expose Hartmann's pouch and Calot's triangle. With the operative field exposed, Hartmann's pouch is grasped with the lateral working grasper inserted via port 3 and pulled laterally to further open up Calot's triangle.



## Figure 4

A dissecting forceps is now passed down the epigastric port and used to dissect out the cystic duct and artery. This involves stripping down any adhesions and the peritoneal covering from Hartmann's pouch, which may consist of tough fibrous tissue in cases of chronic cholecystitis, or during early surgery for acute cholecystitis the stripping down of oedematous tissue. It is essential to strip the tissues away from the gall bladder towards the cystic duct and common bile duct rather than the other way around, and to avoid the use of diathermy until the anatomy has been clearly defined. The cystic duct and artery must be identified, as well as the cystic duct/gall bladder junction and the common bile duct. The dissecting forceps are passed behind both the cystic duct and artery in turn and spread to create a window free of tissue behind each structure.

Figure 3

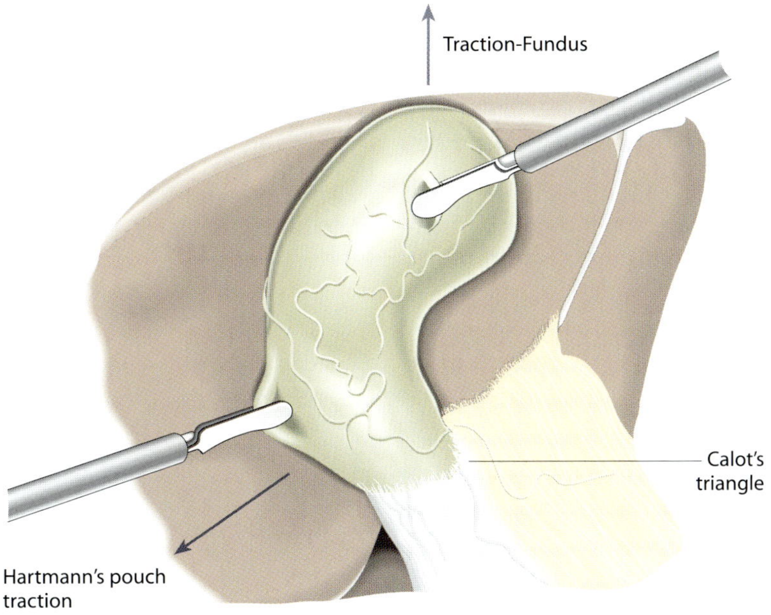


Figure 4

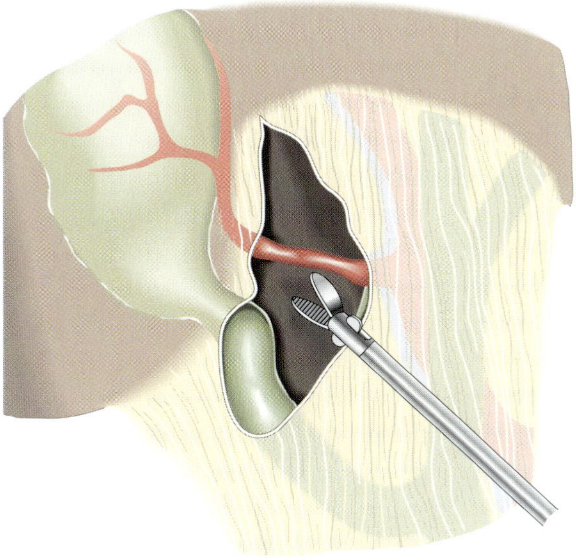

## Figure 5A, B

The routine use of intraoperative cholangiography is controversial with some authors advocating its routine use, whilst others employ a selective policy, only undertaking it in patients with deranged liver function tests, a history of jaundice and/or acute pancreatitis or a dilated common bile duct on preoperative ultrasound scan. Arguments in favour of routine cholangiography include the fact that it clearly demonstrates the biliary anatomy and allows identification of undiagnosed stones elsewhere in the biliary system. The procedure may be carried out using a system similar to that shown here, with a fine catheter (4–5 Fr) with an end hole, passing inside a specially adapted grasper. Alternatively a catheter inserted through a tiny incision in the anterior abdominal wall may be inserted directly into the cystic duct under direct vision.

Figure 5A, B

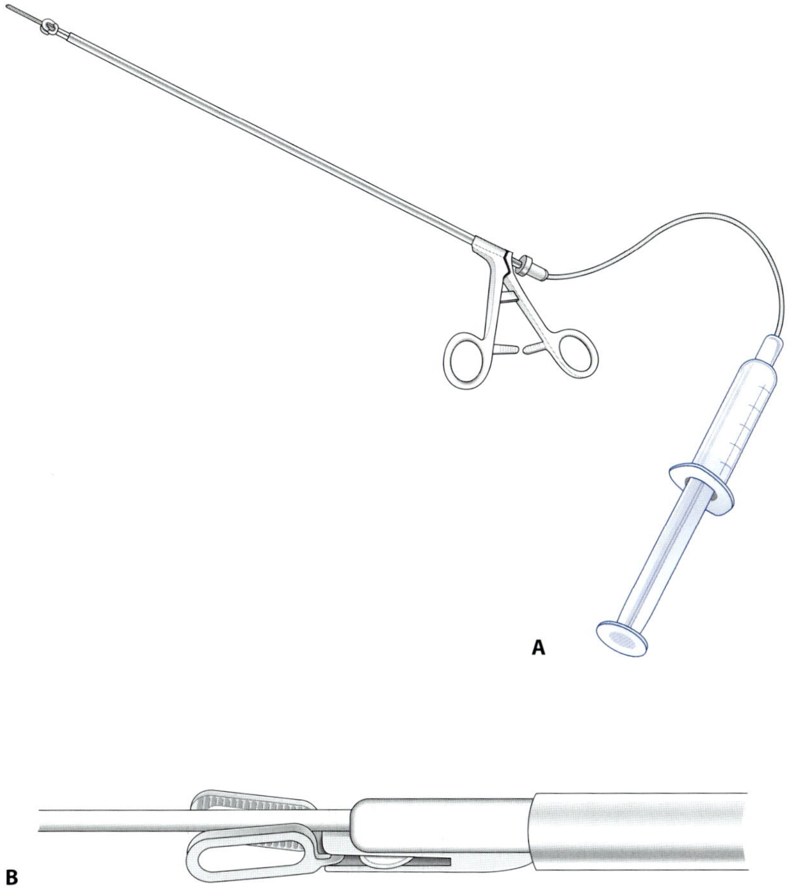

## Figure 6

An endoscopic clip applicator is introduced via the epigastric port and the cystic duct is clipped immediately adjacent to the gall bladder, ensuring that the clip passes across the whole width of the cystic duct. The clip applicator is withdrawn and a small anterior hole is cut in the cystic duct below the clip using endoscopic scissors. The cholangiograsper is inserted via port 3, and with the jaws open the catheter is gently fed down the cystic duct. Once an adequate length of catheter is in place, the jaws of the cholangiograsper are closed over the cystic duct. To ensure the catheter is lying freely within the biliary tree, saline is gently squeezed into the biliary system, which should flow easily, after which bile can be aspirated back into the syringe. The saline is replaced with a syringe containing radio-opaque contrast medium and under fluoroscopic screening the contrast is slowly infiltrated to outline the biliary tree. The pictures obtained are inspected to ensure that there are no filling defects suggestive of gallstones, that there is free flow of contrast into the duodenum, and that the major branches of the intrahepatic biliary tree are all identified. On completion of the cholangiogram the jaws are released and the cholangiograsper and catheter are removed. If a stone is identified floating freely within the biliary tree the operating surgeon may choose to explore the biliary system either laparoscopically or by converting to an open operation, or can continue the operation with a view to endoscopic duct clearance at a later date.



## Figure 7

The clip applier is inserted via the epigastric port and two clips are applied under direct vision across the entire width of the cystic duct below the hole made for the cholangiogram catheter. Endoscopic scissors are used to divide the cystic duct between the clip next to the gall bladder and the two clips on the common bile duct side. This process is now repeated for the cystic artery, with one clip applied next to the gall bladder and two clips applied away from the gall bladder, leaving a gap in the cystic artery at which point it is divided using scissors.

Figure 6

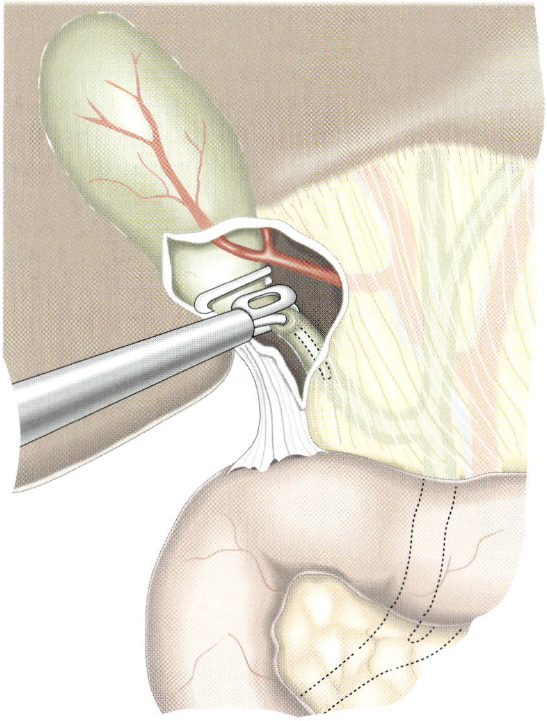

Figure 7

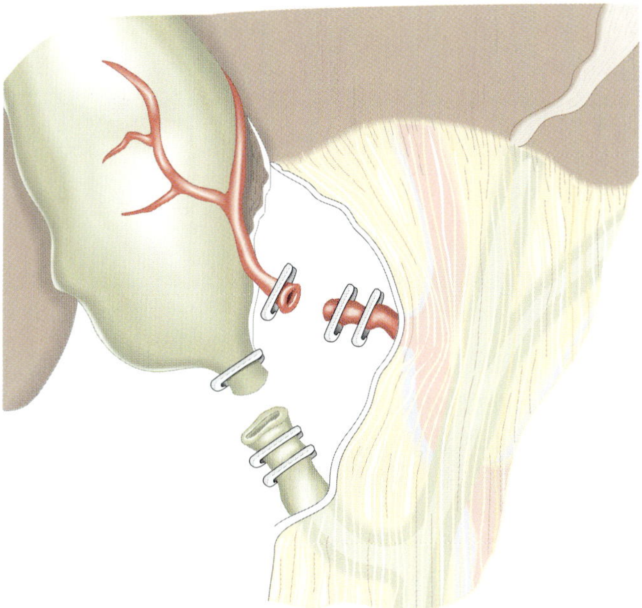

## Figure 8

With the cystic duct and artery divided, Hartmann's pouch is retracted upwards using the grasper inserted via port 3 and the diathermy hook is used to divide the lateral and medial peritoneal covering of Hartmann's pouch and the body of the gall bladder. This in turn allows further upward traction and the plane between the gall bladder and liver bed is displayed and dissected using the diathermy hook. The toothed grasper holding the gall bladder fundus often has to be released to allow the final dissection of the upper part of the gall bladder from the liver bed.

The free gall bladder is now removed from the peritoneal cavity under direct vision via the umbilical port following relocation of the laparoscope to the epigastric port. The gall bladder may be placed in a protective bag before extraction or removed as it is using large toothed graspers. The final stage of the operation is to examine the liver bed for bleeding and irrigate the operative field and surrounding area with saline. Any stones which may have escaped are also removed, after which the trocars are removed in turn, ensuring there is no port site bleeding, and the abdomen is deflated. The 10-mm trocar insertion sites for the subumbilical and epigastric ports are closed with deep polypropylene or nylon sutures to the rectus sheath with skin sutures for all four ports. In selected cases the surgeon may elect to insert a drain to the gallbladder bed via port site 4. This can usually be removed within 24 h.

Figure 8

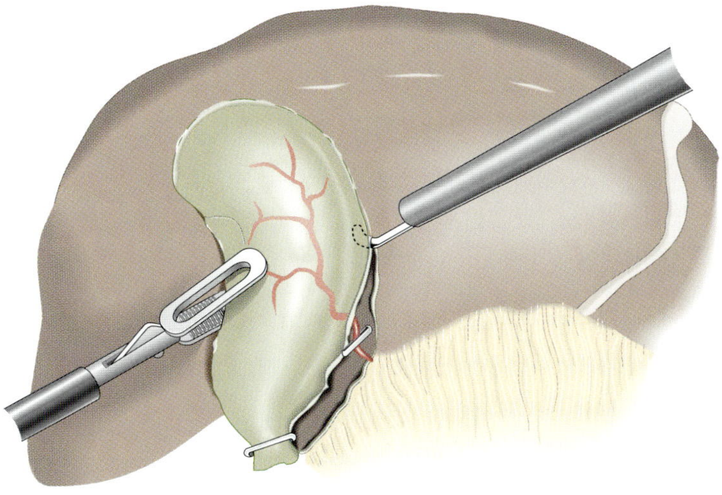

CHAPTER 9

# Mini-Cholecystectomy

Iain C. Cameron, William E.G. Thomas

## INTRODUCTION

The indications for undertaking mini-cholecystectomy are identical to those for laparoscopic cholecystectomy. Mini-cholecystectomy may be preferable in elderly patients with poor cardiac reserve, as the creation of a pneumoperitoneum can cause considerable cardiovascular compromise.

## Figure 1

A transverse skin incision about 6 cm in length is made starting from the midline approximately two finger breadths below the xiphisternum, extending laterally towards the right costal margin. The anterior rectus sheath, rectus muscle and posterior sheath are divided in turn, and the peritoneum picked up with two clips and divided between them. The peritoneum is divided laterally as far as the extent of the incision and medially as far as the falciform ligament, which is sometimes ligated and divided to facilitate access to the structures in Calot's triangle.



## Figure 2

Once the peritoneal cavity is opened, the gall bladder must be located and exposed. This is achieved by the placement of an abdominal swab over the omentum and transverse colon, which are then retracted towards the pelvis by the assistant. A further retractor placed just medially to the gall bladder is then used to retract segment 4 of the liver upwards, thus exposing the common bile duct and porta hepatis. Any adhesions between Hartmann's pouch and the omentum and duodenum are divided carefully under direct vision, and the inferior retractor may be repositioned at this point if necessary.

Figure 1

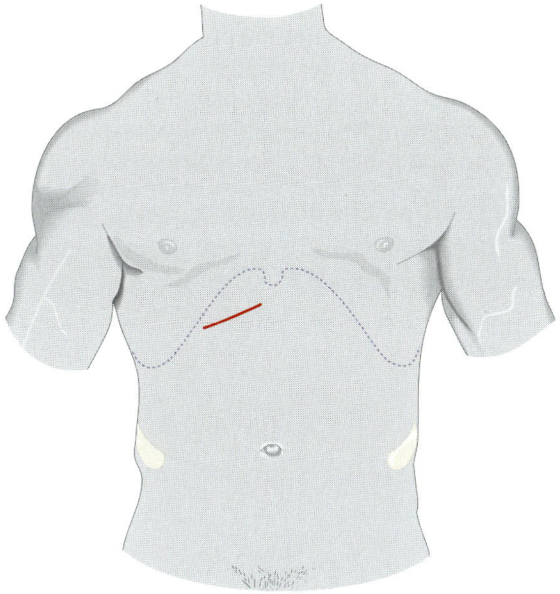

Figure 2

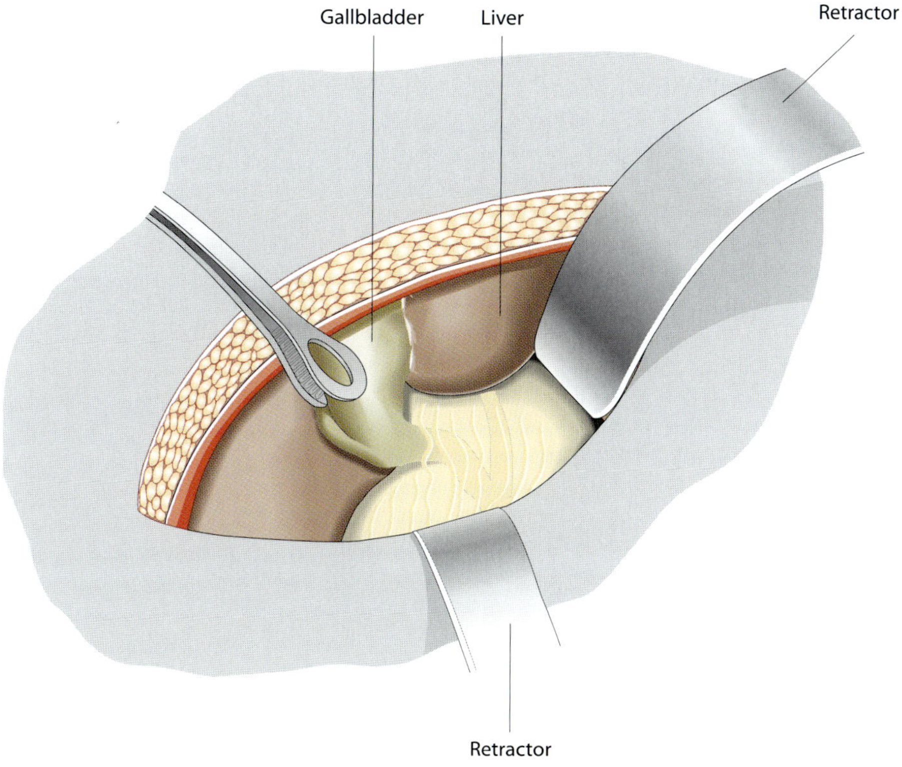

## Figure 3

Hartmann's pouch is grasped with forceps and lifted and retracted laterally to expose Calot's triangle and allow the peritoneal covering over the neck of the gall bladder, cystic duct and artery to be divided. The tissue is swept away from the gall bladder with a pledget and right angled forceps are used to dissect around the cystic duct and artery, ensuring that they are free of all other tissue. If an operative cholangiogram is to be performed, it is undertaken at this point. The procedure is similar to that described for laparoscopic cholecystectomy, with a clip placed across the whole width of the cystic duct next to the gall bladder, following which a small hole is cut anteriorly in the bile duct. The cholangiogram catheter is then fed down the cystic duct and into the common bile duct and held in place with another clip. Saline is slowly injected and if flowing freely, the syringe is aspirated, which should allow bile to be seen in the syringe. Contrast is now injected and a cholangiogram obtained.

Figure 3

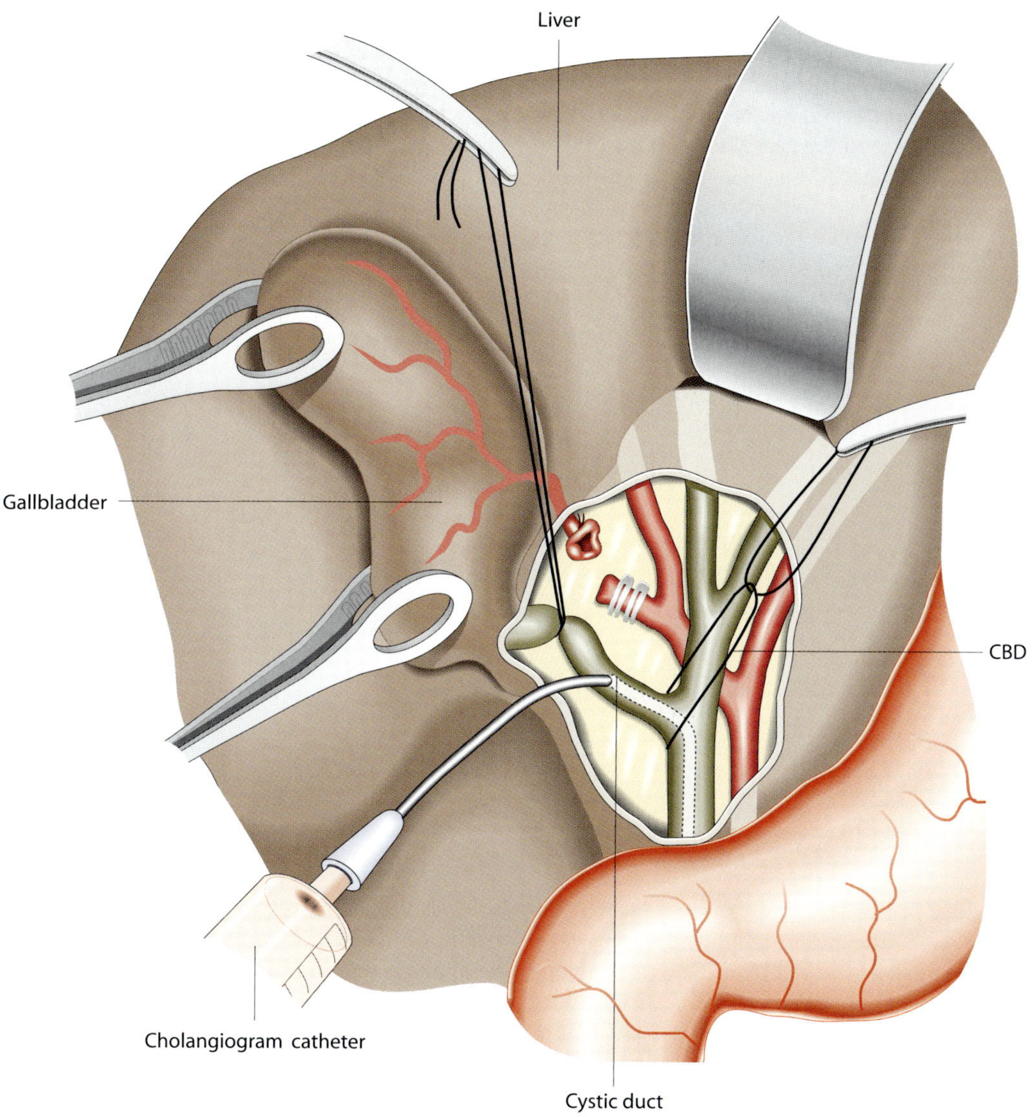
Liver
Gallbladder
CBD
Cholangiogram catheter
Cystic duct

## Figure 4

The clip holding the cholangiogram catheter in place is removed, as is the catheter. Two clips are applied to the cystic duct below the hole, on the side of the common bile duct, and the cystic duct is divided between these and the clip next to the gall bladder. Three clips are now placed on the cystic artery, one next to the gall bladder, and two others away from the gall bladder, with the artery being divided between these clips.



## Figure 5

The gall bladder is now free and can be dissected off the liver bed, with the plane displayed by upward traction on the neck of the gall bladder. On many occasions the authors choose this point to change operating position to the left side of the patient where under direct vision the gall bladder is easily dissected free of the liver bed using diathermy and removed. An alternative approach is to adopt a fundus first dissection which may be beneficial in any cases where the anatomy around Calot's triangle is not absolutely clear or is obscured by dense inflammatory tissue. Meticulous haemostasis is essential and saline lavage may be required. In selected cases a drain may be inserted to the gall bladder bed and brought out through a separate stab incision. A two-layer continuous closure of the posterior and anterior rectus sheath using 0 Prolene is undertaken, with local anaesthetic infiltration of the upper edge of the muscle and wound being administered. The skin is closed with a subcuticular suture.

Figure 4

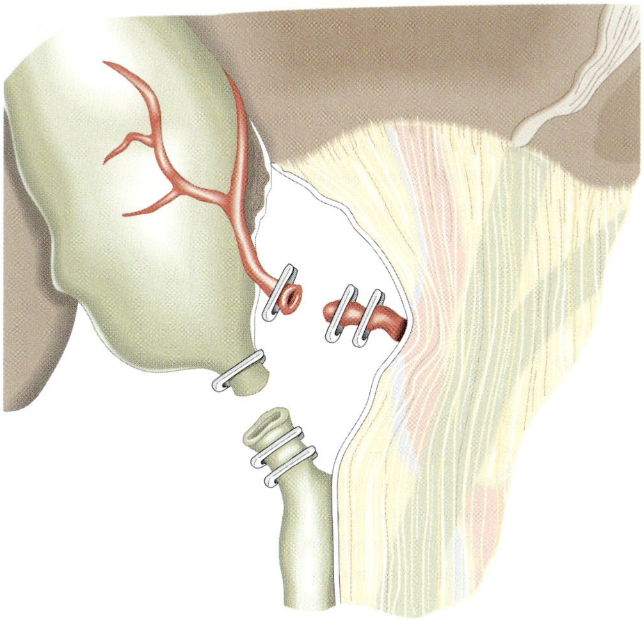

Figure 5

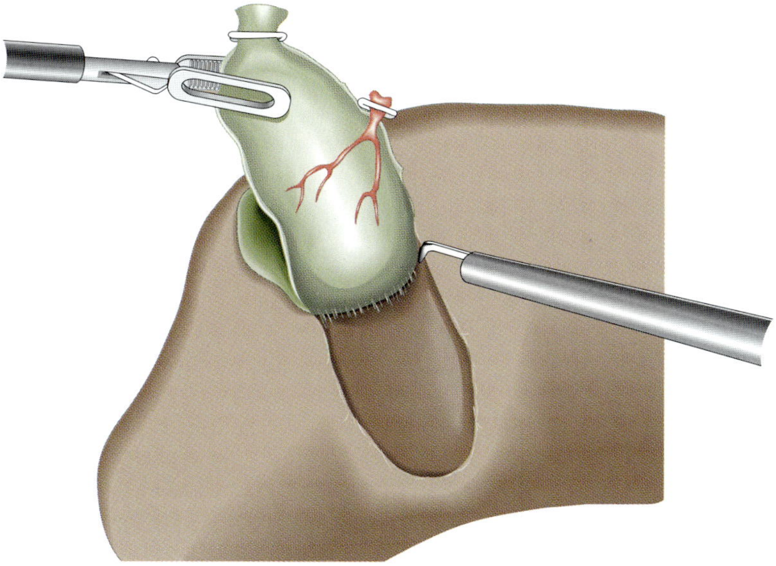

CHAPTER 10

# Open Appendicectomy

Iain C. Cameron, William E.G. Thomas

## INTRODUCTION

The operation of appendicectomy is performed with the patient under general anaesthetic and intubated, using either open or laparoscopic techniques. Preoperatively it is imperative that fluid balance is corrected, especially in children and elderly patients, and renal function thus preserved. Prophylactic antibiotics, usually a single dose of augmentin or a cephalosporin combined with metronidazole, are given at induction of anaesthesia.

## Figure 1

The patient is placed supine on the table and the skin is prepared over the right lower quadrant of the abdomen and right upper thigh. The site of the initial incision is one of personal preference, with some advocating an incision centred on McBurney's point (a point lying two-thirds of the way between the umbilicus and the anterior superior iliac spine), whilst others prefer a lower more transverse (Lanz) incision, especially in young females. The incision should normally be about 5–6 cm in length.

## Figure 2

The appendix can be situated in many different positions as shown, the commonest being the retrocaecal and pelvic positions. This variable position is the main reason why acute inflammation of the appendix can mimic the presentation of many other pathological processes.



## Figure 3

The incision is deepened to expose the external oblique aponeurosis. This is then divided in the line of its fibres in a lateral direction from the edge of the rectus sheath. The edges are retracted and the underlying internal oblique is then split in the line of its fibres from the edge of the rectus sheath laterally towards the iliac crest.

## Figure 4

The transversalis fascia and peritoneum are then lifted between clips and a small hole created in both layers using a scalpel. The clips are immediately reapplied to the edges of the exposed peritoneum and the opening extended under direct vision, with the rectus sheath being opened for 1–2 cm if further exposure medially is required. A swab is taken of any turbid peritoneal fluid in the vicinity and sent for culture.

Figure 1

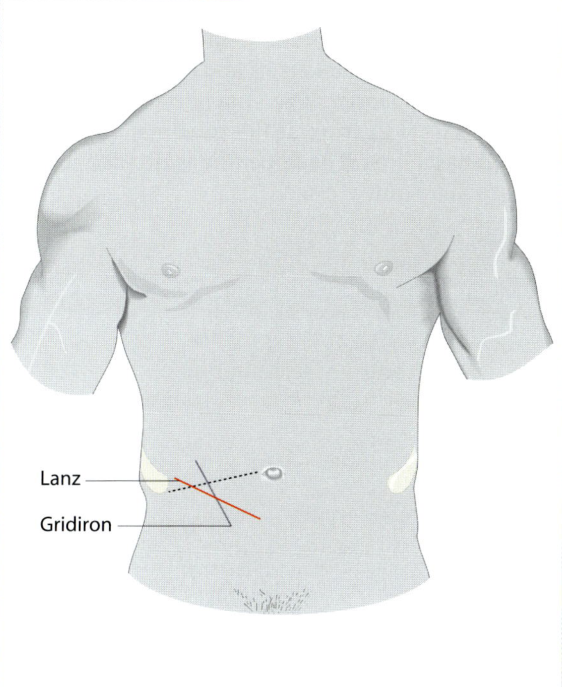


Figure 2

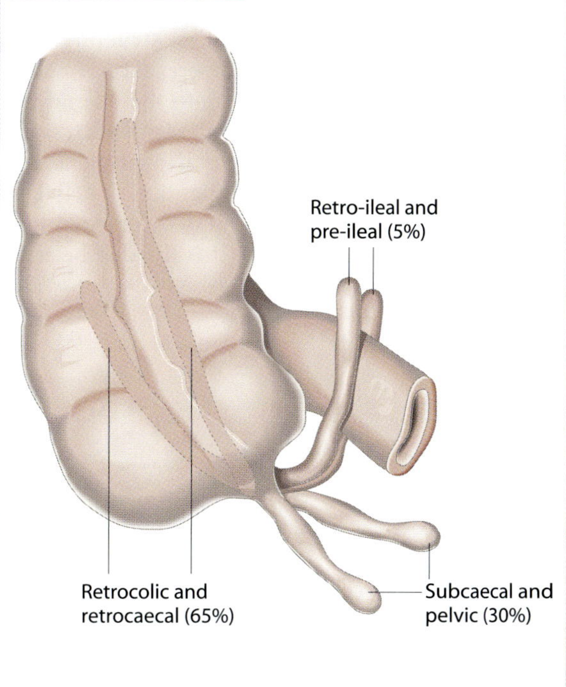


Figure 3

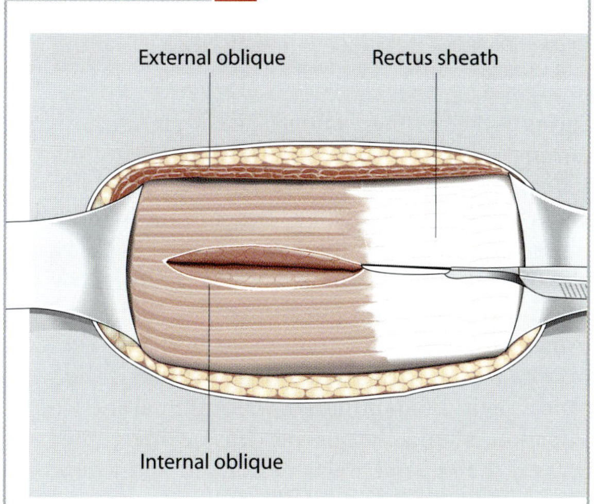


Figure 4

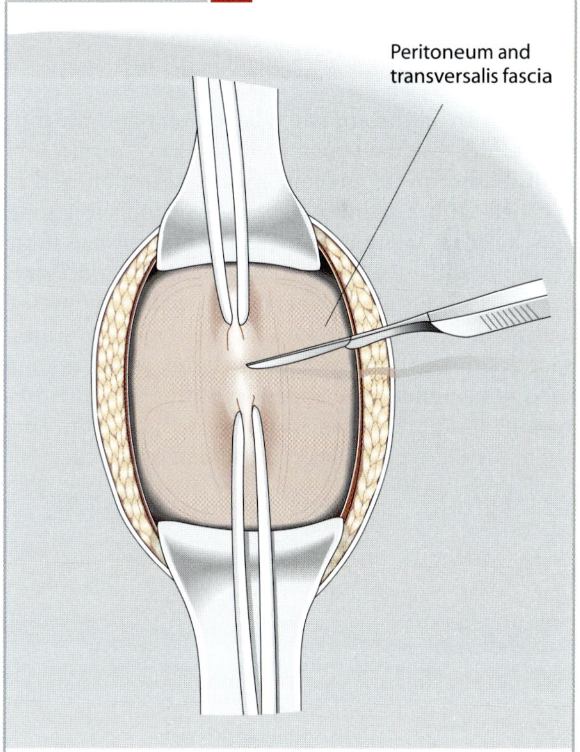

## Figure 5

In most cases the caecum is the first structure to be seen and can be identified by the presence of taenia. The caecum should be elevated into the wound and traced to its base in order to find the appendix, a process which can be facilitated by division of the lateral peritoneal attachments. The appendix is delivered into the wound and the mesentery is grasped near the tip of the appendix, before it is divided between clips and ligated.

## Figure 6

The base of the appendix is then crushed with a clamp, which is then taken off and reapplied 1 cm further up the appendix. The appendix is then ligated with a 0 Vicryl ligature at the proximal edge of the crushed basal area. The appendix is divided just below the clamp and excised.



## Figure 7

The ligature at the appendix base is cut and the mucosa of the residual appendix stump is gently ablated with diathermy to prevent mucus secretion and is brushed with a betadine soaked gauze. The stump may be quite safely left alone at this point but some surgeons still advocate the placement of a 2/0 Vicryl pursestring suture in the caecal wall around the stump. In this case the knot at the appendix stump base is grasped with a straight clamp, which is then used to invaginate the appendix stump into the caecum as the pursestring suture is tied, thus burying the appendix stump inside the lumen of the caecum.

## Figure 8

Saline lavage is then undertaken if significant contamination was present at initial opening of the peritoneum, with care being taken to ensure that the pelvis is thoroughly irrigated, and a drain is rarely required. The peritoneum and transversalis fascia are closed with continuous 2/0 Vicryl, followed by the internal oblique with interrupted 2/0 Vicryl and the external oblique with continuous 0 Vicryl. The skin may be closed with a subcuticular suture if the peritoneal cavity contamination was minimal and wound infection is unlikely, or with clips or interrupted sutures if the appendix was perforated and wound infection is likely. One dose of preoperative antibiotics is sufficient except in cases where the appendix is gangrenous or perforated in which case they should be given for 5 days.

Figure 5

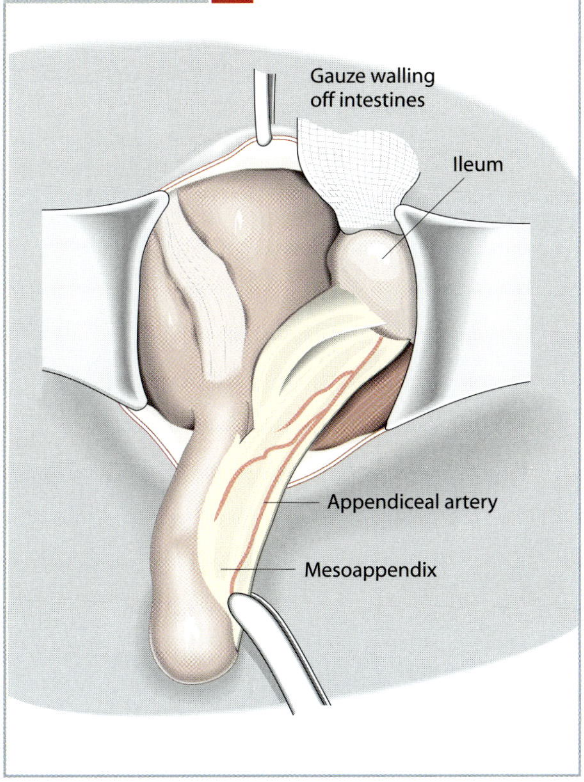


Figure 6

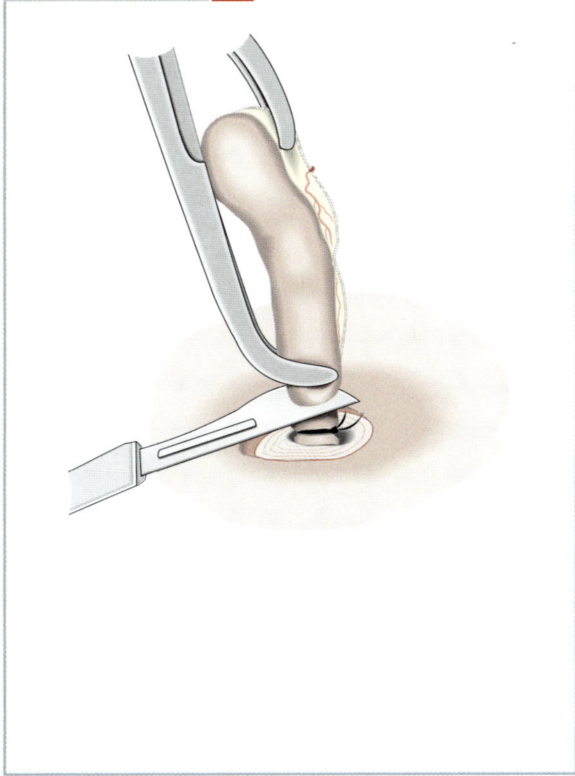

Figure 7

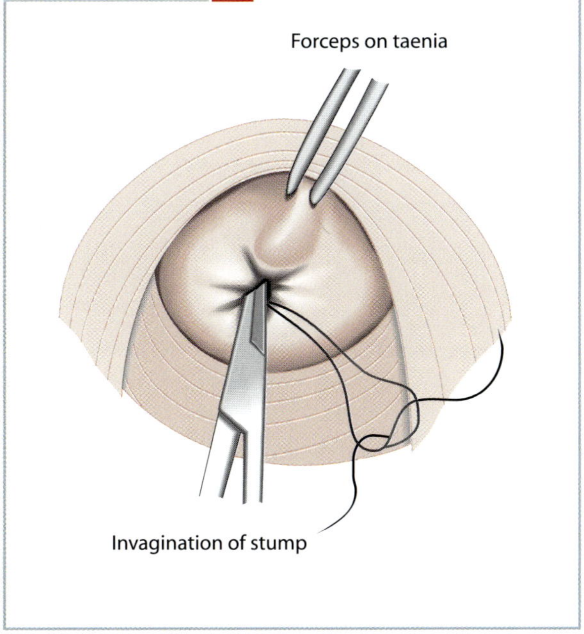


Figure 8

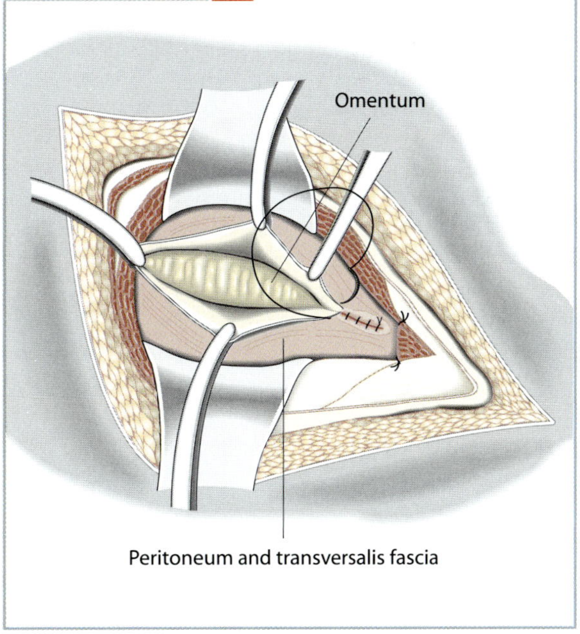

CHAPTER 11

# Laparoscopic Appendicectomy

Iain C. Cameron, William E.G. Thomas

## INTRODUCTION

Laparoscopic appendicectomy has become increasingly popular over the past decade and many centres now favour this procedure, as several studies have shown that patients recover faster and return to full activity more quickly after this procedure compared to open appendicectomy. Another perceived advantage of a laparoscopy in patients with suspected appendicitis is the opportunity to diagnose other conditions which may be the cause of the pain, such as those affecting the gynaecological organs. For this reason a laparoscopic procedure is recommended in young female patients with suspected acute appendicitis. The operation is undertaken under general anaesthesia with tracheal intubation, allowing monitoring of vital CVS functions and maintenance of oxygenation.

## Figure 1

The patient is placed supine on the operating table and the skin sterilised from above the costal margin down to the level of the symphysis pubis. A pneumoperitoneum is created using either the open 'Hasson' technique or a Veress needle, as previously described. The remaining two ports are inserted under direct vision after the camera has been inserted through the umbilical port. The sites of placement of the remaining two ports are shown in the figure. The surgeon stands on the left of the patient with the camera operator stood next to them towards the head end of the patient.



## Figure 2

The first step in a laparoscopic appendicectomy is to undertake a full laparoscopic examination of the entire peritoneal cavity. In female patients the gynaecological organs should be closely inspected and the presence of free fluid or blood in the pelvis should be sought. If the suspected diagnosis of acute appendicitis is confirmed the appendix is removed using the following technique. At this point in the procedure it is useful to alter the position of the operating table so that the patient is head down and slightly rotated to the left. A non-traumatic grasper inserted via the left lateral port is used to grasp the caecum and retract it towards the liver. In many cases this manoeuvre will elevate the appendix into the visual field of the telescope, allowing it to be grasped and lifted up towards the abdominal wall, thus exposing the base of the appendix and the mesoappendix. Occasionally a severely inflamed retrocaecal appendix will prove difficult to visualise. In these cases the caecum may be mobilised by dividing the lateral peritoneum and retracting the caecum medially as well as towards the liver. In some cases it will not be possible to safely expose the appendix and conversion to open operation is required.

**Figure 1**

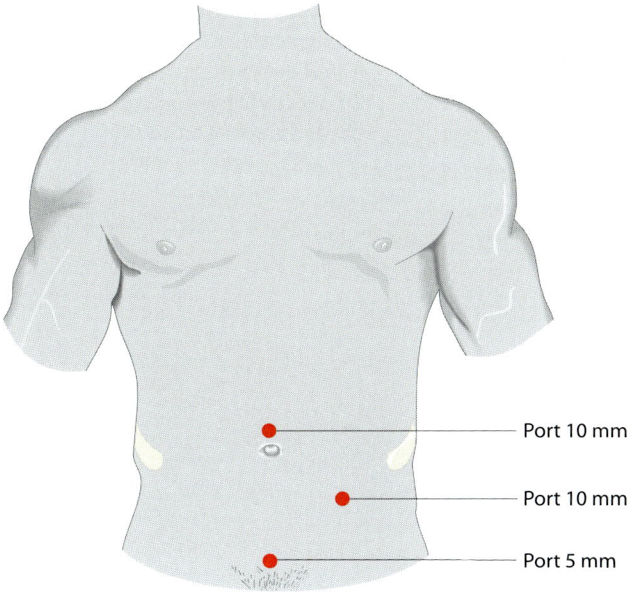


**Figure 2**

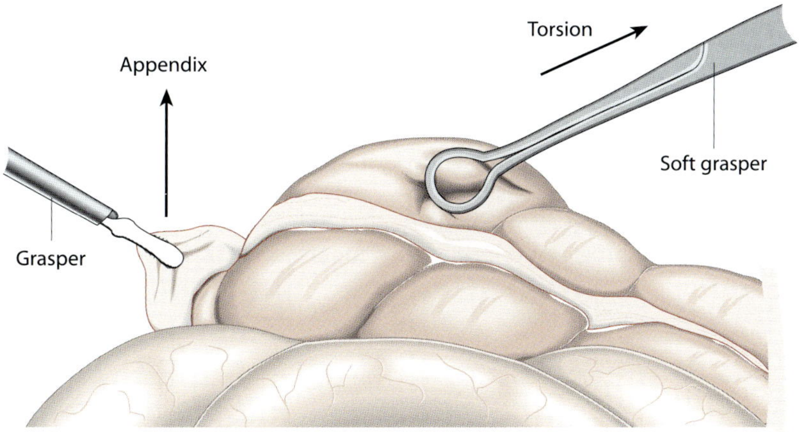

## Figure 3

With the appendix and mesoappendix exposed, the next step is to create a mesenteric window and to divide the mesoappendix. A thin curved grasper is used to create a window in the mesentery next to the base of the appendix. The appendicular artery lies between this mesenteric window and the free edge of the mesentery. The mesoappendix is now gently separated to expose the appendicular artery, which is clipped twice with an endoscopic clip applicator and divided between the metal clips.

## Figure 4



The next step is to divide the base of the appendix. This can be done either using the endoscopic stapler, which inserts two rows of staples and divides between them, or by applying two endoloop sutures around the base of the appendix and dividing between them. The endoloop sutures are fed in through the left lateral port and the appendix is manipulated through the looped catgut suture, which is then tightened around the base. The pushing device is then removed and the suture cut short using endoscopic scissors. A second endoloop suture is then applied to the appendix and tightened approximately 1 cm above the first and the pushing device removed and the suture divided. The appendix is then divided between the two ties using endoscopic scissors.

The appendix is now free of attachments and may be removed via the left lateral or umbilical port. This may be done immediately using toothed forceps to grab the appendix base or the appendix may be manipulated into a retrieval bag and removed. The peritoneal cavity is irrigated thoroughly with normal saline and if the appendix was perforated a drain may be left in place to drain the right paracolic gutter and pelvis. The 10-mm trocar insertion sites are closed with deep polypropylene or nylon sutures to the rectus sheath with skin sutures for all three ports.

Figure 3

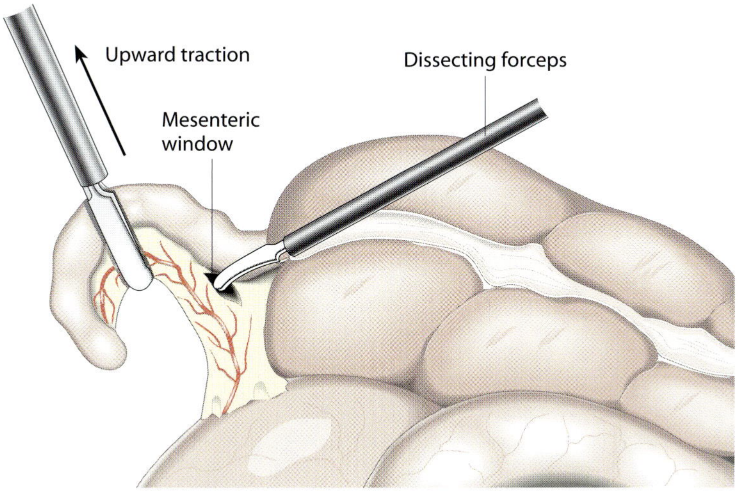
Upward traction
Dissecting forceps
Mesenteric
window

Figure 4

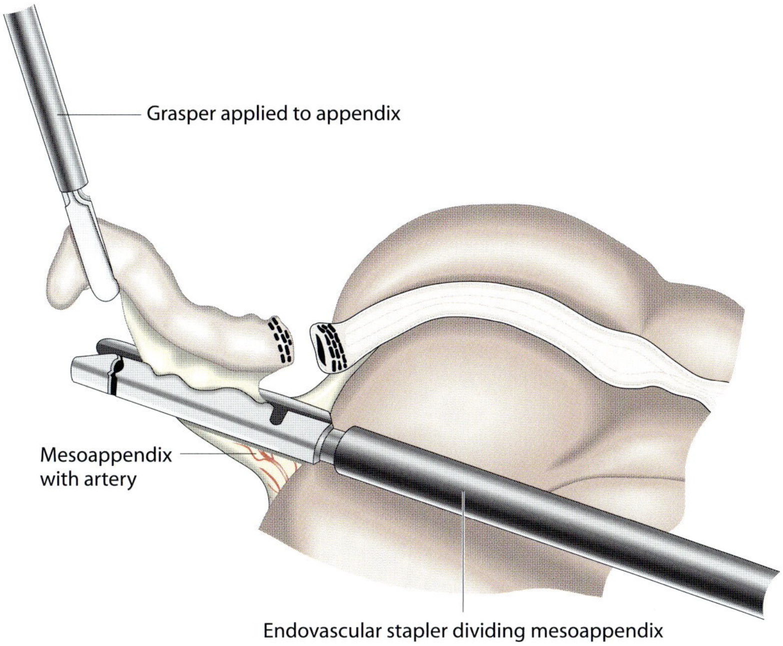
Grasper applied to appendix
Mesoappendix
with artery
Endovascular stapler dividing mesoappendix

CHAPTER 12

# Hernia Repairs: Inguinal, Femoral, and Umbilical

Shoo Yee Wong, Andrew N. Kingsnorth

## INTRODUCTION

Hernias are common surgical conditions. Surgical inpatient waiting lists could be reduced if the majority of hernia repairs were carried out in short stay surgery units. Inpatient beds could then be used for admission of more complex cases such as cancer surgery.

In the United States 750,000 inguinal hernia repairs are performed a year. The Plymouth Hernia Service at Derriford Hospital in Plymouth, UK, provides a service for a pool of hernia patients referred from their general practitioners. Four half-day short stay surgery theatre lists are allocated for hernia repair each week, for seven participating surgeons. About 750 hernias are repaired a year for the population of 0.5 million in Plymouth. Inguinal hernia accounts for more than 90% of the repairs carried out.

Short stay surgery units provide a high turnover of patients. Careful planning is crucial for their success. Patient selection is one important factor. Patients must fulfil certain medical and social criteria, and be willing to and capable of administering their own oral pain relief at home. The Plymouth Hernia Service is operated by a specialist hernia nurse who receives referrals direct from general practitioners. The referred patients attend the nurse's clinic to have their diagnosis confirmed. The nurse assesses the suitability of every patient for short stay surgery unit. The assessment is guided by protocols agreed by the anaesthetic department and the Clinical Governance director. Appropriate investigations are carried out, such as blood tests and ECG, as required. All patients receive a detailed verbal and written explanation of the surgical procedures, and their questions are addressed. Two weeks before their operation patients also receive a copy of an 8-min video explaining the procedures. On the day of surgery patients are well assured and are less anxious. Late cancellations are practically eliminated by asking patients to confirm their attendance for surgery.

Patients for short stay surgery must not exceed ASA (American Society of Anesthesiologists) physical status grade III if general anaesthetic is required, and should not have advanced renal or hepatic disease. Local anaesthesia is a helpful alternative which can be routinely used in inguinal hernia repairs. There is no set age limit, but elderly patients generally have more significant medical conditions and must be more carefully assessed.

Obese patients with a body mass index (BMI) greater than 30 are unsuitable for short stay surgery because of potentially significant concurrent medical conditions. Obese patients may experience greater anaesthetic complications such as longer recovery time from general anaesthesia due to larger tissue distribution; regurgitation of stomach contents; and atelectasis. Postoperative pain may take longer to control. In addition operation times may be prolonged due to technical difficulties such as establishing local anaesthesia, access to the operative site, and securing haemostasis. It is therefore for safety reasons that these patients are unsuitable for the short stay surgery unit.

The social criteria include the need for the patients to have transport to be taken to and picked up from the hospital on the day of surgery; postoperatively the patient must be supervised by a responsible adult in the first 24 h after general anaesthetic or sedation; and the patient must have a working telephone at home to contact the short stay surgery unit for advice or help.

All patients are fasted as for general anaesthetic, according to the guidelines recommended by the Association of Anaesthetists of Great Britain and Ireland and the American Society of Anaesthesiologists:

- 6 h for solid food, infant formula, or other milk
- 4 h for breast milk
- 2 h for clear non-particulate and non-carbonated fluid

Perioperative monitoring includes cardiac monitoring, pulse oximetry, and blood pressure.

General anaesthesia is used in paediatric cases; one parent is encouraged to stay with the child until he/she is anaesthetized. This calms the child and reassures the parents. The child and parent are reunited soon after surgery. In the theatre measures should be taken to prevent hypothermia, using blankets to cover unexposed parts of the body.

## Inguinal Hernia

Infantile inguinal hernia is mostly secondary to failure of closure of the processus vaginalis. It occurs in 4% of male infants; low birth weight and premature birth are particular risk factors and the male to female ratio is 9:1. Ten percent of children with inguinal hernia present as an emergency with irreducible hernias, the incidence being highest in the first 3 - months of life. The probability of strangulation is 1 in 4 for inguinal hernias before the age of 1. Up to a fifth of infantile inguinal hernias are bilateral, particularly in young children less than 6 months old and premature infants. A large prospective study of 656 children found that the development of contralateral inguinal hernias in childhood is particularly high in premature infants and children who have had an irreducible inguinal hernia. Bilateral inguinal hernia repair as prophylaxis for contralateral inguinal hernia may be advisable for these higher risk infants and children.

Prompt elective surgery prevents morbidity secondary to strangulation. It is preferable that very young infants (less than 6 months old) are operated on in units that are appropriately equipped for them. Herniotomy is performed and the hernia contents are reduced. The sac is transfixed and redundant sac excised. Care is taken not to damage the fragile testicular vessels. To avoid damage to the testicular co-lateral blood supply, which can cause testicular ischaemia, the testis should not be dislocated from the scrotum. The wound is closed in layers. At the end of surgery the testis must be checked to ensure it is in the scrotum. A postoperative iatrogenic ascent of the testis should be followed up and treated.

Adult inguinal hernia is secondary to weakened transversalis fascia due to degeneration and/or increased abdominal pressure. In indirect inguinal hernia the weakening is around the internal inguinal ring. The hernia sac passes through the internal inguinal ring, into the canal, leaving through the external inguinal ring to descend into the scrotum or the labia majora. The internal inguinal ring has relatively fixed margins and therefore an indirect inguinal hernia is more likely to strangulate than a direct inguinal hernia.

A direct inguinal hernia protrudes through the weakened transversalis fascia, which constitutes the posterior wall of the inguinal canal. The hernia rarely passes through the external inguinal ring or extends into the scrotum. The risk of strangulation of direct inguinal hernia is relatively low. Surgery therefore is not mandatory if quality of life is not seriously impaired especially in relatively asymptomatic elderly patients.

## Open Inguinal Hernia Repair in Adult

The governing principles are:

- Careful inspection to rule out combined indirect and direct hernias.
- Small hernia sacs may be inverted and returned to the peritoneal cavity.
- Large or inguino-scrotal hernia sacs should be opened and the contents returned into the peritoneal cavity under direct vision. Distal scrotal sacs must be left in situ, to avoid disruption of the vascular supply to the testis.
- The transversalis fascia is repaired and reinforced with mesh.
- The external oblique aponeurosis, superficial fascia and skin are reconstituted.

## Laparoscopic Repair of Inguinal Hernia

Laparoscopic hernia repair is an effective technique in the hands of experienced surgeons. It requires general anaesthesia and is more suitably carried out on younger patients who can then return earlier to physical work. The two common approaches are: totally extraperitoneal (TEP) and transabdominal preperitoneal (TAPP); the mesh is placed at the preperitoneal space in both approaches. The TEP approach is safer but more difficult to learn. This approach does not transgress the peritoneal cavity. The TAPP approach is simpler to learn but carries a small risk of visceral and vascular injuries. Its advantage is that both sides can be examined for the presence and repair of bilateral inguinal hernia.

## Results and Conclusions

The recurrence rate of inguinal hernia has decreased to 1–3% since the widespread introduction of polypropylene mesh. The mesh is sutured securely to aponeurotic tissues so that it cannot shift or wrinkle in the early postoperative period. The Lichtenstein tension-free open repair technique is easily taught and learnt, and is most widely used. As with all successful operations, its success depends on attention to detail, and individual surgeons should not be tempted to corrupt the original procedure.

The results of multicentre randomized trials have indicated that laparoscopic repair is associated with less postoperative pain, quicker recovery and return to activity, but greater expense. Because of the low margin for error, there is a small risk of disastrous complications such as injury to the bladder, bowel or vessels. The recurrence rate is 1–2%. The National Institute of

Clinical Excellence has recommended it is used only for recurrent inguinal hernias or bilateral inguinal hernias in centres with the necessary expertise.

Less frequent complications following inguinal hernia repairs are superficial wound infection, seroma, skin numbness, and testicular atrophy. Incisional hernia of the infra-umbilical port site can be prevented by closing the fascia with a non-absorbable suture.

Inguinal hernias in infants and young children must be treated promptly to avoid strangulation. Bilateral inguinal hernia repairs may be advisable in higher risk children. Mesh has revolutionized inguinal hernia repair, lowering complications and recurrence. Laparoscopic repair is recommended for recurrent and bilateral inguinal hernias.

It is unnecessary for a routine inguinal hernia repair to require prophylactic antibiotics because the operative field is clean, or to soak the mesh in Betadine prior to use.

## Femoral Hernia

The incidence of femoral hernia is about a tenth of that for inguinal hernia. The female to male ratio for femoral hernia is 4:1. In females the incidences of femoral and inguinal hernias are about equal. Femoral hernia is more common in the older population, contributed to by the failure of the transversalis fascia due to aging and secondary factors such as increased intra-abdominal pressure.

The peritoneal sac protrudes through the weakened transversalis fascia, and then descends vertically downwards into the femoral canal. The sac appears below the inguinal ligament, with the fundus bending upwards over the inguinal ligament. The neck of the hernia sac is below the inguinal ligament and lateral to the pubic tubercle, which helps to distinguish this type of hernia from an inguinal hernia. Femoral hernias are often irreducible because of the rigid margins of the femoral ring, contributing to the risk of strangulation. Once diagnosed arrangements for elective repair of a femoral hernia must be prompt.

## Femoral Hernia Repair

The crural or low approach is commonly used for elective femoral hernia repair. It allows direct assess to the hernia sac for reduction and closure with a mesh plug.

The other approaches are:

- Preperitoneal or modified McEvedy, which is commonly used for suspected strangulated femoral hernia. The incision is unilateral Pfannenstiel or lower midline. The transversalis fascia is divided after the rectus muscle is retracted laterally, in order to enter the preperitoneal space where the hernia sac can be found and reduced.
- The inguinal or high approach is now seldom used. The incision is as for inguinal hernia repair, through the floor of the inguinal canal from above to access the femoral canal. The inguinal canal is opened and the transversalis fascia is divided to reach the femoral hernia sac.

Laparoscopic preperitoneal femoral hernia repair is possible. It is not widely practiced as its cost effectiveness has yet to be established.

## Results and Conclusions

Recurrence should be rare following femoral hernia repair with mesh. Morbidity and mortality of strangulated hernias are particularly high in the elderly. Prompt surgery is essential.

## Umbilical Hernia

Minor degrees of umbilical herniation are present in many neonates, the majority regressing spontaneously. Infantile small umbilical hernias, less than 1.5 cm, rarely strangulate – therefore they can be observed during pre-school age. Persisting and enlarging umbilical hernias after that should be surgically repaired. The peritoneal sac protrudes through the umbilical cicatrix to lie in the subcutaneous tissues. It is effectively repaired with the Mayo operation. It is important to preserve the umbilicus for cosmetic reasons.

Adult umbilical hernias are seen in people with obesity and multiparous women. These hernias often have a surprisingly narrow and fibrous aponeurotic defect. In long-standing umbilical hernia the contents adhere to each other forming complex multiloculation, rendering the hernia irreducible. The hernia sac also adheres to the overlying umbilicus and skin; in some cases it may be difficult to preserve the umbilicus. Strangulation is common in large umbilical hernias, whereby patients present with abdominal pain and subacute small bowel obstruction.

The Mayo repair is the standard for infantile or small hernias. Larger aponeurotic defects of more than 4 cm will require reinforcement with an onlay mesh.

## Results and Conclusions

Weight reduction preoperatively and mesh for larger fascia defects reduce recurrence.

## Figure 1

Groin hernias, namely indirect and direct inguinal, and femoral, may be misdiagnosed prior to surgery. Ten percent of femoral hernias are misdiagnosed as inguinal. Three landmarks help to distinguish the hernias: pubic tubercle, femoral artery, and inferior epigastric vessels (Fig. 1: relation of inguinal and femoral hernias).

The indirect inguinal hernia sac passes through the internal inguinal ring, into the inguinal canal, and may or may not exit through the external inguinal ring to lie medial and inferior to the pubic tubercle. When examining an inguinal hernia, the internal inguinal ring can be found 1 cm caudal to the pulsatile femoral artery at the groin. A finger over the internal ring successfully blocking the occurrence of hernia confirms the diagnosis of an indirect hernia.

Direct inguinal hernia sac protrudes through the posterior wall of the inguinal canal, medial to the inferior epigastric vessels. The inferior epigastric vessels are located closely to the medial border of the internal inguinal ring. They can be injured and bleed.

Femoral hernias descend almost vertically from the peritoneal cavity into the femoral canal, which lies between the femoral vein laterally and the medial part of the inguinal ligament (Gimbernat's ligament) medially. The neck of the femoral hernia sac is palpable below the inguinal ligament and lateral to the pubic tubercle.

Figure 1

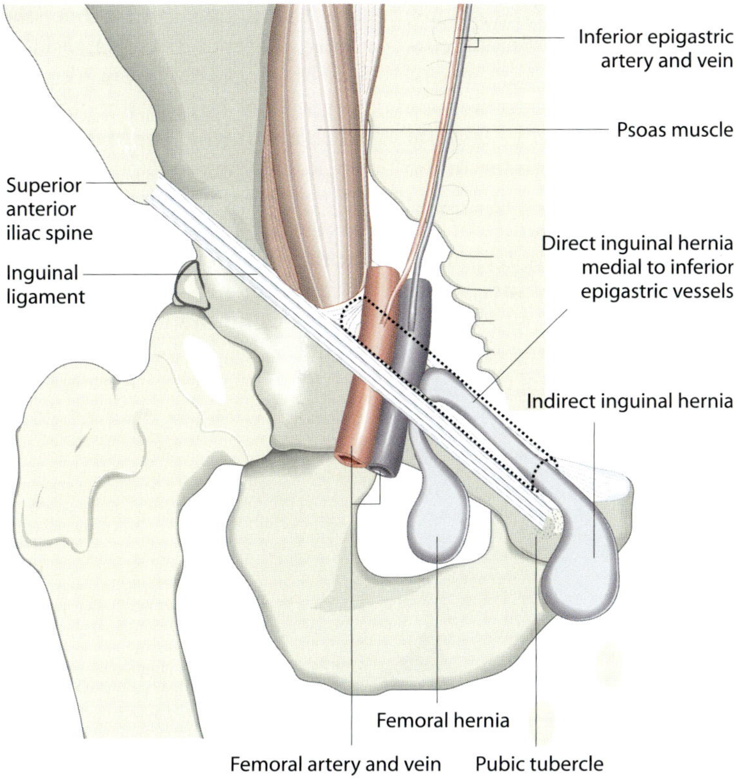
Inferior epigastric artery and vein
Psoas muscle
Superior anterior iliac spine
Inguinal ligament
Direct inguinal hernia medial to inferior epigastric vessels
Indirect inguinal hernia
Femoral hernia
Femoral artery and vein
Pubic tubercle

## Figure 2

The groin has a rich overlap of sensory innervations; supplying the lower abdominal wall are T12 subcostal, iliohypogastric and ilio-inguinal nerves; the genital branch of the genitofemoral nerve supplies the cord structure and anterior scrotum, and its femoral branch supplies skin and subcutaneous tissue in the femoral triangle. To achieve effective local anaesthesia during groin hernia repair, large volumes of anaesthetic agent described as the flooding technique must be injected widely along the line of incision as well as close to the nerves.

A combination of short and long acting local anaesthetic with epinephrine is ideal for short stay surgery. This allows instant anaesthesia as well as providing postoperative analgesia. The maximum safe dose of lignocaine is 3 mg/kg, and with epinephrine 7 mg/kg. For bupivacaine it is 2 mg/kg, and 4 mg/kg with epinephrine. The local anaesthetic mixture used is of equal volume 1% lignocaine, and 0.25% bupivacaine with epinephrine. Up to a total volume of 60 ml per person is safe. An additional infiltration of 1% lignocaine may be used during the repair should the patient experience any discomfort, commonly to the tissue around the pubic tubercle and the peritoneal sac.



## Figure 3

The patient walks into the anaesthetic room and is asked to lie supine, with one pillow behind their head, on the operating table. Obtain and secure intravenous access. A small dose of intravenous midazolam, 2–10 mg, may be given for sedation without suppressing respiration. Apply the arm cuff for blood pressure monitoring and the finger probe of the pulseoximeter to monitor oxygen saturation. Shave the pubic hair on the operative site. Local anaesthetic is given prior to cleaning and draping.

The incision is oblique and 1 cm above and parallel to the medial half of the inguinal ligament, extending slightly over and medial to the pubic tubercle. Another incision favours a horizontal course (dotted black line). Having established a mental image of where this incision should be made, infiltrate 20–30 ml of the combined local anaesthetic using a 21-gauge needle into the skin and subcutaneous tissue, along the incision line. It is important a safe and sufficient volume is used to anaesthetise the overlapping nerve supplies. This is followed by marking the incision line with a pen or a light scratch mark with the injection needle.

Next insert the injection needle, with a 20-ml syringe of the anaesthetic mixture, 1 cm medial and superior to the ASIS. At this position inject 5 ml subcutaneously around this point to block the subcostal (T12) nerve. Reposition the needle to point at the pubic tubercle and at a 45° angle to the skin; gently inject as the needle advances. The iliohypogastric and ilio-inguinal nerves run between the internal oblique muscle and external oblique aponeurosis. When the needle reaches the external oblique aponeurosis a resistance is felt; advance the needle in a little further and inject 20–30 ml of the anaesthetic mixture into this plane. The needle may be left in situ, while another 20-ml syringe of anaesthetic is attached to the needle and injected. The patient is then transferred to the operating theatre.

Figure 2

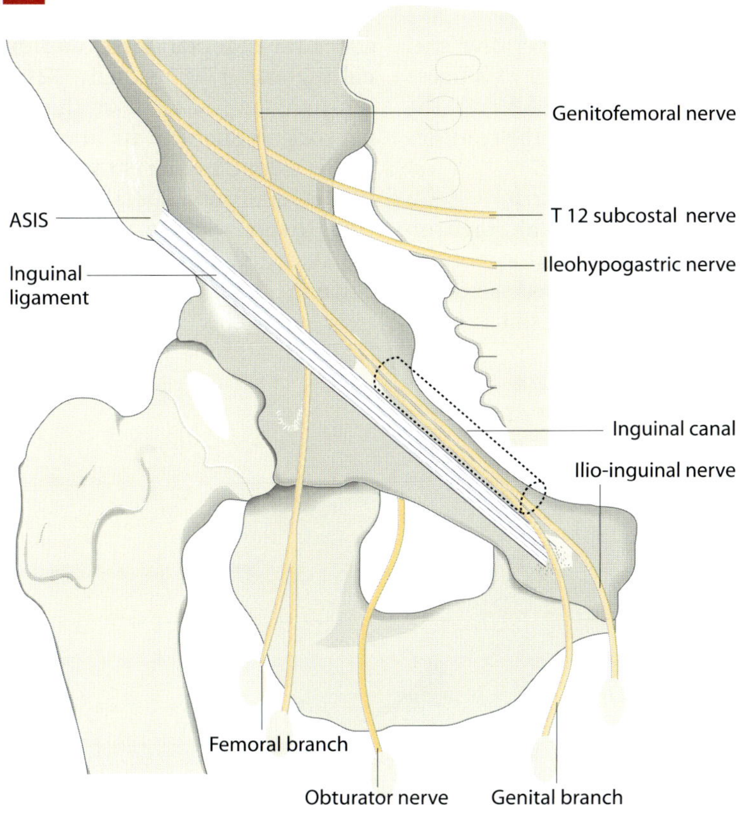
Genitofemoral nerve
ASIS
T 12 subcostal nerve
Inguinal ligament
Ileohypogastric nerve
Inguinal canal
Ilio-inguinal nerve
Femoral branch
Obturator nerve
Genital branch

Figure 3

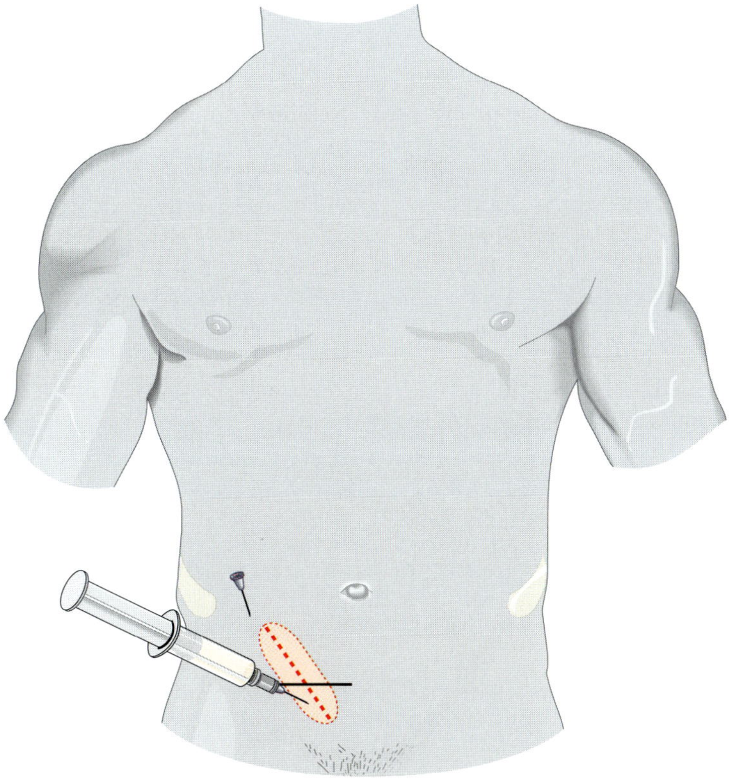

## Figure 4

Drape the patient, exposing only the operative site. The patient is reassured by the company of a nurse throughout the procedure, who also observes the patient's comfort level and takes note of the readings of blood pressure and oxygen saturation.

■ **Lichtenstein Mesh Repair.** Make the incision along the marked line. Ensure haemostasis every step of the way with ties and diathermy. At the external oblique aponeurosis gently dissect out a plane above the inguinal canal, and dissect out the external inguinal ring medially. Retract the skin with a self-retainer. Cut a slit on the external oblique aponeurosis in line with its fibre. Open the inguinal canal by extending the slit with scissors to its external ring medially and laterally over the internal inguinal ring. Dissect the two aponeurosis flaps from the canal structure and reposition the self-retainer to include the two flaps.



## Figure 5

Additional 1–2 ml of 1% lignocaine is injected into the soft tissue around the pubic tubercle.

**Figure 4**

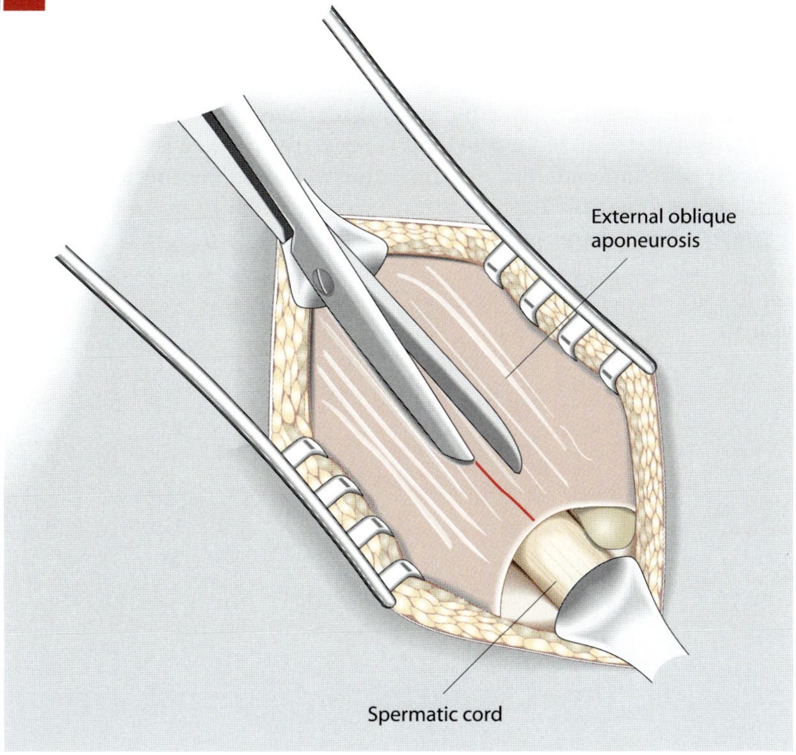


**Figure 5**

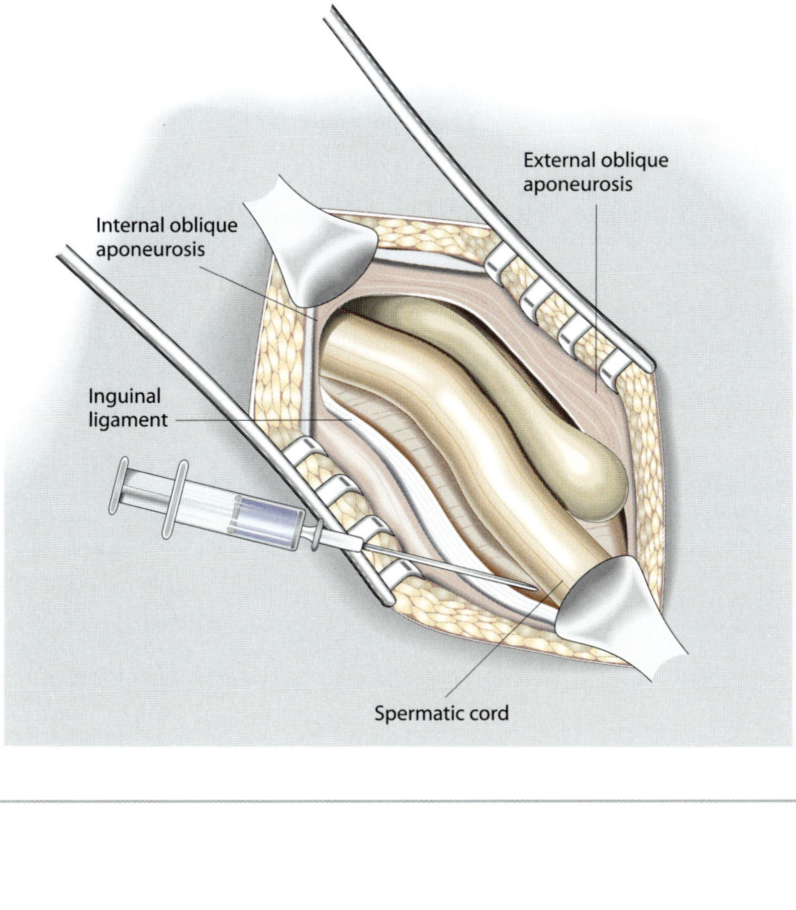

## Figure 6

The spermatic cord is carefully dissected out of the inguinal canal by dissecting a tunnel between the cord and the pubic tubercle. The cord is lifted up from the inguinal canal by sharp dissection toward the internal ring. Apply the inguinal hernia ring around the cord which helps to isolate the cord from the deeper tissues of the inguinal canal. Examine both the posterior wall of the inguinal canal for any direct hernia sac and the cord for an indirect hernia. Fenestrate the cremasteric muscle of the cord, to look for an indirect hernia sac.



## Figure 7

Lift up the cord tissue and, with the help of the light to trace the outline of the sac, dissect around it. Dissect towards the internal inguinal ring. Reposition the clips along the way to help to identify the sac.

Figure 6

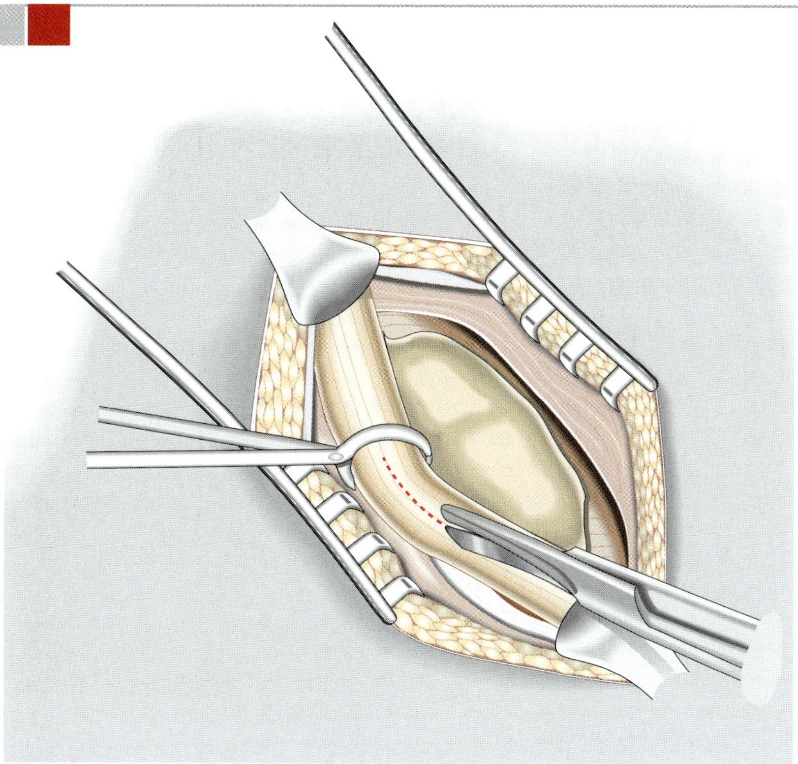

Figure 7

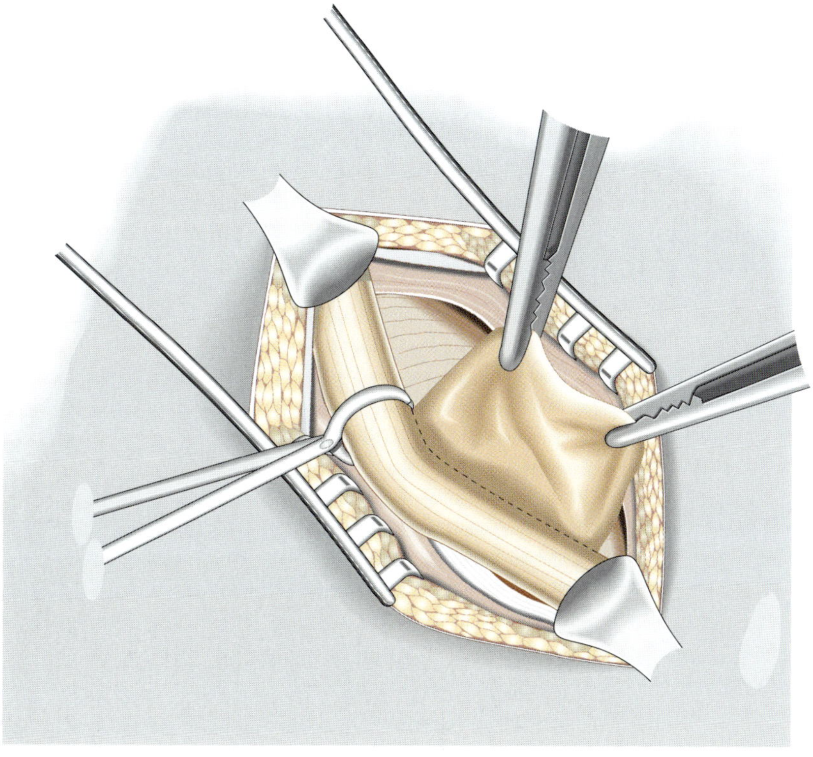

## Figure 8

For a direct inguinal hernia, if the defect of the posterior wall is large, plicate the transversalis fascia before placing the mesh over it.

This is the area where in performing shouldice operation, the whole transverse fascia should be duplicated as "first line of defense".



## Figure 9

For an indirect inguinal hernia, identify and dissect the hernia sac from the cord to the internal ring. Invert the sac into the abdomen through the internal ring. For a large inguino-scrotal hernia, dissect the hernia sac to the internal ring but do not disturb the distal sac in the scrotum; reduce the hernia contents into the abdomen. Open the sac to examine that all structures are reduced before transfixing and ligating the sac at its neck, leaving the open distal sac in the scrotum. If the hernia sac was accidentally opened during dissection, continue to dissect the sac to the internal ring; ligate and excise at the neck. The internal ring may be reinforced with a Vicryl stitch to reduce its size.

Figure 8

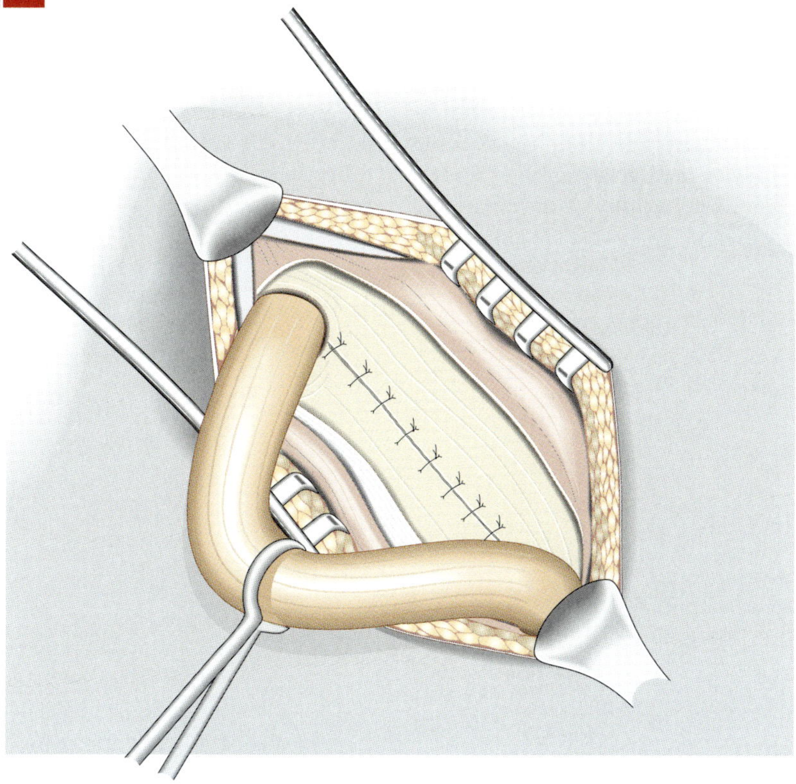

Figure 9

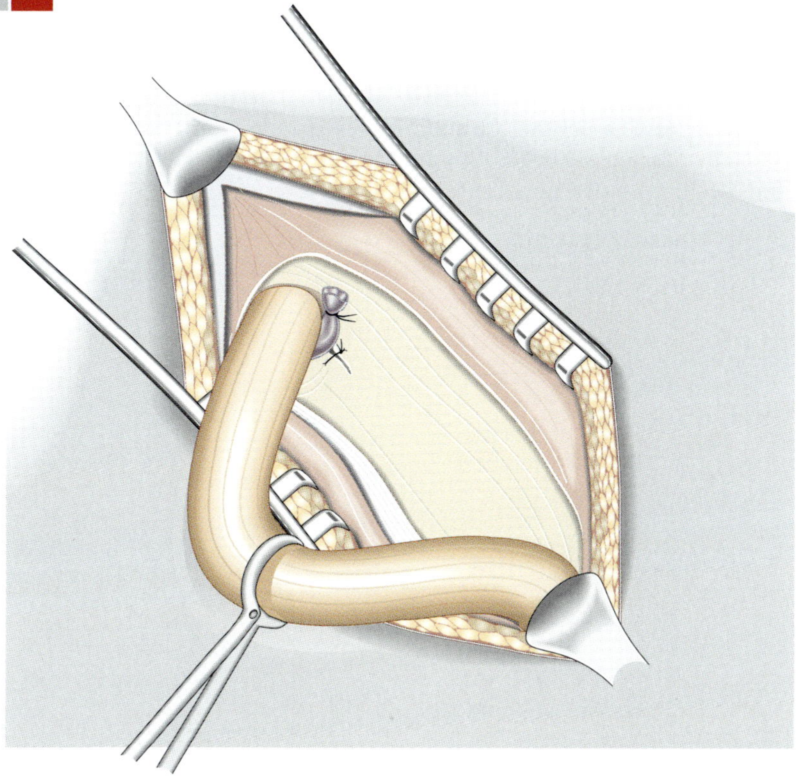

## Figure 10

A polypropylene mesh is used to reinforce the repair. Its top medial corner is trimmed to fit better under the external oblique aponeurosis. The inferior border of the mesh is placed side by side along the inguinal ligament, and the inferior medial corner overlaps the pubis tubercle by 1 cm. A continuous non-absorbable monofilament suture with a J needle, for easier access to the corner, is used to fix the mesh. Avoid stitching the pubis tubercle or its periosteum, because that is painful. The suture begins from medial to the pubic tubercle to as far as the lateral margin of the internal ring.



## Figure 11

Make a horizontal slit from the lateral border to accommodate the cord. The upper flap is brought down and around the cord to suture together with the lower flap to the inguinal ligament. The tightness around the cord can be checked by passing the head of a clip through the encircling two flaps. Interrupted sutures are used to secure the mesh flatly onto the underlying aponeurosis. The mesh must be tension-free and lie flat on the posterior wall of the inguinal canal. The tails are then trimmed and tucked laterally beneath the external oblique aponeurosis.

Figure 10

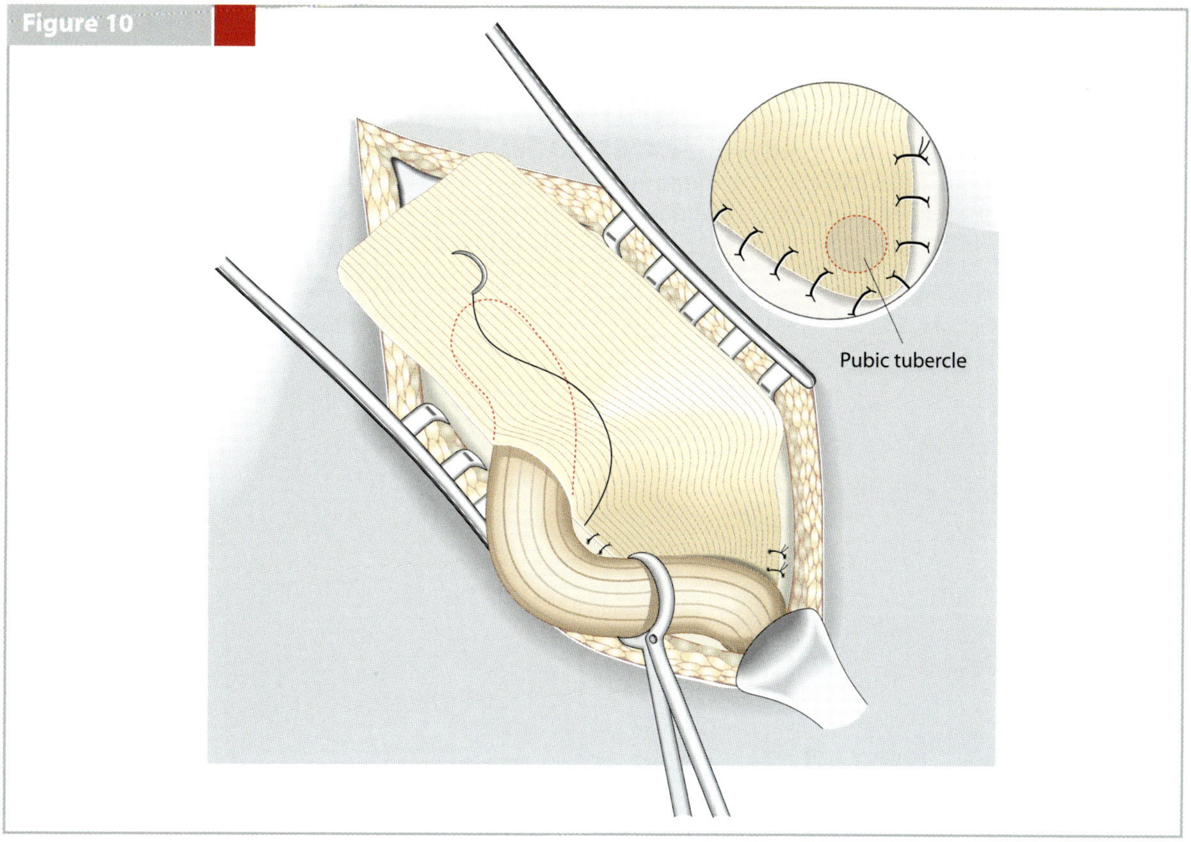


Figure 11

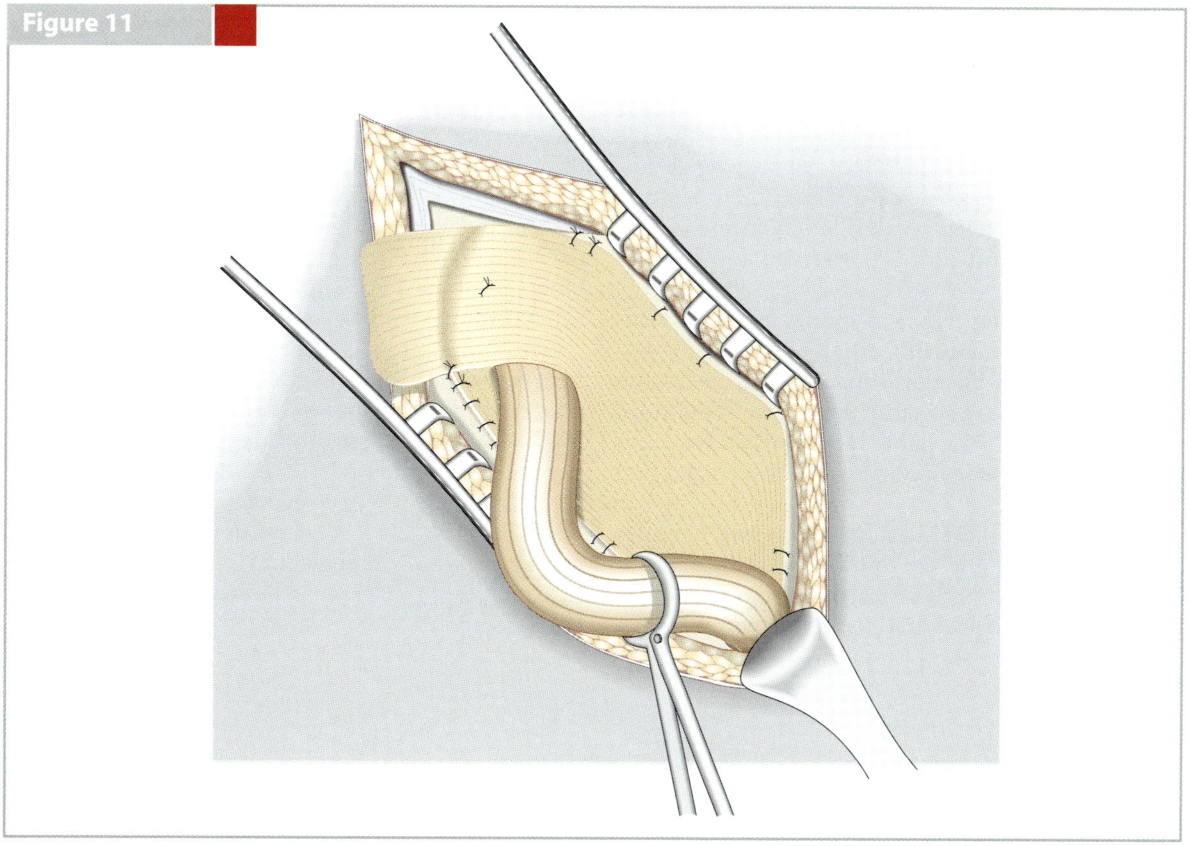

## Figure 12

Close the external oblique aponeurosis with a continuous absorbable suture. The subcutaneous fat may be brought closer with a few interrupted sutures. The skin is closed with an absorbable subcuticular suture. The wound is cleaned with water, dried, and covered.

At the recovery bay, the patient is offered food and drink. Prior to discharge the patient must have passed urine and received instructions for postoperative care such as analgesia regime, wound care, and a reminder of the telephone number to contact the unit with any queries in the first 24 h. Follow-up is usually not necessary.



## Figure 13

Patients for laparoscopic inguinal hernia repairs are asked to empty the bladder before going to the anaesthetic room, to avoid injury and obscuring the operative view. The patient is supine on the operating table, and given general anaesthetic and muscle relaxation. The TV monitor is positioned at the end of bed.

The totally extraperitoneal approach (TEP) is safer but technically more difficult. It is gaining in popularity. Three mid-line port sites are used: one 10 mm infra-umbilical and two 5 mm ports, one is one-third of the way between the pubic symphysis and the umbilicus and the other one halfway between the first two sites.

The infra-umbilical incision is deepened to under the rectus muscle and the thin fascia of the anterior layer of the transversalis fascia, on the operative side. Using a balloon or by blunt dissection with a finger, this plane is expanded where repair is to be carried out. Inferior epigastric vessels and fat are found in this plane. Underneath this space is: a thicker posterior layer of the transversalis fascia, the posterior rectus sheath (thins out below the arcuate line), and the peritoneum. The trocar is inserted into the infra-umbilical port site and secured in place with a stay suture. Insufflate with $CO_2$ to 10 mmHg.

The laparoscope is inserted and under direct vision the other two port sites are inserted. Extend the operative plane further to the midline medially and the psoas muscle laterally. Identify the vessels and nerves. The hernia sac is dissected from the surrounding structure and reduced. Also look for combined hernias. A 10 × 15 cm mesh is secured in placed covering the area of dissection including the internal inguinal ring. The transversalis fascia is reinforced as in open repair.

Figure 12

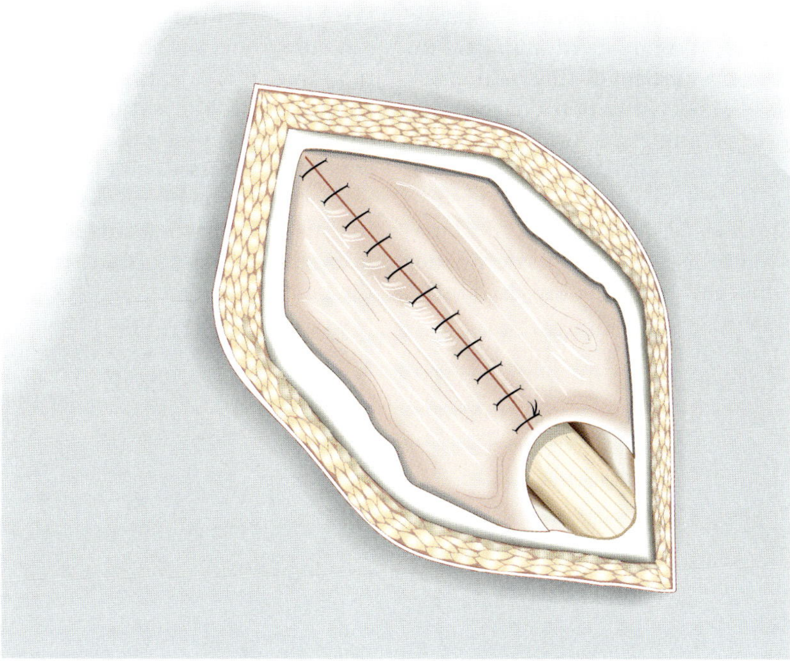

Figure 13

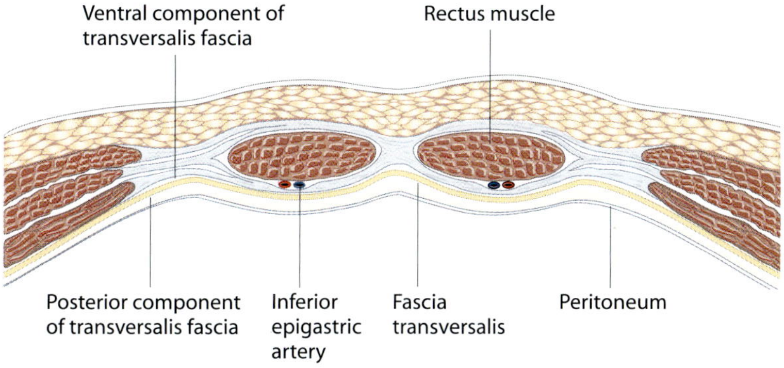

## Figure 14

In the transabdominal preperitoneal (TAPP) approach the pneumoperitoneum is created with the conventional technique. Make an infra-umbilical incision and insert the tip of a small finger to check that bowel has not adhered to the peritoneal lining. Once it is safe, insert a 10-mm blunt trocar and insufflate with $CO_2$. The pneumoperitoneum is maintained at 10–12 mmHg and the trocar is secured to the abdominal wall with stay sutures. Insert the laparoscope, and insert the other two trocars safely under direct vision. Maintain the pressure at 10–12 mmHg. Identify and reduce the hernia content.

Enter the preperitoneal space by cutting the peritoneum at the neck of the hernia; dissect and identify the vessels and nerves. As in open repair, the internal ring of an indirect inguinal hernia may be reinforced with a stitch, and the transversalis fascia of the direct inguinal hernia may be plicated. The repair is reinforced with a mesh which spreads out flat and secure in place with sutures to cover the repair. Close the peritoneal opening with sutures, to avoid direct contact of the mesh and the bowel, which may result in erosion of the bowel and formation of fistula, and internal hernia when small bowel protrudes into the preperitoneal space. After removing all instruments, the port site of more than 1 cm in size must have its fascia closed to prevent incisional hernia. Figure 14 shows the posterior view of the lower abdomen when the peritoneum is lifted.



## Figure 15

The 'low' or crural operation is commonly used for uncomplicated femoral hernias. General anaesthetic is preferred. Local anaesthetic is possible, and the nerves involved are as in inguinal hernia repair. Infiltrate the skin and subcutaneous tissue over the incision line. The femoral branch of the genitofemoral nerve may be infiltrated under direct vision.

The patient is placed in the supine position, cleaned and draped, exposing the shaved operative site. An oblique skin incision is made 1 cm below and parallel to the medial third of the inguinal ligament, overlying the swelling. Haemostasis is maintained every step of the way.

Figure 14

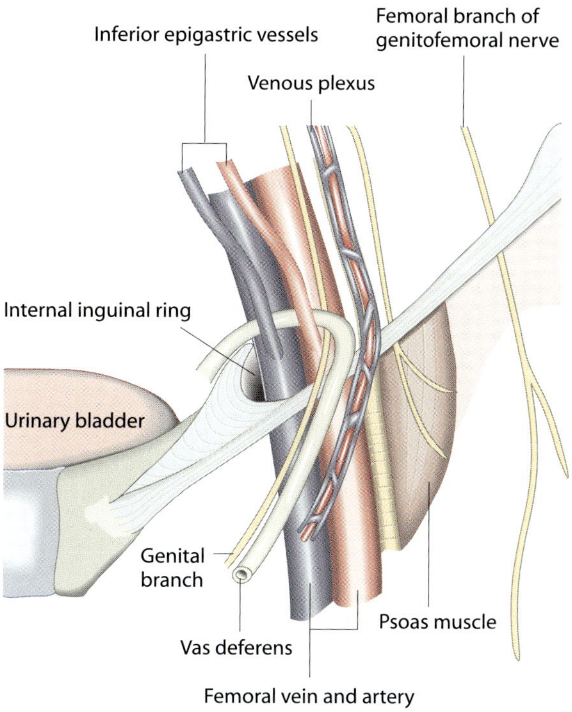
Inferior epigastric vessels
Femoral branch of genitofemoral nerve
Venous plexus
Internal inguinal ring
Urinary bladder
Genital branch
Vas deferens
Psoas muscle
Femoral vein and artery

Figure 15

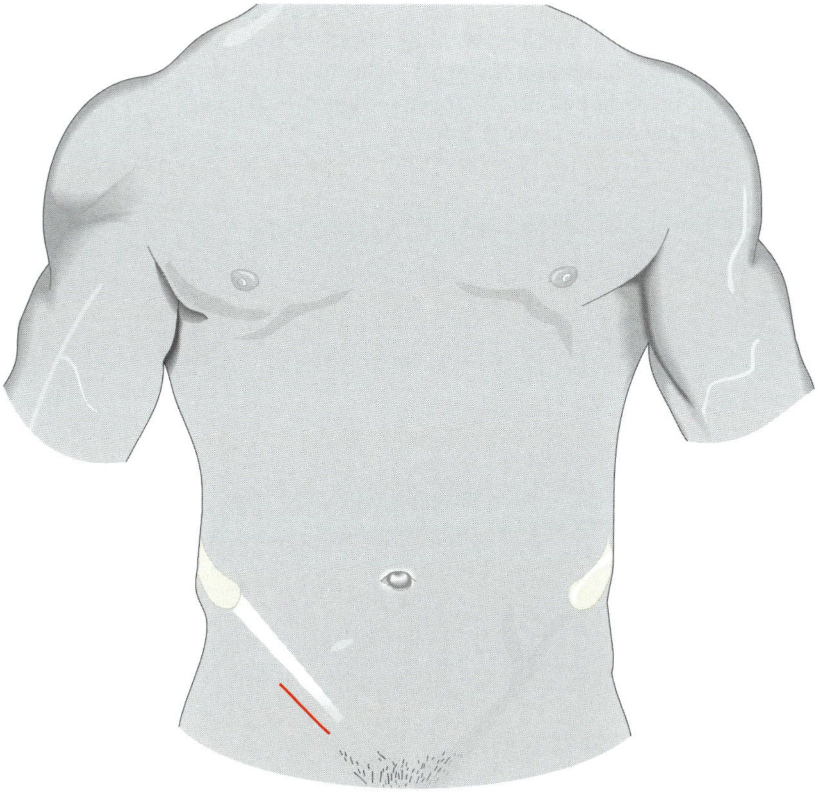

## Figure 16

The hernia sac is covered by fascia and preperitoneal fat. Use blunt dissection by wiping the fascia aside with a gauze swab to get to the sac. Excessive preperitoneal fat may be excised. Carefully dissect the sac from its surrounding tissue down to the neck of the sac, and free the neck from its surrounding structures.



## Figure 17

A small hernia sac is inverted and reduced. A larger hernia sac is opened from the lateral side to avoid injuring any herniated viscus, e.g. bladder on the medial side. The hernia content is examined for evidence of strangulation. Reduce the normal content under direct vision. Often a small pedicle of strangulated omentum is found, which is ligated and excised. The hernia sac is then ligated at its neck, and the redundant sac excised.

Figure 16

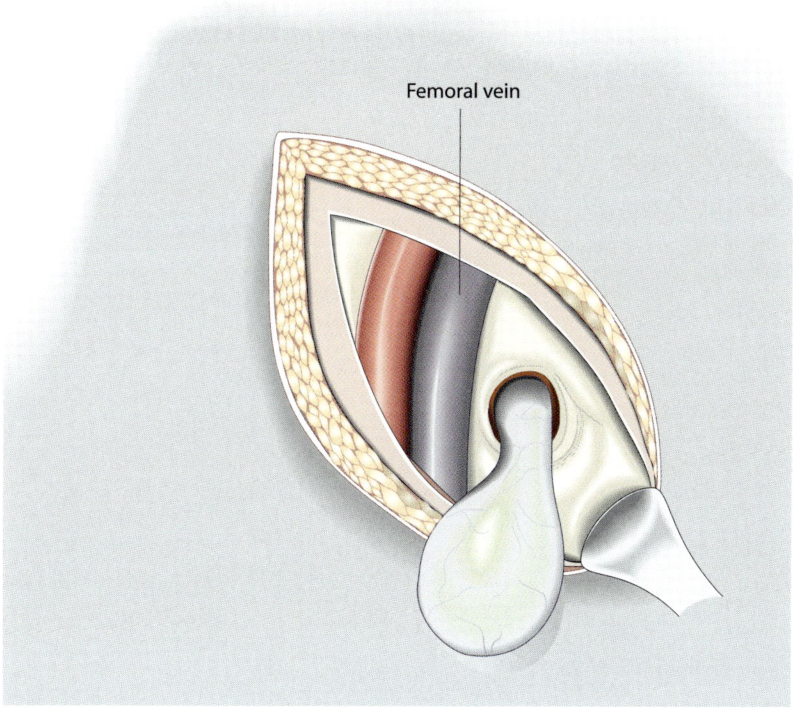


Figure 17

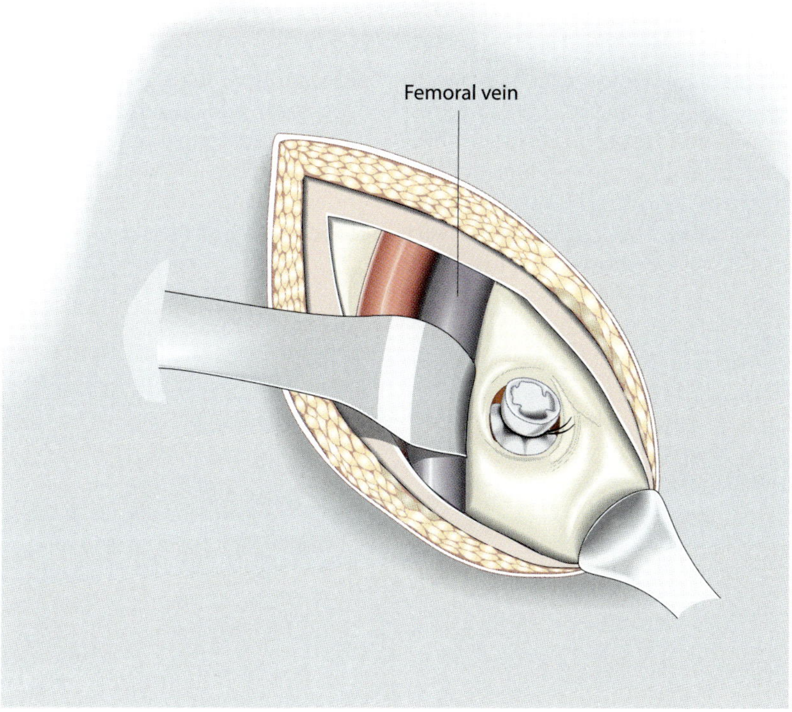

## Figure 18

To close the canal a rolled-up mesh, i.e. 'cigarette stub', is inserted in the femoral canal, over the hernia stump, and sutured in place with 2/0 Prolene to its surrounding fibrous tissue. Avoid injury to the femoral vein. The skin is closed with absorbable subcuticular suture.



## Figure 19

Patients are encouraged to reduce weight prior to their umbilical hernia repair. A curved infraumbilical transverse incision is made to preserve the umbilicus. For very large umbilical hernias an elliptical incision is made to remove the overstretched skin and subcutaneous fat, including the umbilicus. A very large hernia is unsuitable for short stay surgery as postoperative ileus is common and a drain may be necessary, which requires inpatient hospital care. Care should be taken not to excise too much skin, as it can result in high wound tension. Avoid excessive undermining of the skin as that can compromise blood supply to the skin, risking wound failure.

Figure 18

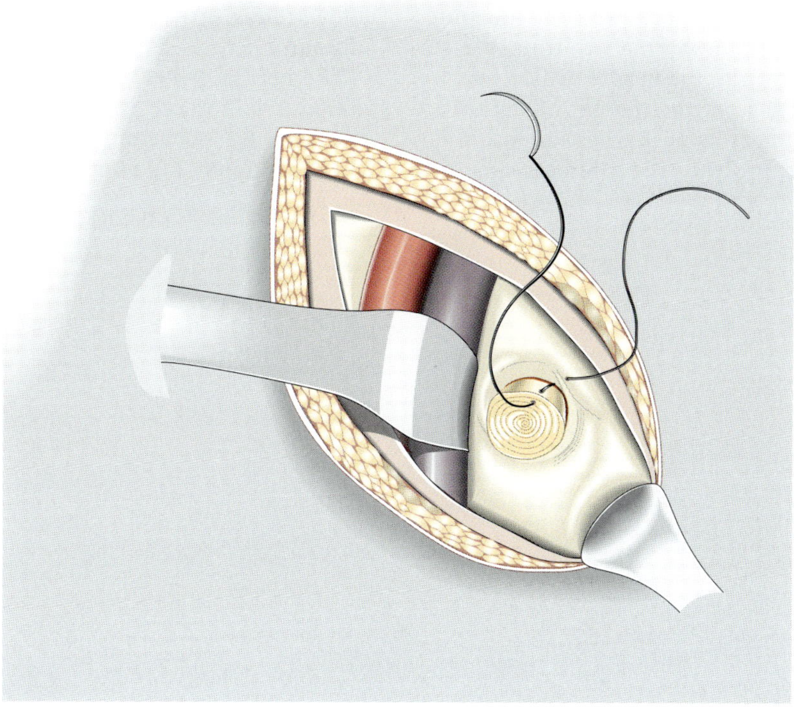

Figure 19

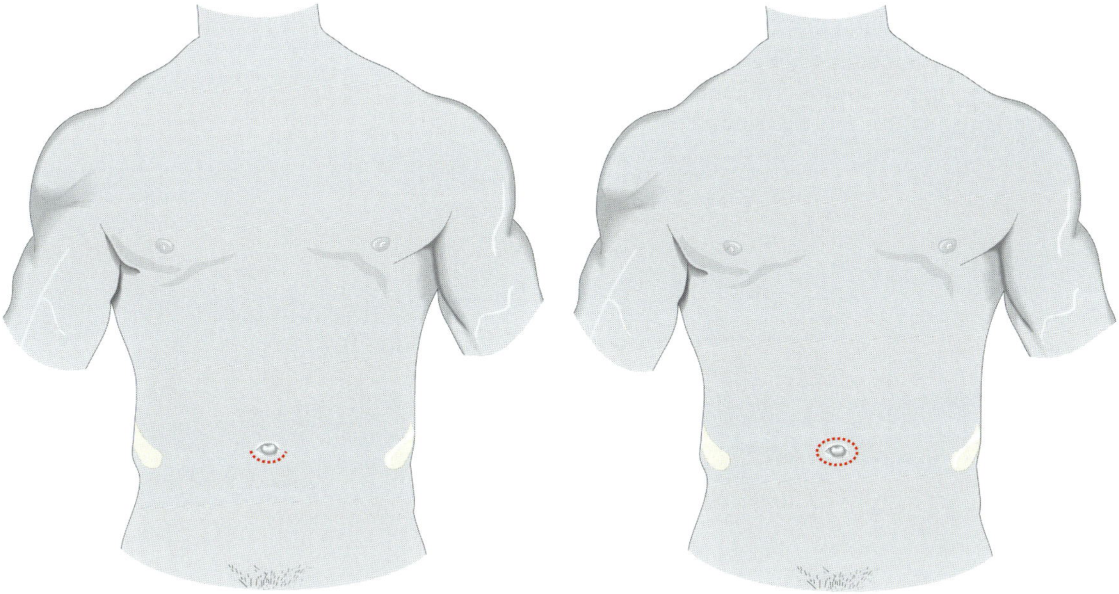

## Figure 20

Careful dissection is made to allow the skin flap and the umbilicus to be pulled back exposing the underlying hernia. Dissect the hernia sac from the surrounding tissue down to the hernia orifice, and free the neck of the sac from the margin of the orifice. The sac is opened near its neck where adhesions are least likely to be present. The contents are often densely adhered to the lining of the sac particularly at the fundus. Insert a finger into the sac to break any adhesions before extending the cut.

The hernia content is carefully examined for viability; viable tissue is reduced into the peritoneal cavity. Partly ischaemic omentum and irreducible densely adherent omentum are ligated and excised.



## Figure 21

The undersurface of the umbilicus is stitched to the linea alba, the subcutaneous fat being brought together with interrupted suture. The skin is closed with a subcuticular suture, and the wound covered.

Figure 20

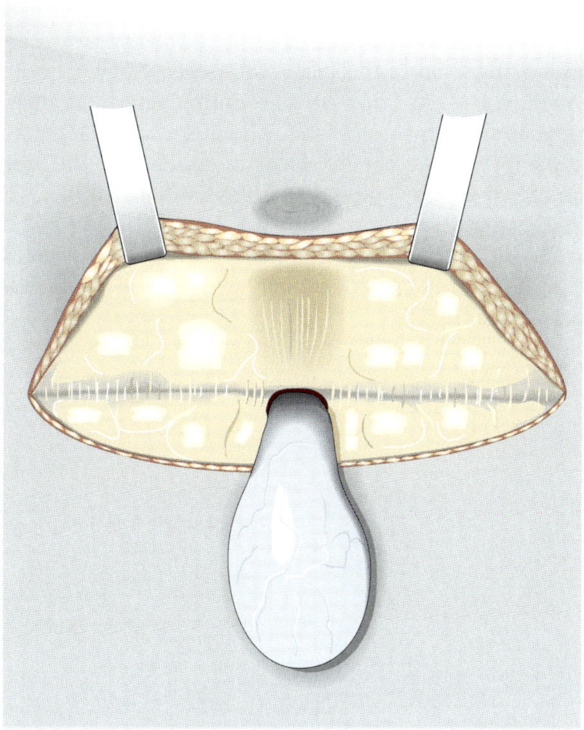

Figure 21

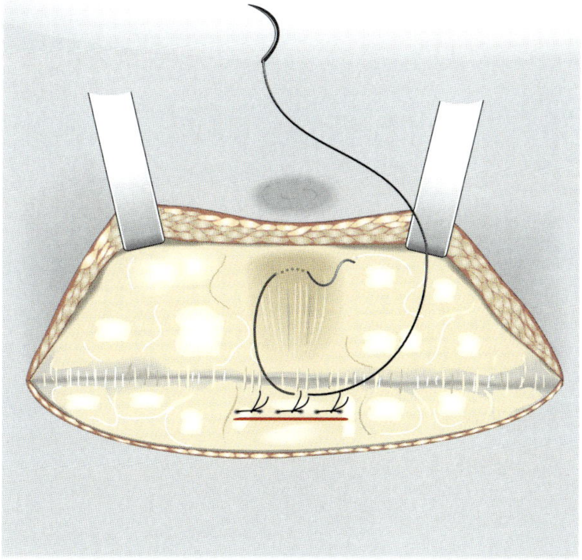

## Figure 22, 23

Prepare the adjacent anterior rectus fascia by dissecting the surrounding tissue away from it, to provide a clear surface for Mayo repair. The hernia orifice may be enlarged to allow a Mayo repair with a 2–3 cm overlap of the two flaps. Non-absorbable or slow absorbable PDS suture may be used to make interrupted stitches. The fascias and peritoneum are closed as one layer. The needle comes through the top flap, 2–3 cm from its margin, and takes a stitch of the bottom flap, 1–2 cm from its margin. The needle then exits from the undersurface of the upper flap, ending with the two ends of the stitch on the outer side of the upper flap. Give allowance for tying, then clip and cut the suture after each stitch. Continue the same stitching for the entire length of the opening at 0.5 cm intervals. The more sutures that are put in, the easier it is to close the fascia, and the more evenly is the tension distributed. When the stitching is completed, the two flaps are brought together with the upper one overlapping the lower flap. Each set of sutures is tied individually to close the fascia defect.



## Figure 24

Larger fascia defects greater than 4 cm would require reinforcement with placement of an onlay mesh. The mesh is sutured on the anterior rectus sheath, and laterally to the external oblique aponeurosis. The mesh must overlap the fascial closure by at least 3 cm in all directions. The mesh must lie flat with no folding of the edges or tension.

Figure 22

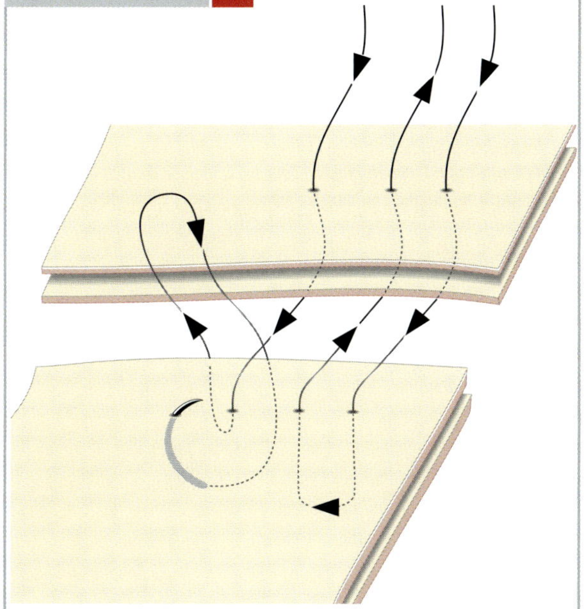

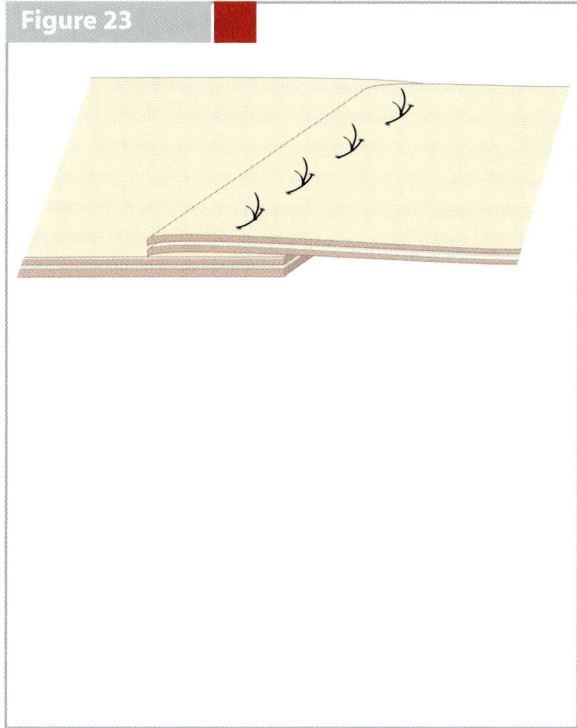

Figure 23

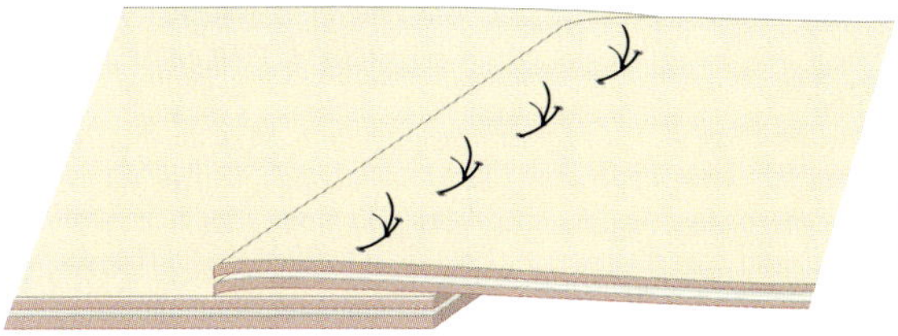

Figure 24

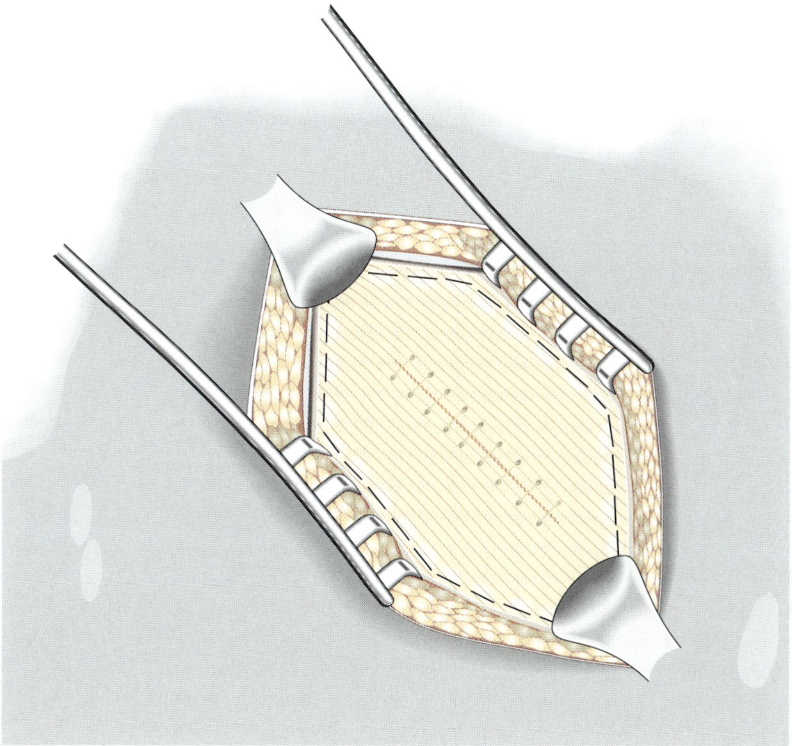

## SELECTED REFERENCES


1. Kingsnorth AN, deBlank KA (2003) Management of abdominal hernias, 3rd edn. Chapman & Hall Medical, London
2. Lange JF et al. (2002) The preperitoneal tissue dilemma in totally extraperitoneal (TEP) laparoscopic hernia repair: an anatomo-surgical study. Surg Endosc 16(6):927–930
3. National Good Practice Guidance on Pre-operative Assessment for Day Surgery (2002) www.modern.nhs.uk/theatre programme/preop
4. Tackett LD et al (1999) Incidence of contralateral inguinal hernia: a prospective analysis. J Paediatr Surg 34:684–687
5. National Institute of Clinical Excellence (2001) Guidance on the use of laparoscopic surgery for inguinal hernia. Technical Appraisal Guidance No. 18. NICE, London
6. McCormack K (2003) EU Hernia Trialists Collaboration et al. Laparoscopic technique versus open technique for inguinal hernia repair. Cochrane Database Syst Rev 1:CD001785

CHAPTER 13

# Haemorrhoids

Franz Raulf, Christian F. Krieglstein,
Norbert Senninger

## INTRODUCTION

The basis of haemorrhoid disease is the corpus cavernosum recti. This apparatus is composed of arteriovenous vascular formations and provides a highly sensitive closure function for the anus and is an important part of the anorectal continence organ. Dependent on the localisation of the arterial inflow, enlarged haemorrhoidal cushions are usually found at the 3, 7 and 11 o'clock lithotomy positions. The corpus cavernosum recti in the closed state of the anal canal therefore shows a star-shaped configuration between the three main cushions [6].

## Figures 1–5: Pathophysiology

The haemorrhoidal cushions are held in position by a scaffold of muscular and elastic fibres in the upper anal canal. Long standing trauma to this suspensory apparatus of the haemorrhoids may cause damage that is followed by distal migration of the corpus cavernosum recti, leading to a different anatomical arrangement in the anal canal. At the same time as this distal movement, shearing forces affect the vessels, causing damage to the vessel wall with thrombosis and a potentially changed vascular architecture in the cushions. This causes "haemorrhoidal disease". Therapy is not targeted at the haemorrhoids as such but at the haemorrhoidal disease process.

The stages of haemorrhoidal disease therefore take into account both the increase in size and the degree of distal dislocation of the haemorrhoidal tissue. First degree haemorrhoids are slightly elevated cushions in the upper anal canal that can only be shown proctoscopically and protrude into the lumen of the proctoscope.

Second degree haemorrhoidal cushions (Fig. 1) protrude into the distal anal canal and at times externally following defecation. They spontaneously retract into the anal canal after defaecation finishes.

Third degree cushions (Fig. 2) no longer have any retractile capacity. They have to be reduced and repositioned digitally or can be seen for a significant period of time outside the anal canal.

Fourth degree haemorrhoids are no longer reducible and are permanently prolapsed (Fig. 3). A prolapse that is fixed at the anal edge can make reduction impossible. Very frequently this is accompanied by acute bouts of pain due to thrombosis or incarceration of the protruded cushion. Following conservative management of such a situation for a couple of days reduction may once again be possible. Then a definitive judgement should be taken as to the clinical classification into second or third degree haemorrhoids. Figure 4 shows relative indications for operation because early excision does not necessarily cause a defect of the anoderm leading to incontinence. However, in the presence of a circular haemorrhoidal prolapse with thrombosis, excessive resection of the anoderm can provoke sensory incontinence. Therefore in this situation a strictly conservative approach is recommended. If only a segment is affected, then excision may shorten the course of the disease and the defect of the anoderm is small enough to cause only minimal consequences relating to incontinence. However, there is no indication for an emergency haemorrhoidectomy.

Knowledge of the position of the dentate line is important for differential diagnosis. Anal prolapse is the protrusion of the lower anal canal distal to the dentate line, which is covered by anoderm. In these forms of prolapse the dentate line is still located intra-anally and the mucosa-covered corpus cavernosum recti is not usually visible from outside. On the other hand, haemorrhoidal prolapse by protrusion of tissue from above the dentate line is very often associated with an eventration of the anoderm and the dentate line (Fig. 3).

## Figure 1

Enlarged haemorrhoidal tissue seen in the proctoscope (stage 2). The enlarged cushions are found at the preferential sites according to the arterial supply at the 3, 7 and 11 o'clock lithotomy positions (patient in left sided position).

## Figure 2

Prolapse in haemorrhoidal disease stage 3 (manually reducible); (patient in left sided position).

## Figure 3

Circular anal and haemorrhoidal prolapse (disease stage 3) demonstrates the typical positions at the 3, 7 and 11 o'clock lithotomy positions. The dentate line appears eventrated in a circular fashion (patient in left sided position).

## Figure 4

Segmental haemorrhoidal thrombosis on the right side from the 7 to 10 o'clock lithotomy positions. The patient is lying on his left. A small thrombosis is visible in the area of the prolapsed mucosa. Accompanying oedema of the anoderm. Normal left side and ventral circumference of the anus. Relative indication for operation. During excision, a small anoderm defect should be expected (patient in left sided position).

Figure 1

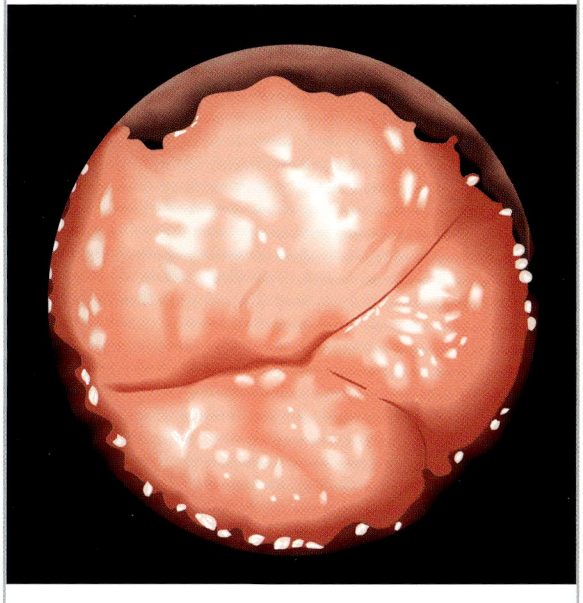

Figure 2

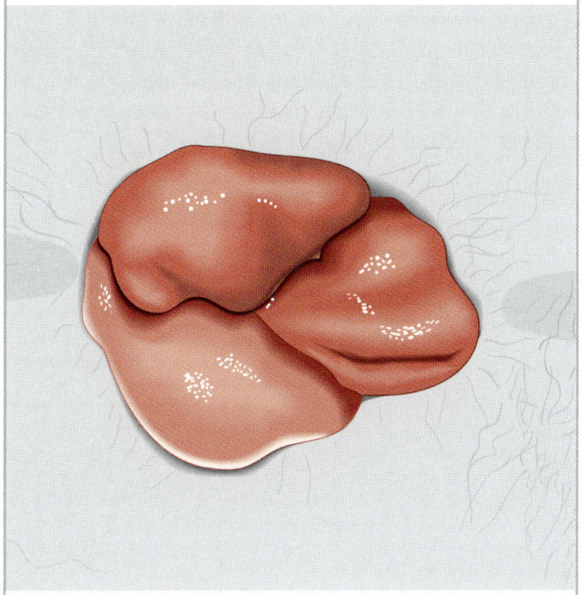

Figure 3

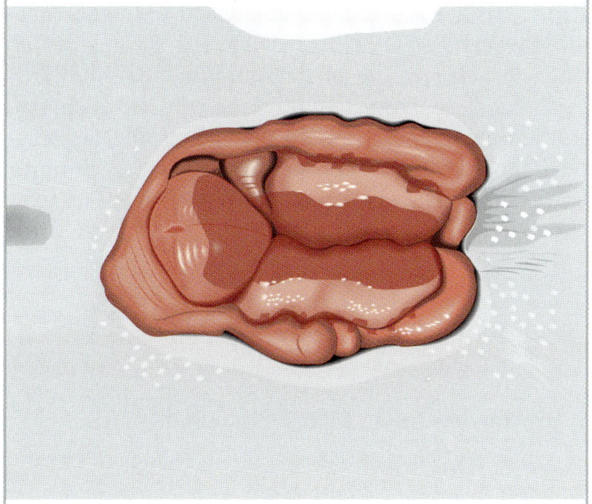

Figure 4

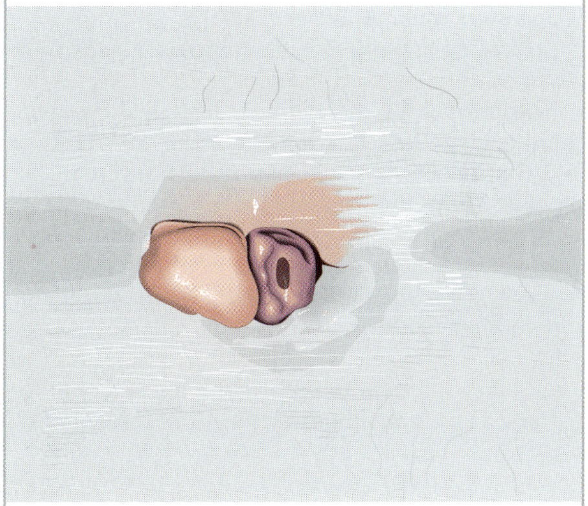

## Figure 5A, B

**A** Acute, oedematous anal prolapse. A circular prolapse of the anoderm is shown; the dentate line is not visible from outside (patient in lithotomy position). **B** Circular anal prolapse: chronic appearance without oedema (patient in lithotomy position)

## Figures 6, 7: Conservative Therapy of Haemorrhoidal Disease

The application of haemorrhoidal ointments or suppositories may favourably influence the symptoms in the early stages of haemorrhoidal disease. In some cases this topical treatment can be considered as an adjuvant treatment to surgery.



Sclerosing therapy of haemorrhoids is performed with two different modifications:

The essence of the therapy described by Blanchard [2, 6] is the reduction of the arterial supply by injecting an oily substance paravasally next to the artery just above the haemorrhoidal cushion. This injection is supposed to create an inflammatory reaction with subsequent shrinkage of the perivascular tissue. The readiness to bleed is thereby reduced and a reduction of the haemorrhoidal cushion size is achieved. As a rule, injections of sclerosant are undertaken adjacent to each supplying artery at the 3, 7 and 11 o'clock lithotomy positions, every 3 or 4 weeks. The substance of choice in most cases is phenol in almond oil (5%). This technique has received the widest acceptance internationally.

Sclerotherapy as described by Blond [3] utilises stronger sclerosants injected directly into the haemorrhoidal tissue using a detailed dosage which leads to a shrinkage of haemorrhoidal tissue. This method carries some danger due to the use of chinin-containing substances with the risk of allergic reactions and systemic consequences. This technique, however, is performed quite frequently in Germany.

### Fig. 6

Sclerosing treatment according to Blanchard.

Figure 5A

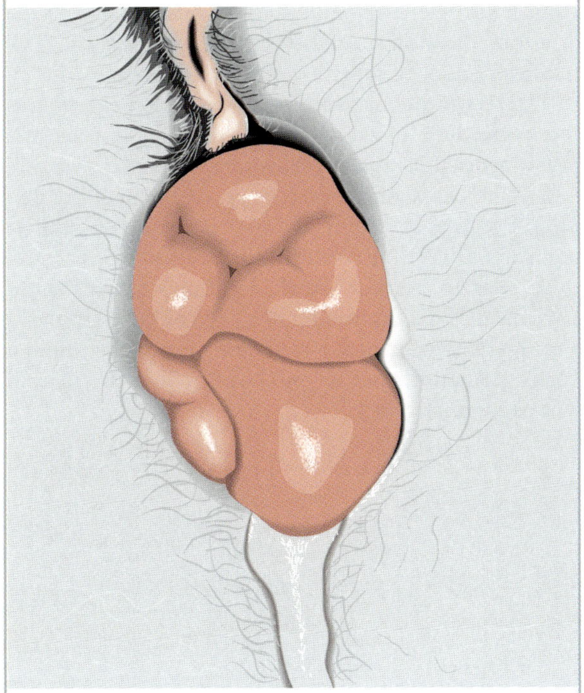

Figure 5B

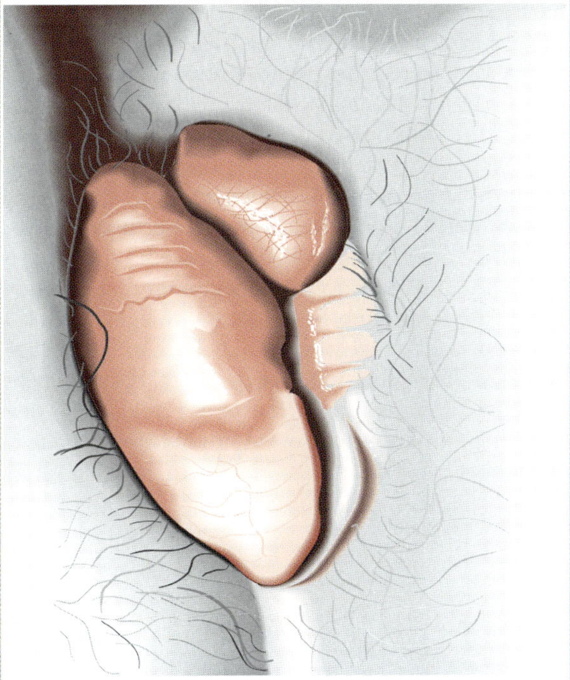

Figure 6

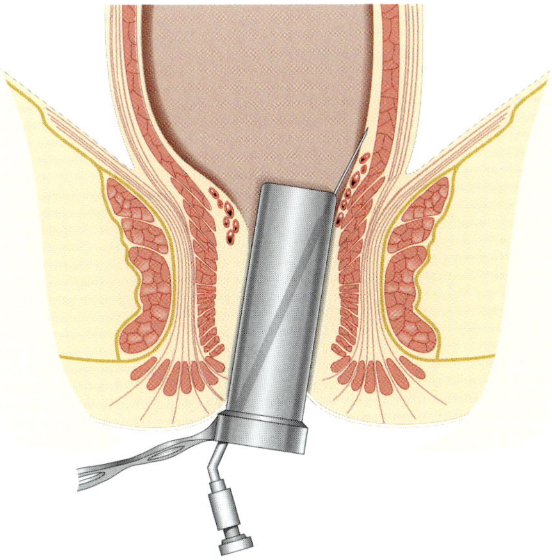

## Figure 7A, B

Elastic rubber band ligatures as described by Barron [1, 10] may also be used in the treatment of haemorrhoidal disease. By means of a simple instrument, the haemorrhoidal tissue is pulled proctoscopically into the ligature cylinder, from which a tight ring of rubber is applied to the base of the tissue. Alternatively, instruments are available which suck the tissue into the cylinder. The tissue cushion will become necrotic and fall off after 10–20 days. This procedure is very effective in the reduction of haemorrhoidal cushion size. At the same time, by applying the ligature in the upper part of the haemorrhoidal tissue or in the lower part of the rectum mucosa, the distal tissue may be retracted proximally into the upper anal canal and fixed there. In order to prevent premature slippage of the rubber ring, it may be useful to inject a small quantity of sclerosing oil into the ligated cushion. One or more cushions can be treated per session. The treatment may be repeated every 3–4 weeks.

The technique has similar side effects to an operative procedure in which bleeding and pain are the most frequently observed sequelae. Bleeding occurs in 0.5% of cases, and therefore systemic bleeding disorders or major haemorrhoidal bleeding should be regarded as relative contraindications.

**A** Elastic rubber band ligation according to Barron (using a suction ligator). **B** Rubber ligature in situ. The ligated cushion is visible after insertion of a Parks retractor. After a few days the ligated cushion will become necrotic.

Figure 7A

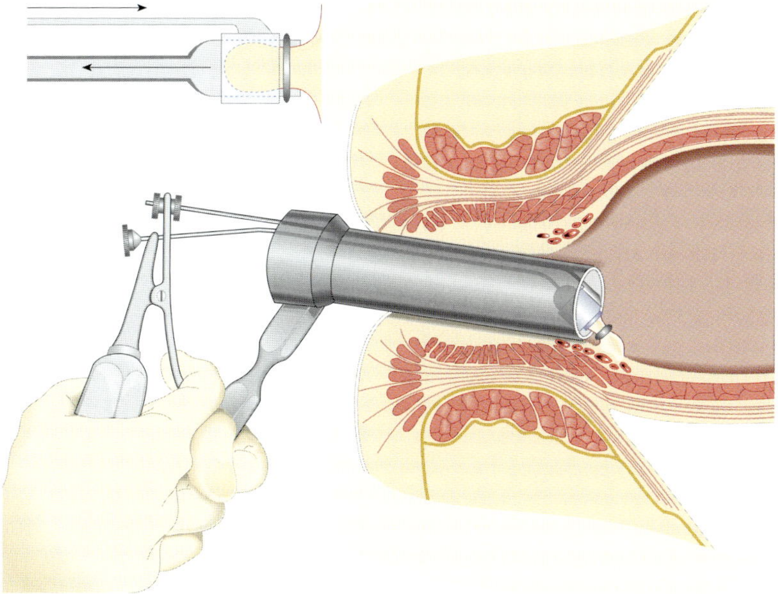

Figure 7B

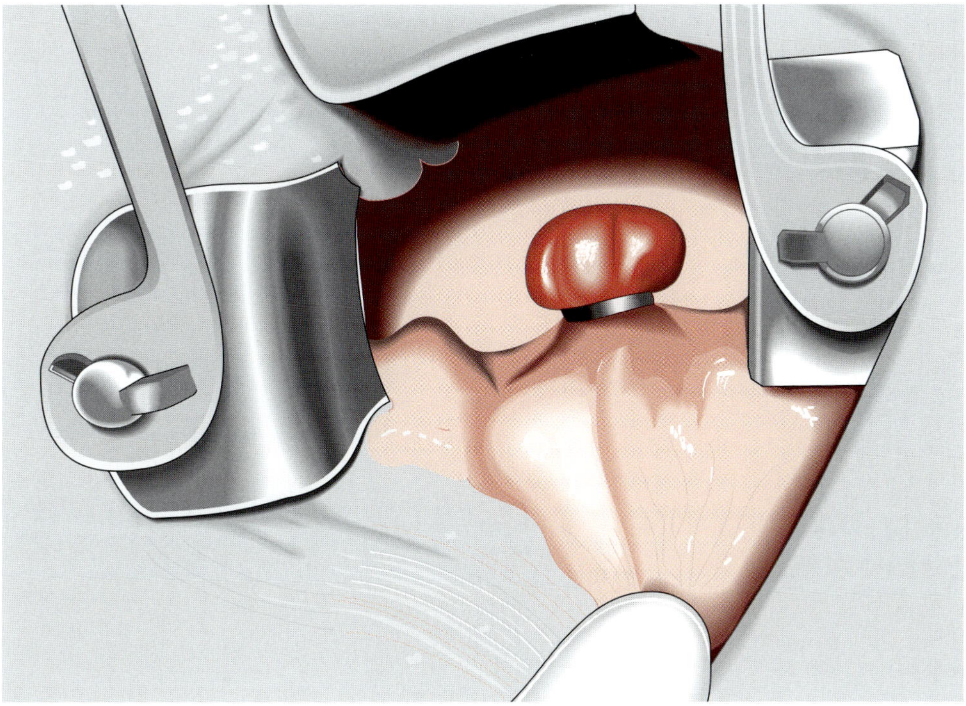

## Figure 8: OPERATIVE TREATMENT OF HAEMORRHOIDAL DISEASE

Morinaga [12] described the Doppler sonographic-guided haemorrhoidal artery ligature (HAL) in 1995. The supplying arteries are identified by means of a special proctoscope with a Doppler transducer. Distally to the Doppler probe there is a window in the side of the proctoscope. This window enables suture ligation of the vessel. The disappearance of the arterial signal demonstrates the successful ligation. This treatment is possible without anaesthesia, although occasionally sedation is required. This method has been described by only a few workers in the field. However, a success rate of 93% is to be expected without any significant complications, making it a very effective type of therapy.

There are no long-term results available concerning the question of whether third degree haemorrhoids can be effectively reduced in size by HAL. It is of interest that, apart from the main branches of the arteries at the 3, 7 and 11 o'clock lithotomy positions, additional arteries can be found and ligated. Some authors have described an application of more than ten ligatures in the area of the upper anal canal. Since HAL can be done without anaesthesia on an outpatient basis, it is very likely that it will become an important technique alongside conservative and operative treatment.

### Fig. 8A–C

**A** Instruments for HAL. Doppler probe at the shaft of the proctoscope distal to the side window with, in addition, a needle holder and pusher. **B** Stitch ligation through the window proctoscope after localisation of the Doppler signal of the artery. **C** View through the proctoscope during ligation of the vessel.

Figure 8A

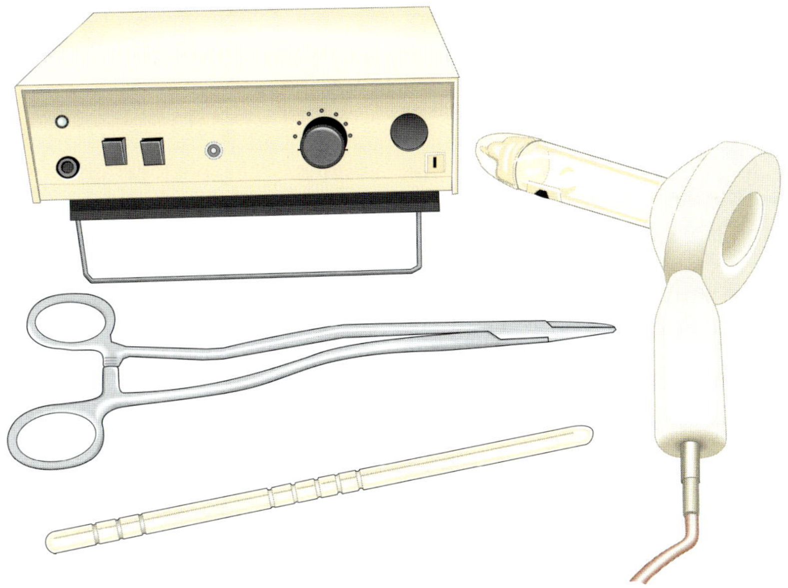

Figure 8B

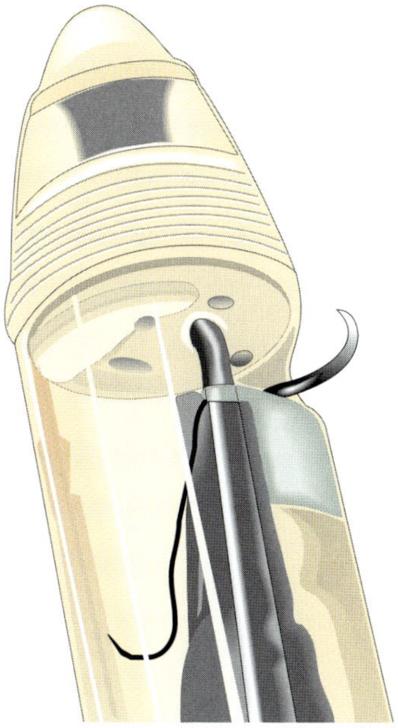

Figure 8C

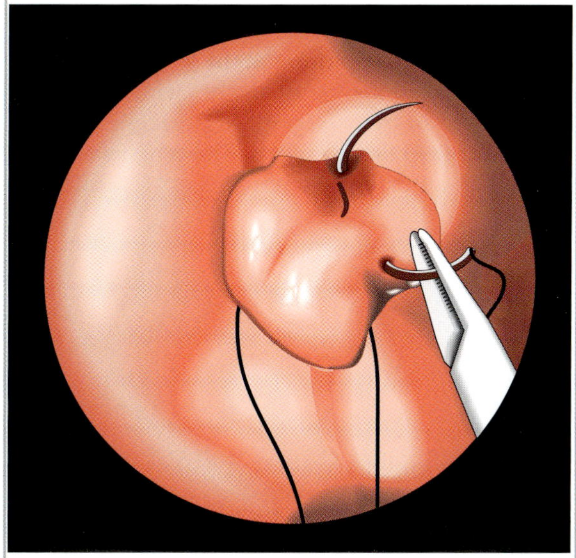

## STANDARD PROCEDURES FOR THE OPERATIVE TREATMENT OF HAEMORRHOIDAL DISEASE

In a more advanced stage of the disease process, when the haemorrhoidal tissue becomes irreducible, operative treatment is indicated. In principle there are two different procedures competing with each other. On the one hand, open excision with subsequent secondary healing of the operative defect (the Milligan-Morgan procedure) has been established for many years. On the other hand, operative procedures are often recommended where a closed technique is applied and the haemorrhoidal tissue is dissected out from underneath the anoderm. The anoderm which has not been destroyed is then fixed in the anal canal by absorbable sutures (as described by Parks).

The open excision of Milligan-Morgan tends to be recommended in single enlarged haemorrhoidal cushions. The postoperative functional results are excellent in these cases. In the presence of a circular prolapse of haemorrhoidal tissue and especially in the presence of a prolapse of the total anoderm (anal prolapse), a closed procedure is mandatory to prevent sensory incontinence.

## Figure 9: The Milligan-Morgan Haemorrhoidectomy

In this operation [11] the enlarged cushion is separated segmentally from the underlying internal anal sphincter muscle starting externally. The base is then stitch-sutured, thereby ligating the supplying artery. This stitch ligation is undertaken using absorbable suture material, e.g. Vicryl 3-0. The defect is left open and heals by secondary intention. If this procedure is applied in all three positions at the 3, 7 and 11 o'clock lithotomy positions, sufficiently wide anoderm bridges need to be preserved. In principle only the enlarged segments are excised. The prophylactic excision of an un-enlarged cushion is not indicated.



### Fig. 9A–E

**A** Segmental excision of the haemorrhoidal cushion at the 11 o'clock lithotomy position using the Milligan-Morgan technique. Start of the excision from outside. After separation of the cushion from the internal sphincter ani muscle, the base is displayed with placing of the arterial suture ligation (Vicryl 3-0). **B** The defect following complete excision of the cushion at 11 o'clock. The open defect will heal by secondary intention. **C** Segmental haemorrhoidectomy of a cushion at 3 o'clock. Display of the internal sphincter muscle and external sphincter muscle, preservation of the internal sphincter muscle during the dissection of the cushion. **D** Stitch ligation of the base of the cushion. The ligature is inserted by pulling the mobilised cushion distally. **E** Completion of the ligation of the base. The haemorrhoidal cushion is excised.

Figure 9A

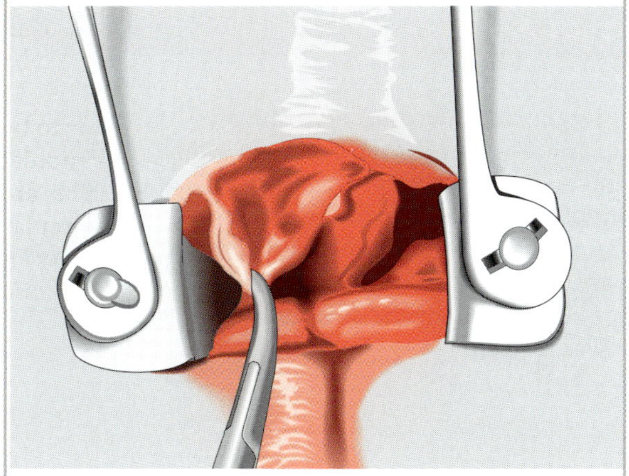

Figure 9B

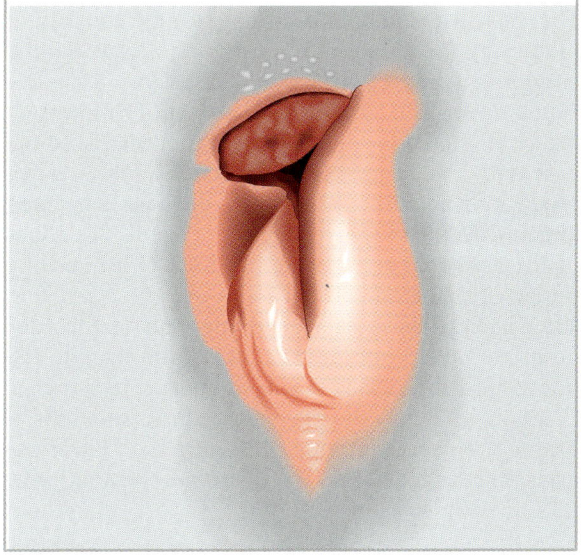

Figure 9C

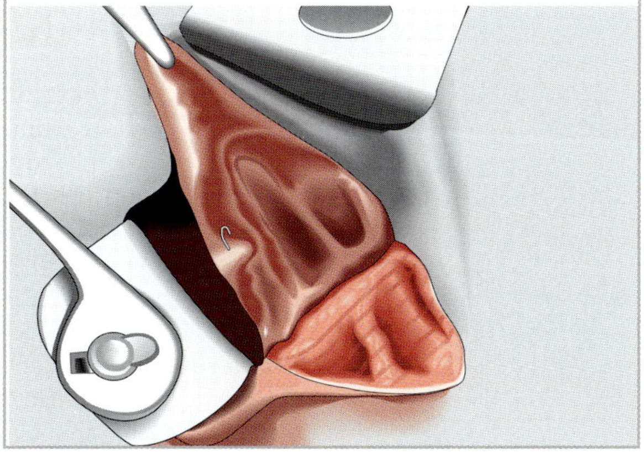

Figure 9D

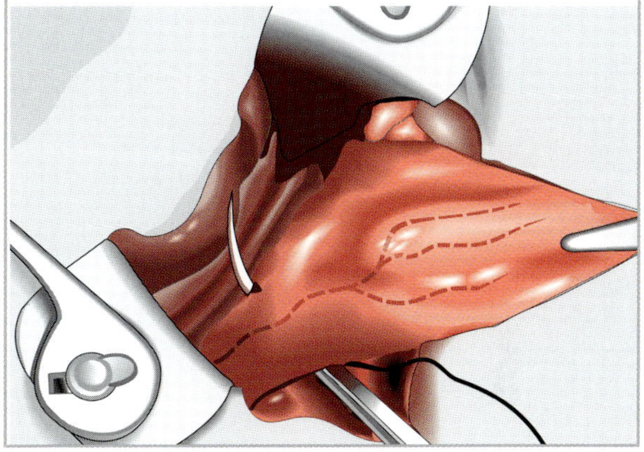

Figure 9E

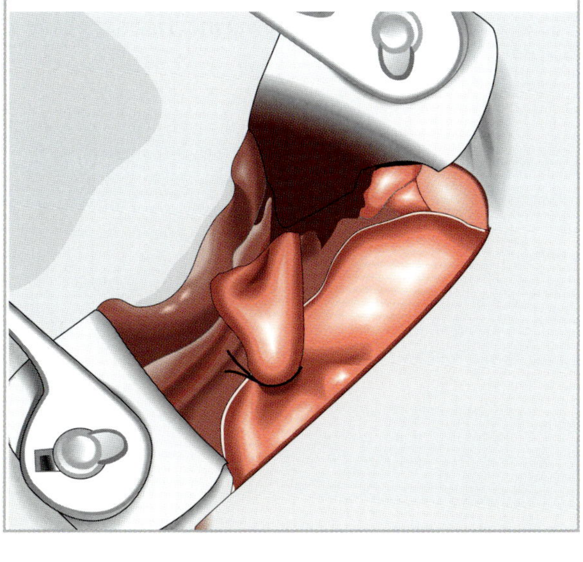

## Figure 10A–F: The Parks "Closed" Haemorrhoidectomy

The closed haemorrhoidectomy [10, 13] consists of modifying the excision of a cushion in a way that the anoderm is incised in a radial direction. Excessive skin at the anal edge is excised as well. The haemorrhoidal tissue of the dentate line is mobilised and the base is divided in several small sections. In this way, a big ligation nodule in the area of the base is avoided and a wide, flat mucosal edge is the result. The edges of the anoderm are elevated on both sides and the underlying haemorrhoidal parts are dissected out. After haemostasis is achieved, the rims of the anoderm are pulled into the anal canal and fixed to the upper mucosal edge by means of interrupted stitches (Vicryl 3-0). Below the fixed anoderm, a small distal drainage defect is left open. The aim is to cover the excisional defect by preserved parts of the anoderm.

### Fig. 10A, B

**A** Haemorrhoidectomy according to Parks (schematic). Incision lines of the anoderm, which is preserved and undermined according to the size of the haemorrhoid. **B** Mobilisation of the anoderm and excision of the haemorrhoidal tissue followed by ligature of the base. The mobilised anoderm is advanced intra-anally and fixed by means of sutures to the mucosa of the lower rectum.

**Figure 10A, B**

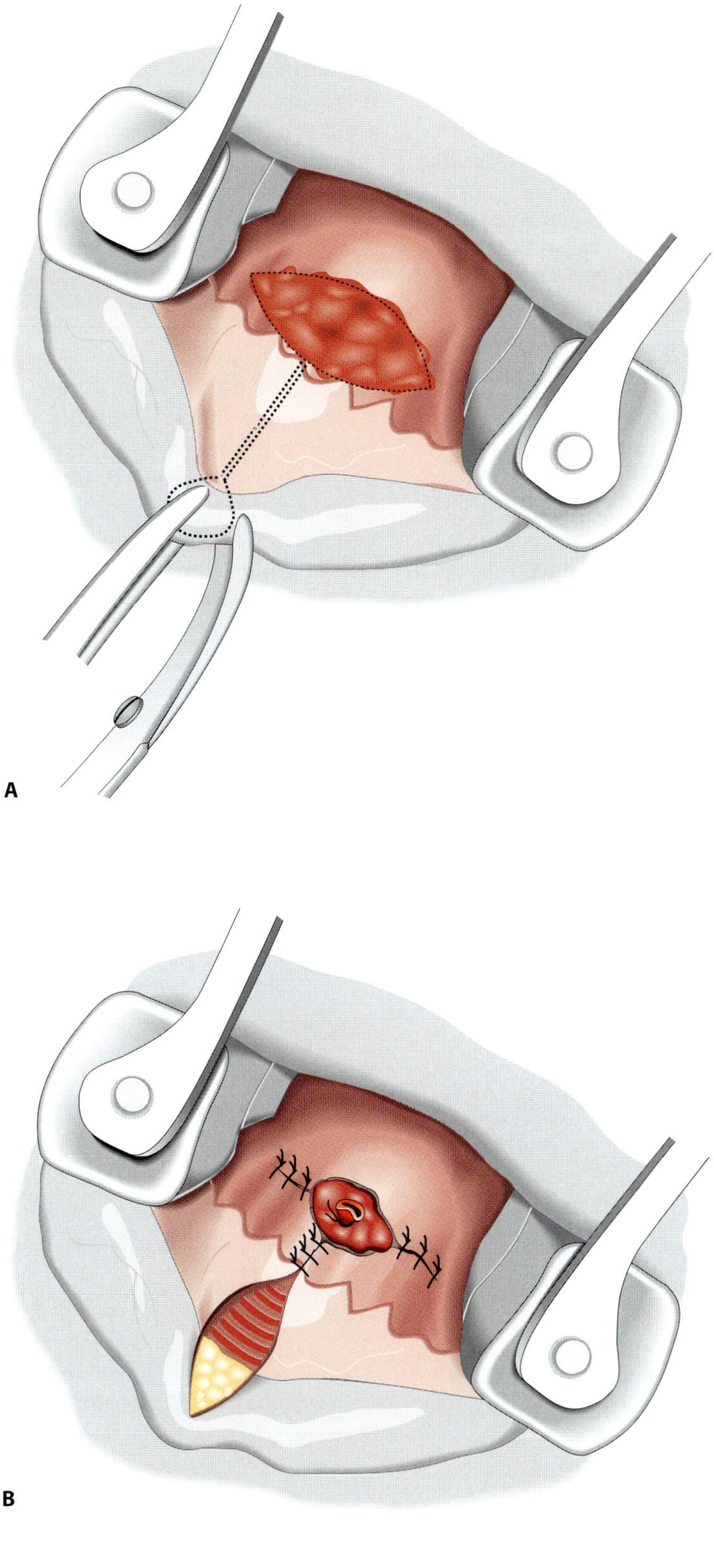

A

B

## Figure 10C–F

**C** The sections of the anoderm are mobilised and folded to the outside. Mobilisation of the proximal parts of the haemorrhoidal plexus. **D** Suture ligation at the base of the mobilised haemorrhoidal plexus. The ligated haemorrhoidal plexus is then exised. **E** Situation following complete excision of the haemorrhoidal plexus. Coagulation of residual bleeding at the mucosal edge. Subsequent folding in of the anoderm flap and fixation by sutures. **F** Situation following complete suture fixation of the mobilised anoderm flap. The external drainage opening is visible.

## HAEMORRHOIDECTOMY AS DESCRIBED BY FERGUSON

This method [5] modifies the Milligan-Morgan procedure in a way that the excisional wound of the anoderm is made smaller and subsequently closed with a running suture in a sagittal direction. By doing so, the anoderm is not undermined and mobilised as in the Parks procedure, but instead is sutured under a degree of tension. This procedure therefore fulfils the criteria of a semi-closed haemorrhoidectomy [10], because the anoderm is not preserved to the same extent as in the Parks technique.

There are further procedures for closed haemorrhoidectomy which are modifications of the procedures described above. In Germany during the 1970s, Arnold resurrected the procedure of closed haemorrhoidectomy according to Fansler/Anderson [4]. It is still of some value [14].

Figure 10C–F

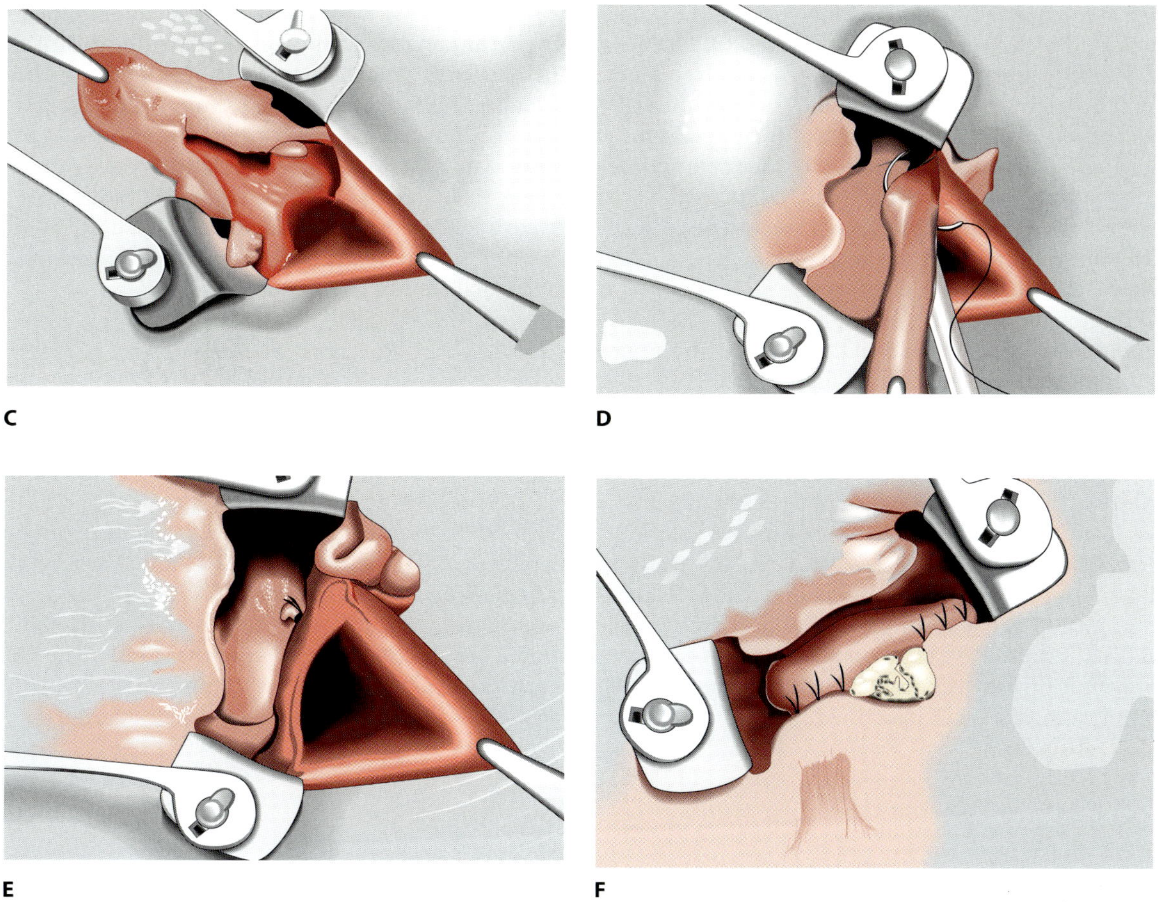

## Figure 11A–J: Recent Developments

The stapled haemorrhoidectomy (or stapled haemorrhoidopexy) as described by Longo [8] has been performed since 1998 with increasing frequency. Here the haemorrhoidal tissue and the neighbouring mucosa of the rectum are resected in a circular fashion. The first step is the creation of a circular purse-string suture 3 cm above the dentate line, in the area of the base of the haemorrhoidal segments. An instrument for the positioning of the haemorrhoidal tissue and the subsequent placing of the suture is commercially available. The purse-string suture is tied around the central bar of the anvil. Then the stapler is closed, and the cutting mechanism is fired. A circular cuff with haemorrhoidal and rectal mucosa is excised and the defect is closed at the same time with a circular staple line. The advantage of this procedure is that, despite removal of the cranial parts of the haemorrhoidal tissue, no operative wound is created in the area of the anoderm. This leads to highly improved patient comfort and a shorter period of postoperative healing. Several prospective randomised studies have been undertaken that come out in favour of the technique. The procedure-related complications are well described [7].

The ideal indication for stapled haemorrhoidectomy is the circular, completely reducible prolapse of the anoderm and the haemorrhoids. For segmental prolapse, Milligan-Morgan excision is more suitable and much cheaper. In the case of an irreducible prolapse, the stapled haemorrhoidectomy cannot achieve satisfactory results, since the tissue that is fixed outside cannot be adequately reduced in size and repositioned intra-anally, and the contours of the anal canal cannot be normalised.

### Fig. 11A–D

Stapled haemorrhoidectomy. **A** Positioning of the purse-string suture (schematic). **B** Application of the purse-string suture. Alternatively, the instruments depicted in **H** can be used. **C** Tying down of the purse-string suture (schematic). **D** By pulling on the purse-string suture, the haemorrhoidal tissue is drawn around the central bar of the stapler. The situation is depicted using the commercially available system for the execution of the stapler operation.

**Figure 11A–D**

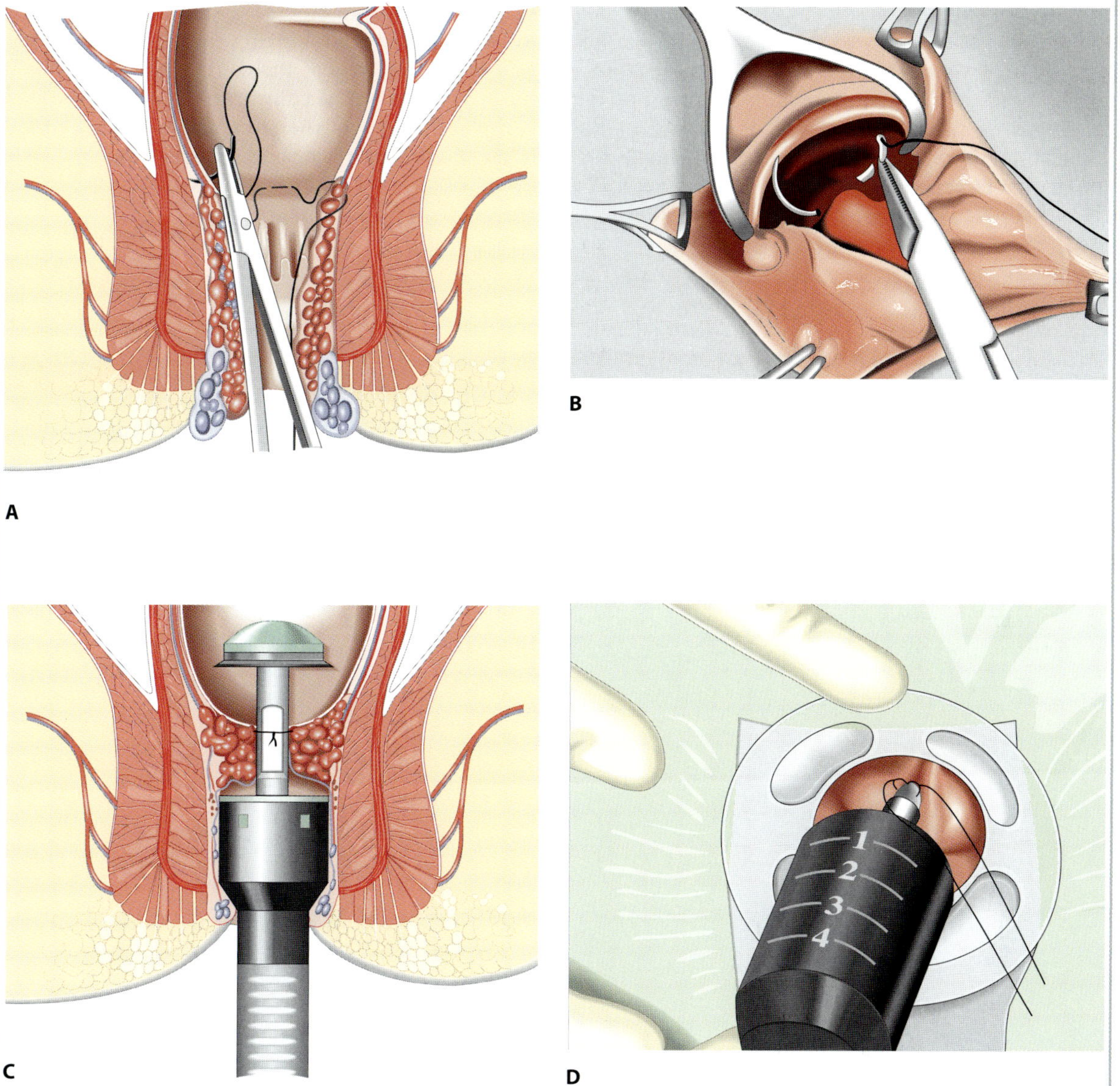

## Figure 11E–I

**E** Closure of the stapler, thereby enveloping the haemorrhoidal tissue. The next step is to fire the stapler mechanism with circular resection of the haemorrhoidal tissue and rectal mucosa and closure of the neighbouring tissue (schematic). **F** Closure of the stapler thereby repositioning the tissue intra-anally. The degree of repositioning is seen from the scales on the outside of the stapler. **G** View of the suture line in the lower rectum following removal of the stapler (schematic). **H** View of the completed suture line in the lower rectum. The commercially available system is in place. **I** View of the circular excisional cylinder of haemorrhoidal tissue and rectal mucosa.

**Table 1**

| STAGES OF HAEMORRHOIDAL DISEASE | |
|---|---|
| Stage 1 | Haemorrhoidal cushions proctoscopically visible and enlarged |
| Stage 2 | Prolapse during defecation with spontaneous retraction |
| Stage 3 | Prolapse manually reducible |
| Stage 4 | Irreversible prolapse due to fibrosis and/or thrombosis |

**Figure 11E–I**

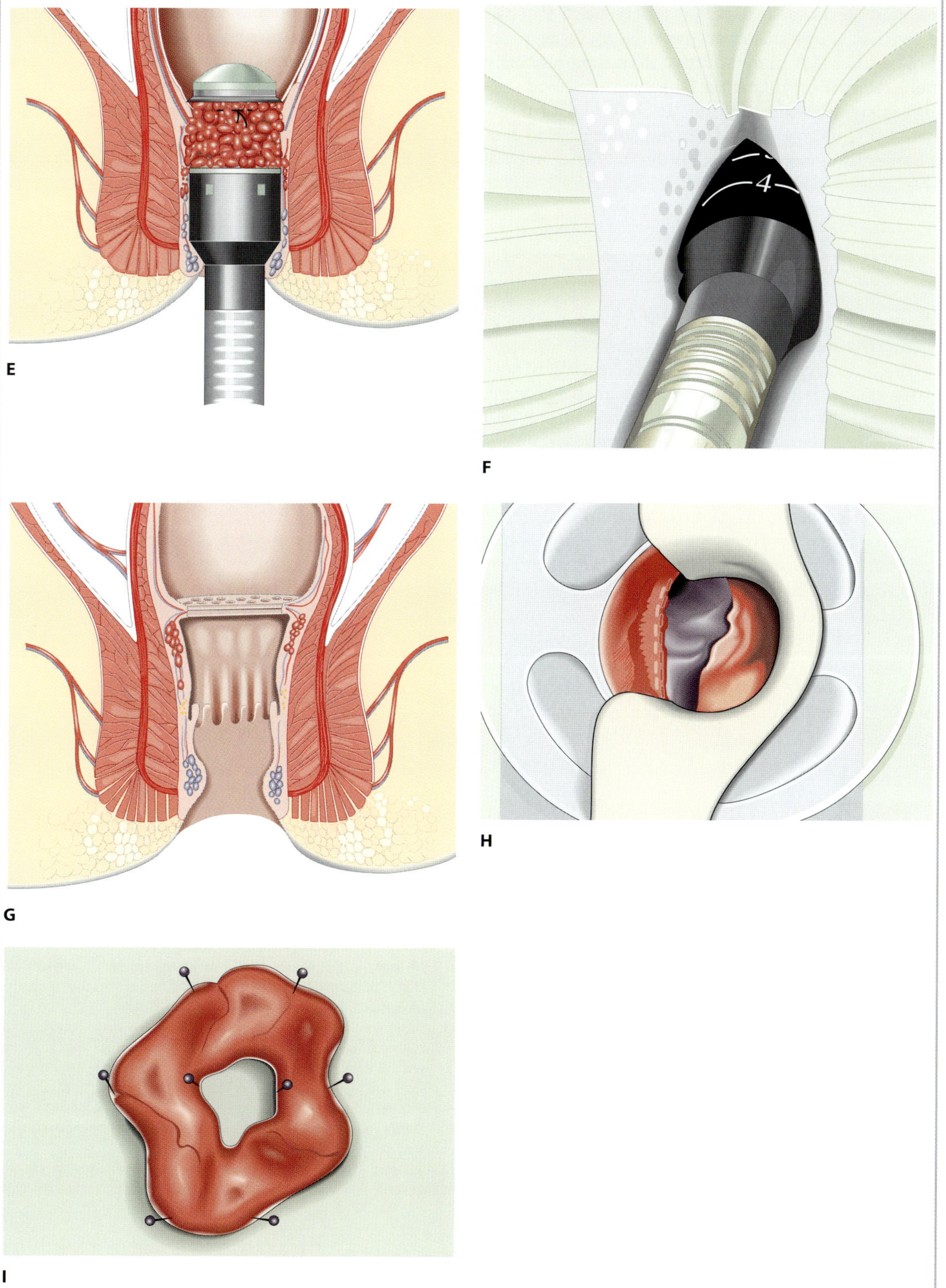

## RESULTS OF OPERATIVE THERAPY

A meta-analysis undertaken by MacRae and McLeod in 1995 [9] shows that operative therapy of haemorrhoidal disease is more effective than the previously preferred manual dilatation. The success rate of surgery is significantly superior to conservative treatment (96% vs. 77%). However, the complication rate is higher (18% vs. 6%) and so is the incidence of pain (83% vs. 10%). Rubber band ligation is more effective than sclerosing treatment for all stages of the disease. Third degree haemorrhoids are still usually dealt with operatively, but rubber band ligations can be the first step, followed by operation if the desired therapeutic effect is not achieved.

## PERIOPERATIVE MANAGEMENT

The preoperative preparation of the patient prior to haemorrhoidectomy usually only involves a saline enema. Since many patients may receive a colonoscopy for diagnosis, total bowel prep is available in some instances. Although this anal operation is done in a potentially infective environment, septic complications are relatively rare. Thus disinfection of the operative field in excess of normal cleansing procedures and antibiotic prophylaxis are not necessary.

Postoperatively, swabs with disinfectant ointments can be placed on open wounds. Local shower cleansing or baths with disinfectant additives can be helpful. Some surgeons recommend digital exploration of the anal canal starting on the first postoperative day, but this is painful. The rationale behind this painful procedure is that the intra-anal wound edges are dilated and potential retention of secretions is prevented. Premature wound closure may be regarded as a precursor for septic complications and stenosis. By digital exploration, any impaction of stool in the rectal ampulla can be detected and the application of a laxative suppository or enema may be indicated. Oral laxatives are neither required nor useful since liquefaction of bowel contents can cause increased pain without preventing distal stool impaction. On the other hand, stools of normal composition induced by a fibre-rich nutrition are desirable.

The so-called closed operative techniques carry an increased risk of disturbed wound healing and submucous abscesses. If digital examination finds intra-anal localised pain or reveals purulent secretion on the finger, a proctoscopic wound inspection is obligatory.



## SELECTED REFERENCES


1. Barron J (1963) Office ligation treatment of hemorrhoids. Dis Colon Rectum 6:109–113
2. Blanchard C (1928) Textbook of ambulant proctology. Medical Success Progress, Youngstone, Ohio p 134
3. Blond K, Hoff H (1936) Das Hämorrhoidalleiden. Deutike, Leipzig, Wien
4. Fansler WA, Anderson JK (1933) A plastic operation for certain types of haemorrhoids. JAMA 101:1064–1066
5. Ferguson JA, Heaton JR (1959) Closed haemorrhoidectomy. Dis Colon Rectum 2:176–179
6. Hansen H, Stelzner F (1987) Proktologie, 2nd edn. Springer, Berlin, Heidelberg, New York
7. Herold A, Kirsch JJ (2001) Komplikationen nach Stapler-Hämorrhoidektomie – Ergebnisse einer Umfrage in Deutschland. Coloproctology 23:8–16
8. Longo A (1998) Treatment of hemorrhoids disease by reduction of mucosa and hemorrhoidal prolapse with a circular suturing device: a new procedure. Sixth World Congress of Endoscopic Surgery. Manduzzi, Rome, pp 777–784
9. MacRae H, McLeod R (1995) Comparison of hemorrhoidal treatment modalities: a meta-analysis. Dis Colon Rectum 38:687–694
10. Marti M-C, Givel J-C (eds) (1990) Surgery of anorectal diseases. Springer, Berlin, Heidelberg, New York
11. Milligan ETC, Morgan C, Naughton Jones LF, Officer RR (1937) Surgical anatomy of the anal canal and the operative treatment of haemorrhoids. Lancet II:1119
12. Morinaga K, Hasuda K, Ikeda T (1995) A novel therapy for internal hemorrhoids: ligation of the hemorrhoidal artery with a newly devised instrument (Moricorn) in conjunction with a Doppler flow meter. Am J Gastroenterol 90:610–613
13. Parks AG (1956) The surgical treatment of haemorrhoids. Br J Surg 43:337–351
14. Raulf F (1989) Indikationen, Technik und Ergebnisse der geschlossenen Hämorrhoidektomie. Akt Chir 24:211–215

CHAPTER 14

# Anal Fissure

**Franz Raulf, Christian F. Krieglstein, Norbert Senninger**

## INTRODUCTION

The diagnosis of anal fissure is easily made by digital examination and/or proctoscopy. Nevertheless, fissure disease is often only recognised after a prolonged clinical course and accordingly treatment is often delayed.

## Figure 1: Anatomy and Pathophysiology

An anal fissure is a longitudinal ulcer in the lower anal canal in the area of the anoderm. Due to its location, fissures are characterised by pain associated with bleeding. Fissures most commonly occur in the area of the posterior commissure (90%), less frequently in the anterior commissure, with about 5% of patients having two fissures. The aetiology is unclear. The common perception is that a fissure is related to a hypertonic state of the internal anal sphincter muscle. However, more recent hypotheses relate the fissure to the existence of an infection of the anal crypts. The passage of constipated stool can injure the area, causing oedematous swelling followed by scar formation and fissure. An intersphincteric abscess may also penetrate into the anal canal and cause similar scar tissue. The common issue for both hypotheses is a septic underlying process. This coincides with the frequency of localisation of the fissure in the posterior and, less frequently, the anterior commissure, because crypts are represented here in higher numbers. Such local infection is also an explanation for the scarring tendency of the fissure with the development of so-called secondary changes. The hypertensive status of the sphincter muscle may then be looked upon as a secondary phenomenon.

Clinically one needs to differentiate between an acute and a chronic fissure. It is not clear, however, whether this represents progression of the same disease entity. An acute fissure shows a superficial lesion of the tissues, which may heal or take a more chronic inflammatory course. The chronic fissure needs to be defined according to its secondary changes:



Secondary changes are:

- A deep epithelial defect with exposed muscle fibres of the internal sphincter and callous edges of the fissure
- Hypertrophy of the anal papilla at the upper fissure edge
- A sentinel tag on the outside
- Signs of local chronic inflammation involving the intersphincteric area (fistula or active abscess)
- The development of an inflammatory and scarred anal stenosis

There is no clear correlation between the duration of the disease and the degree of secondary changes. A fissure that exists for a longer period of time without secondary changes should be interpreted as a recurrence of an acute fissure.

Primary fissures need to be differentiated from secondary ones, which are indicative of different inflammatory diseases of the anal region. These diseases include Crohn's disease, anal tuberculosis and manifestations of AIDS disease. These types of fissure are mainly dealt with by treating the underlying disease, and local interventions are usually ineffective if used alone. Of importance is the differentiation to the so-called "rhagade". This is a lesion of the skin which can also protrude into the anal canal.

**Conservative Therapy.** The acute fissure normally disappears spontaneously and only requires symptomatic therapy. This is usually done by local application of an appropriate ointment. Additives such as local anaesthetics and adstringent and disinfectant substances can enhance this symptomatic therapy. The application of an anal dilator for the treatment of anal stenosis due to a hypertonic sphincter is potentially useful, although the value of this has not been confirmed by studies. More specific recommendations involve botulinum toxin and ointments containing nitroglycerin as locally effective substances for the treatment of the fissure. The local injection of botulinum toxin into the external sphincter ani causes a reversible palsy of this muscle (by inhibiting acetylcholine liberation), which leads to a decreased muscle tone in the anal canal and enables a healing of the fissure. Usually an injection of 15–25 units is required. The effect on the muscle is spontaneously reversed after 8–12 weeks.

There are conflicting study results concerning the use of nitroglycerin containing ointments in the treatment of chronic fissures. These preparations are usually given in a concentration of 0.2% (up to 0.4%) and may decrease the internal sphincter tones, improve local perfusion and by doing so improve the utilisation of oxygen, thereby leading to the healing of the fissure. Side effects are headaches which may be dose dependent. There are several studies in chronic fissure patients that show a decreased operative frequency and a lower rate of recurrence. Multicentre studies, however, have not been able to reproduce these results. In more recent studies the local application of nifedipine has been investigated. In total, local treatment as described is recommended as an alternative to lateral sphincterotomy. A definitive judgement as to the role of such conservative therapy is not possible at the moment. It has to be stressed, however, that the therapeutic approach of lowering the sphincter tone is contrary to the pathophysiological concept of the origin of fissures being related to a septic mechanism involving the anal crypts.

### Figure 1

Posterior fissure. View with Parks retractor in place. The undermining of the distal edge of the fissure is visible leading to the development of the sentinel tag. In the proximal part of the fissure a hypertrophied anal papilla is visible. Outside one can see the external opening of an associated fistula

Figure 1

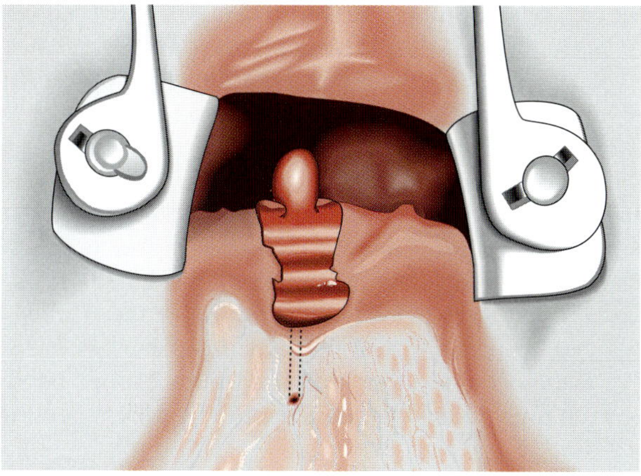

## Figures 2–9: Operative Therapy

The established operative approaches are based on two different hypotheses concerning the pathophysiology of the fissure disease.

Operative manipulation at the internal anal sphincter aims to reduce increased sphincter tone thus initiating the healing process. Manual dilatation of the sphincter apparatus has been abandoned due to the danger of uncontrolled tearing. Internal anal sphincterotomy involves incision of the muscle fibres either using a closed technique [5] or an open technique [6]. However, many would stress that besides a sphincterotomy, excision of the fissure also needs to be undertaken if marked secondary changes are present.

The procedure of fissurectomy is aimed at the fissure directly. The scarred tissue of the fissure and any secondary changes are excised, taking care not to injure the underlying muscle. Eisenhammer [2] combined this treatment with sphincterotomy in the base of the fissure (dorsal sphincterotomy).

The *lateral sphincterotomy as described by Notaras* is usually performed using local anaesthesia. After a small radial incision of the skin at 3 o'clock on the anal margin, the intersphincteric area is identified by means of digital examination (closed operation). A special scalpel similar to that used for cataract surgery is introduced into the intersphincteric area and then turned 90 degrees with the cutting edge towards the internal sphincter thus dividing the muscle fibres. This division of the fibres is also possible by means of scissors. The recommendation of how much of the muscle should be cut differs between authors. At least the distal third of the muscle should be cut, and in severe cases this division should be extended up to the dentate line.

14

The involuntary opening of a crypt with the subsequent creation of a fistula is a procedure-related complication. Using the finger in the anal canal during the cutting process should help to avoid this. This technique was described by Notaras to be used under local anaesthesia as an outpatient procedure.

The *lateral sphincterotomy described by Parks* is done using local, regional or general anaesthesia. This procedure always requires a retractor in the anal canal. A curved incision over the palpable introitus to the intersphincteric cleft is made. The incision is made long enough to allow visualisation of the internal anal sphincter muscle. By opening the blades of the scissors, the intersphincteric cleft and the subanodermal area are separated. Following this, the internal anal sphincter can be incised openly under vision with a pair of scissors. As in the Notaras procedure, the degree of muscle incision varies between authors. The incision is closed at the end by skin sutures.

Both procedures yield an effective lowering of sphincter pressure and permit healing of the fissure. A meta-analysis done by Nelson [4] demonstrated that both procedures achieve the same results with a rate of incontinence of 0–20% and a rate of recurrence of fissures or persistence of fissures of between 3% and 29%. The lateral sphincterotomy is therefore the treatment of choice for the uncomplicated fissure if conservative treatment has failed. It has to be stressed, however, that excision of the scarred tissue of the fissure with its secondary changes has to be undertaken or else this procedure cannot be regarded as the gold standard for the treatment of chronic fissures.

### Figure 2

Lateral sphincterotomy as described by Notaras. Radial incision at the 3 o'clock lithotomy position. Visualisation of the internal anal sphincter. Cutting the muscle with scissors (closed procedure). During the incision, the left index finger should be inside the anal canal to help avoiding an inadequately deep incision.

### Figure 3

Lateral sphincterotomy as described by Parks (I). Bow-shaped incision over the palpable entrance into the intersphincteric cleft

### Figure 4

Lateral sphincterotomy as described by Parks (II). Visualisation of the internal anal sphincter and mobilisation of the intersphincteric cleft and the subanodermal area

### Figure 5

Lateral sphincterotomy as described by Parks (III). Incision of the internal anal sphincter muscle under vision (open procedure) with scissors. The incisional wound is closed by skin stitches

### Figure 6

Fissurectomy (I). Segmental excision, starting far outside

### Figure 7

Fissurectomy (II). Separation of fissure base and internal anal sphincter muscle

Figure 2

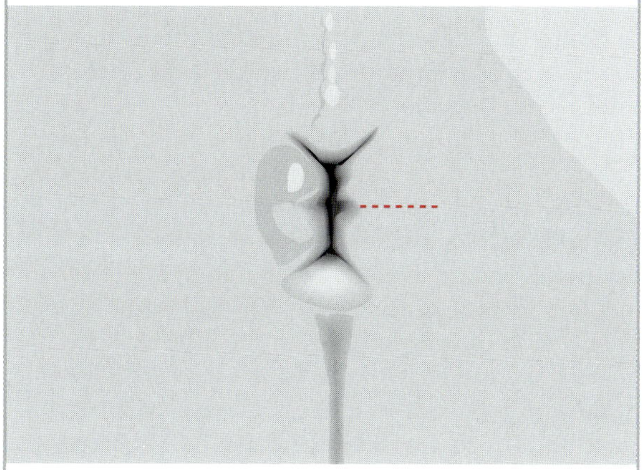

Figure 3

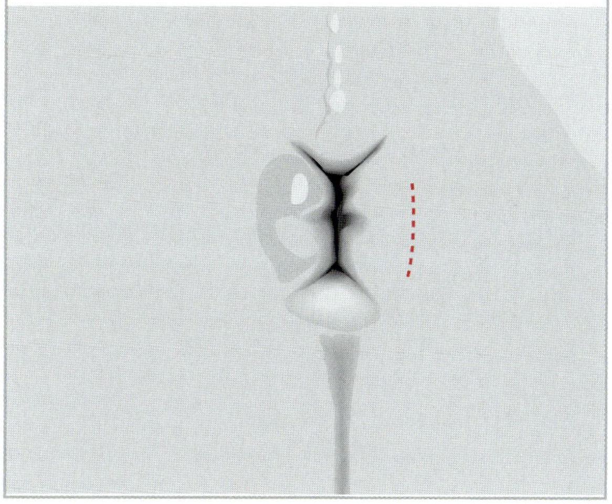

Figure 4

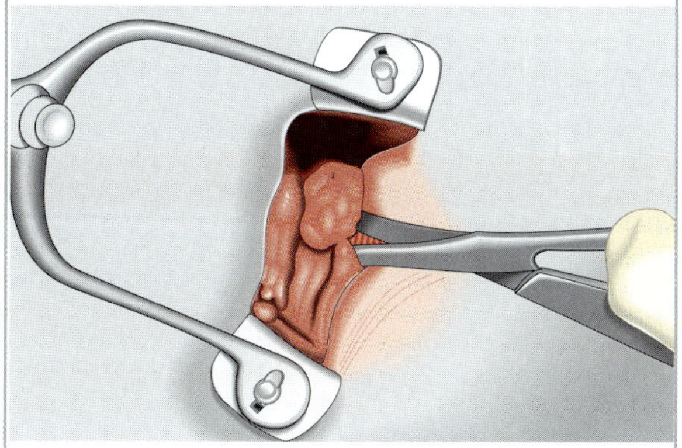

Figure 5

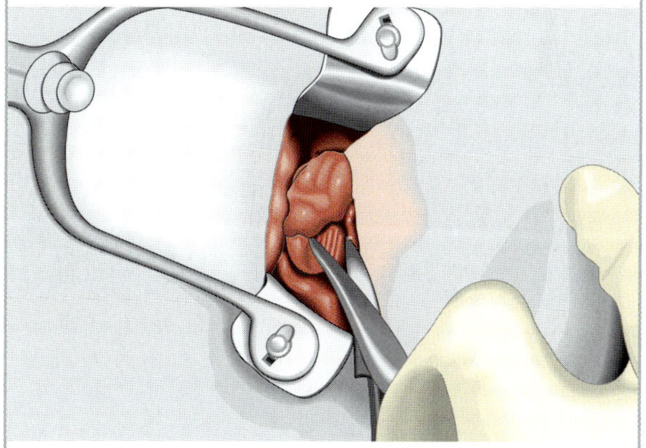

Figure 6

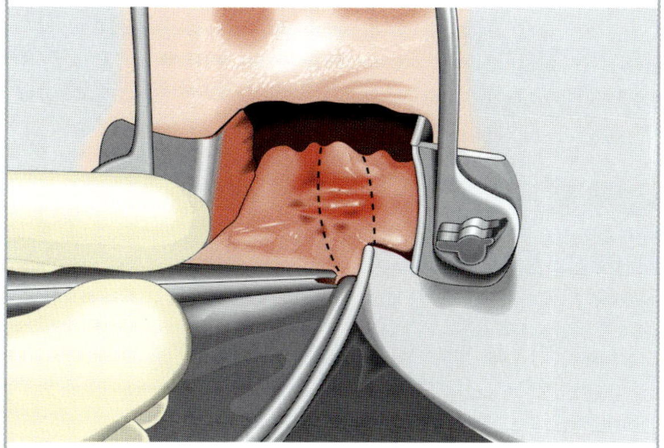

Figure 7

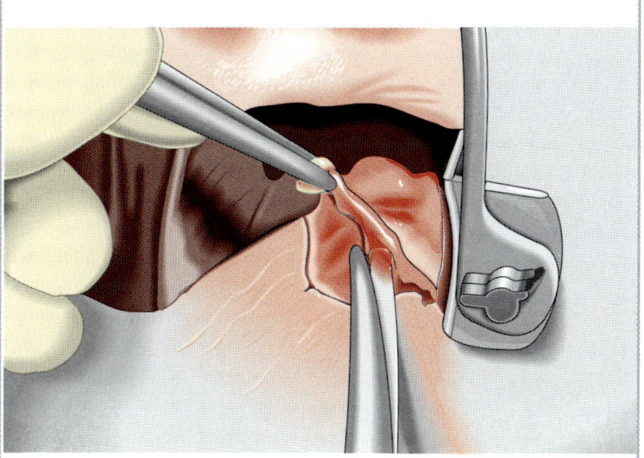

Excision of the fissure as desribed by Eisenhammer, when combined with a dorsal sphincterotomy on the base of the fissure, remains popular in the treatment of chronic fissure with secondary changes [3]. However, there are no recent studies which have investigated this procedure. A study by Bennett and Goligher [1] found a high rate of incontinence (34%), but this related to the first few weeks postoperatively. The late results were much better, with 13% being incontinent for flatus after 3 years. In principle, one has to keep in mind that intra-anal wounds cause an irritation of the sphincter muscle early postoperatively and therefore it is the late results that are decisive.

Intervention usually requires regional or general anaesthesia. Excision of the fissure is done in segments, starting outside the anal edge. The perianal skin is excised superficially and then the intra-anal scar is cut free, preserving the internal sphincter. The separation of the base of the fissure from the internal muscle can be quite difficult due to cicatrised adhesions.

Proximally, the neighbouring parts of the crypt line including any fibroepithelial polyps (hypertrophied papillas) are excised as well. The defect is left open. By excision of a wide skin area, a "mock recurrence" is prevented. The external aspects of the wound show a faster scar development than the intra-anal areas. This results in the potential risk of an obliquely running scar that can be undermined by stools, leading to a new inflammatory process in the wound at the anal edge. As mentioned previously, at the end of the operation the internal anal sphincter in the base of the wound can be incised with scissors (dorsal sphincterotomy).

Gabriel has described fissure excision without concomitant sphincterotomy. When an anal retractor is used, its dilating effect has to be taken into account. In the case of a chronic fissure with secondary changes the excision of the scar tissue without sphincterotomy may be a suitable option. In several studies comparing short distance sphincter incision vs. sphincter incision up to the dentate line, the latter option is not recommended as routine. From the surgical point of view, the division of muscle fibres in the internal sphincter below the distal edge of the fissure appears advisable. At the end of this short incision the anal canal is sufficiently elastic to minimise the danger of recurrence of the fissure. The danger of incontinence following a so called "key-hole deformity" is virtually zero.

**Figure 8**

Fissurectomy (III). Excision of the proximal part of the fissure excising the hypertrophied papilla and the neighbouring anal crypts

**Figure 9**

Fissurectomy (IV). Wound at the end of the procedure

Figure 8

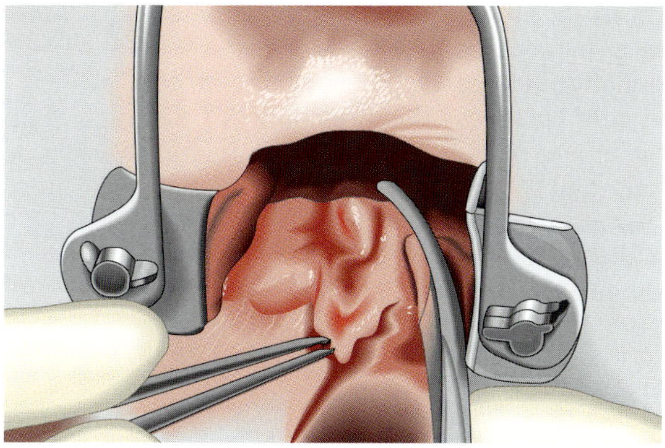

Figure 9

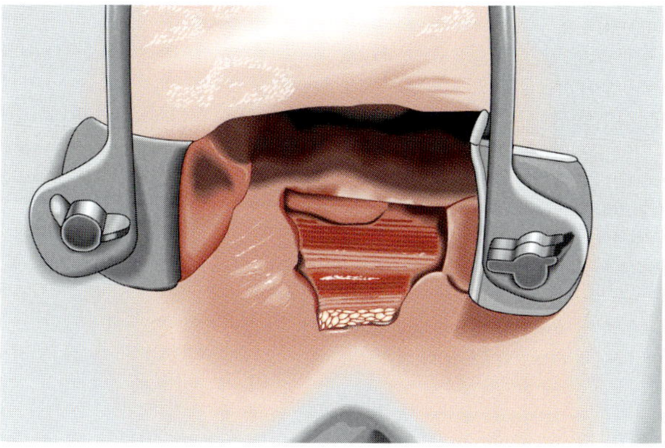

## Figure 10: Complications and Postoperative Care

For the postoperative management of a lateral sphincterotomy or fissurectomy, the principles of open wound management in a potentially infected area are mandatory. The administration of laxatives is contraindicated since soft stools favour the development of a scarred stenosis. The anal canal should be dilated daily and later weekly by means of digital dilation. This prevents a premature closure of the wound. The definitive healing process lasts several weeks.

### Figure 10

Fissurectomy (V). Secondary healing of the fissurectomy wound: situation 3 weeks postoperatively

Figure 10

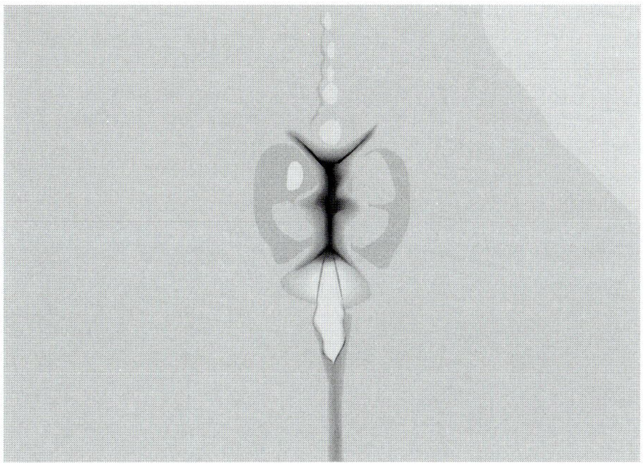

## SELECTED REFERENCES


1. Bennett RC, Goligher JC (1962) Results of internal sphincterotomy for anal fissure. BMJ 2:1500–1505
2. Eisenhammer S (1951) The surgical correction of chronic internal anal (sphincteric) contracture. S Afr Med J 25:486–489
3. Kraemer M, Bussen D, Leppert R, Sailer M, Fuchs K-H, Thiede A (1998) Bundesweite Umfrage zum therapeutischen Vorgehen bei Hämorrhoidalleiden und Analfissur. Chirurg 69:315–318
4. Nelsen RL (1999) Meta-analysis of operative techniques for fissure-in-ano. Dis Colon Rectum 42:1424–1431
5. Notaras M (1969) Lateral subcutaneous sphincterotomy for anal fissure: a new technique. Proc R Soc Med 62:713
6. Parks AG (1967) The management of fissure in ano. Hosp Med 1:737–739

CHAPTER 15

# Surgical Procedures for Perianal Sepsis: Ischiorectal Abscesses, Fistulas, and Pilonidal Sinus

Christian F. Krieglstein

## Figure 1: Anatomy of the Anus

- Internal sphincter = smooth muscle
- External sphincter = striated muscle
- Mucosa of upper third of anal canal: no somatic sensation
- Mucosa of lower two-thirds of anal canal: somatic innervation from inferior rectal nerves
- Anal glands occur in the intersphincteric plane and open at the level of the dentate line within the anal canal

Before any anorectal surgical procedure is performed, digital and sigmoidoscopic examinations are mandatory. Since these examinations may be painful in patients with local inflammation, it may be necessary to perform them with the patient under some kind of anaesthesia. Digital examination should always precede sigmoidoscopy and proctoscopy as it relaxes the sphincters and detects any obstruction that may cause injury during proctosigmoidscopy. It also provides helpful information on the strength and muscular symmetry of the sphincter muscles.

The pigmented perianal skin is separated from the pink transition zone by the anal verge. Since the anal verge can be readily seen during inspection, it serves as the reference line for the position of all other structures found on examination.

Before examination the gloved index finger is lubricated. The finger is then inserted so that the distal interphalangeal joint is at the anal verge and the subcutaneous portion the external (voluntary) sphincter is felt as a tight ring around the distal half of the distal phalanx. With the tip of the finger the pectinate line of anal valves can be palpated roughly 2 cm above the anal verge. Above the valves the anal columns (Morgagni) also may be detected. External haemorrhoids, polyps, and hypertrophied anal papillae in this region can now be readily felt. Of great importance in males is the palpation of the prostate gland.

Further insertion of the finger to the level of the middle interphalangeal joint allows palpation of the anorectal ring, which is formed by the deep component of the external anal sphincter, the puborectalis loop, and the upper margin of the internal sphincter. The ring can only be palpated posteriorly and laterally, and not anteriorly.

Further penetration of the finger to the level of the metacarpophalangeal joint allows the distal phalanx to enter the lower third of the rectum. Often the left lower rectal fold may be reached. At this level the pelvirectal space lies lateral and the rectovesical or rectovaginal space lies anterior. Anterior to the rectum one can palpate the prostate gland in men and the upper vagina and cervix in women.

The proctosigmoidoscope should be inserted at an angle that aims at the patient's umbilicus. At 5 cm from the anal verge, the tip will be at the anorectal ring. With the obturator removed, the left lower rectal fold should be visible. At about 8 cm from the verge, the middle rectal fold may be seen. This is the level of the peritoneal reflection. The superior rectal fold is reached at between 10 and 12 cm and once beyond this, passage of the scope is easy.

The area between the middle and superior rectal folds, just above the peritoneal reflection, needs to be treated with respect since this is the level at which perforation by the sigmoidoscope may occur.

Figure 1

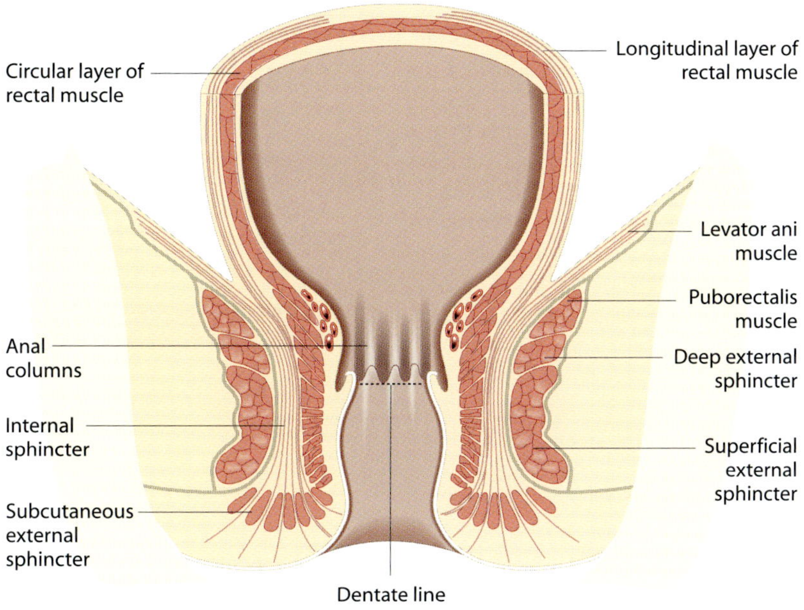
Circular layer of rectal muscle
Longitudinal layer of rectal muscle
Levator ani muscle
Puborectalis muscle
Anal columns
Deep external sphincter
Internal sphincter
Superficial external sphincter
Subcutaneous external sphincter
Dentate line

## Figure 2–4: Abscesses: Incision and Drainage

Perianal sepsis is a relatively common surgical problem and yet the contribution of rare aetiological factors, the frequency of fistula formation complicating perianal abscess, the significance of bacteriological findings and the optimum treatment of fistula in ano are poorly understood. It is important that patients with anorectal sepsis have complete medical and surgical assessments at the time of their first admission. Some abscesses may arise from intersphincteric sepsis (cryptoglandular hypothesis). Perianal sepsis requires abscess drainage with minimal tissue trauma.

### Figure 2

Incision of an ischiorectal abscess for drainage

### Figure 3

Digital exploration of the abscess cavity

### Figure 4

Light packing of the abscess cavity with iodoform gauze



**Table 1**

**Classification and procedures for abscesses**

| | |
|---|---|
| Classification | Submucosal/Subcutaneous |
| | Ischiorectal |
| | Intersphincteric/extrasphincteric |
| | Supra-levatoric |
| Preparation | One to two enemas |
| Position | Prone |
| Anaesthesia | Local, in most cases, as an office procedure |
| Procedure | Initial surgery should simply be incision and drainage. Avoid looking for a fistula at initial surgery. Endoanal ultrasound is recommended at approximately 5 days, especially if gut related organisms are found on culture. The incision can be radial or parallel. It must be long enough to allow drainage of the cavity. The incision should be close to the anus if possible, depending of course on the localized maximum swelling and tenderness. Perform intracavitary digital examination to break possible septa and allow pus to drain (see Figs. 2–4). Light packing with, e.g. iodoform gauze, should be removed after 24 h |
| Remember: | Eighty percent of recurrent abscesses are associated with a fistula. If fistulas require excision, they will be close to the anal verge |

Figure 2

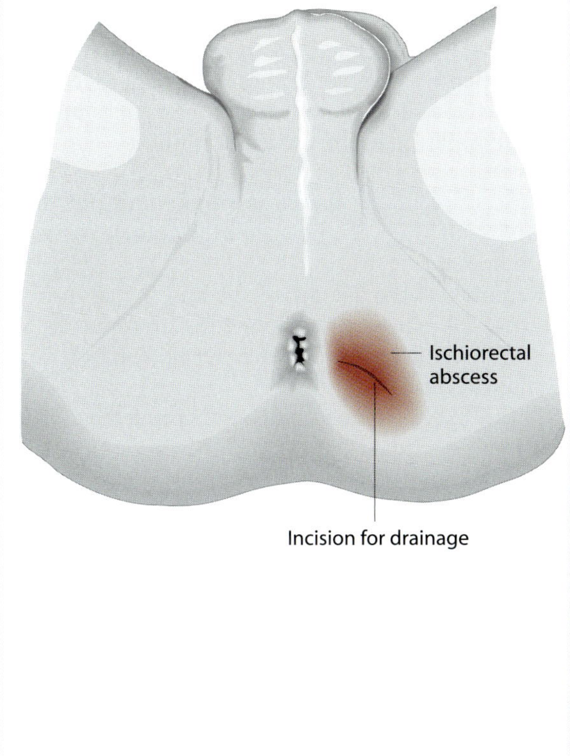


Figure 4

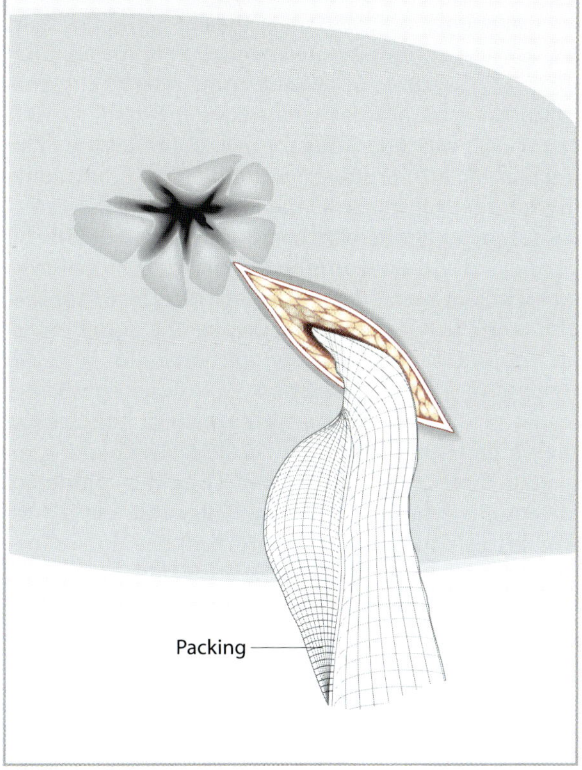


Figure 3

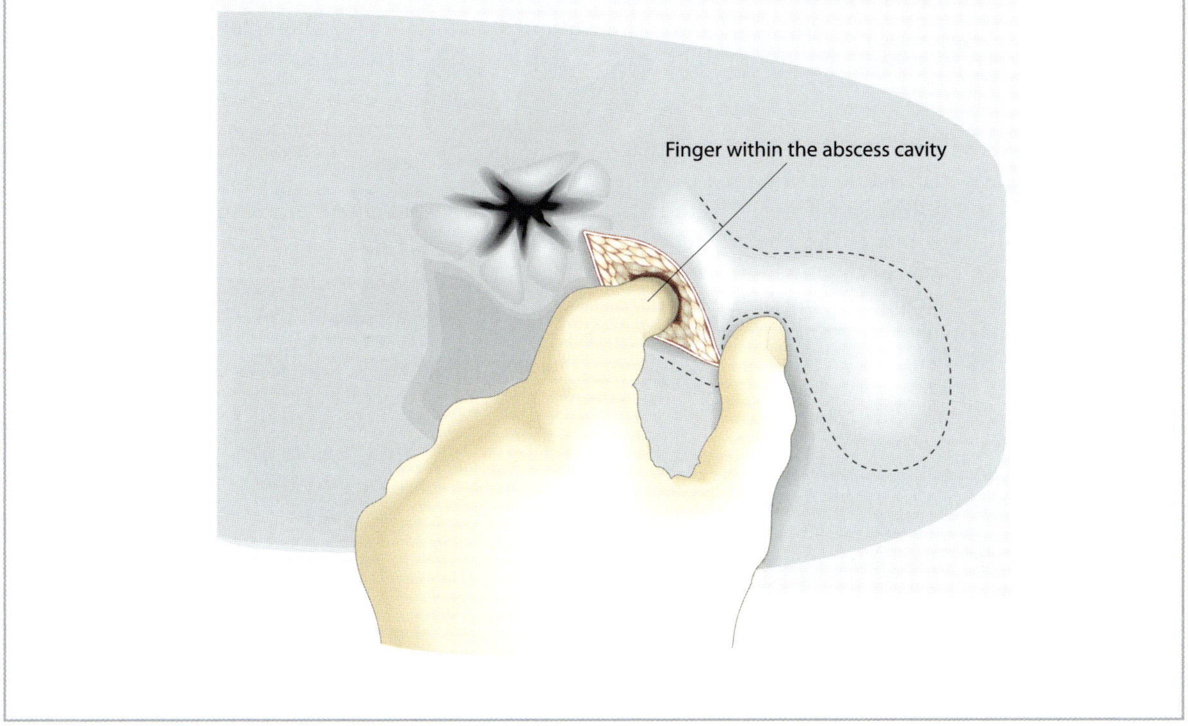

## Figure 5–7: Anal Fistulectomy

It is generally accepted that the laying-open technique constitutes the only effective cure for anal fistulas. The sacrifice of at least some part of the anal sphincter apparatus is therefore the inevitable consequence of every operation for fistula. In the case of an intersphincteric or low-transsphincteric fistula, only the internal sphincter or the lower half of the external sphincter needs to be incised. This may usually be performed without running the risk of postoperative faecal incontinence. High transsphincteric or suprasphincteric fistulas, however, involve the entire external sphincter and/or the puborectalis muscle. Straightforward transsection of these sphincters would result in faecal incontinence. For this reason such high fistulas should be progressively laid open in staged procedures, after encircling the sphincters for some weeks with a seton. The same procedure should also be employed for complex horseshoe-shaped fistulas. Contrary to traditional teaching, anal fistulas in Crohn's disease are no exception to these general therapeutic guidelines. Exploration for an underlying fistula and, if possible, immediate fistulotomy are advocated for all patients with an acute perianal abscess.

- Preparation: one to two enemas
- Position: prone
- Anaesthesia: general or spinal
- Examination: digital, dilatation, retractor of choice and very careful external and internal probing. Methylene blue staining (with or without use of $H_2O_2$) may be of great help.
- Remember: most fistulas in ano are midline and lie posteriorly

15

*Goodsall's rule* states that an external opening situated behind the transverse anal line will open into the anal canal in the midline posteriorly. Goodsall-Salmon's rule of fistulas relates the internal location of the fistula to its external opening, and must be kept in mind. If the external opening of the fistula is anterior to an imaginary transverse line across the anus, the tract of the fistula is usually a straight line terminating in the anal canal. Thus an anterior opening is usually associated with a radial tract. If the external opening is located more than 3 cm anterior to the transverse line, then the tract may curve posteriorly, terminating in the posterior midline.

- **Procedure.** If the fistula is simple and not deep, the fistulous tract can be excised in toto, leaving the wound open (Fig. 6).

Remember: the subcutaneous and the superficial external sphincter can be divided with impunity, but be very careful with the deep external sphincter and the puborectalis.

If the fistula is deep, the seton procedure is the treatment of choice (Fig. 7).

- Fistulas may be classified as:
  - Intersphincteric (70%)
  - Transsphincteric (25%)
  - Suprasphincteric (5%)
  - Extrasphincteric (<1%)
- Extrasphincteric fistulas are usually not associated with intersphincteric sepsis
- Consider inflammatory bowel diseases like Crohn's or ulcerative colitis and neoplasia

### Figure 5

Typical sites of anorectal fistulas and abscesses: (1) intersphincteric, (2) ischiorectal (transsphincteric), (3) extrasphincteric, (4) submucosal

### Figure 6

Laying open a subcutaneous fistula using a probe

### Figure 7

The seton procedure

Figure 5

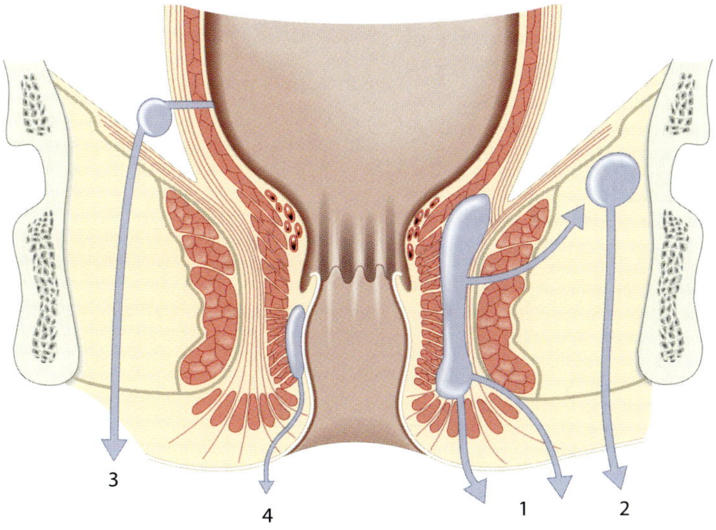


Figure 6

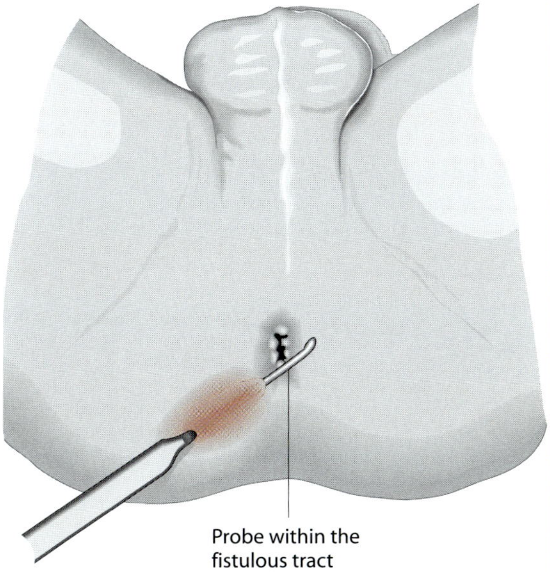


Figure 7

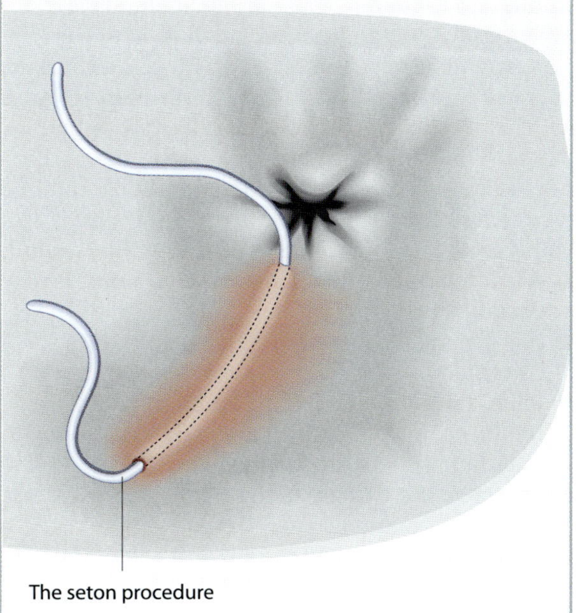

## EXCISION OF PILONIDAL SINUS

Sacrococcygeal pilonidal disease is a common and well recognized entity. For many years the cause of sacrococcygeal pilonidal sinus has been a matter of debate. With regard to treatment, there was a frequent lack of success following surgical excision with significant morbidity, delayed healing, recurrence and failure to heal or cure. Karydakis attributed the hair insertion process to three main factors: the invader, i.e. the loose hair; the force, which causes the insertion; and the vulnerability of the midline skin at the depth of the natal cleft to the insertion of hair. The sinus is initiated from a small midline opening lined by stratified squamous epithelium. Additional sinuses are frequent and have lateral openings. Options for treatment of an acute pilonidal abscess include aspiration, drainage without curettage, and drainage with curettage. The choice of a particular surgical approach depends on the surgeon's familiarity with the procedure and perceived results in terms of low recurrence and rapid healing of the resulting cavity or surgical wound. Conservative non-operative management, closed methods, laying open of any track, wide excision and open drainage, wide excision and primary closure, and limited excision are the methods currently in use. From the profusion of studies, it is apparent that various methods are still under evaluation and no one method is universally accepted. Recurrence rates vary with the technique, operator and length of follow-up. Primary closure with a lateral approach (Karydakis procedure or Bascom's modification) appears to give the best results (Fig. 8) because it produces a shallow midline furrow free from scar or suture holes which is less vulnerable to hair penetration than a midline wound.

- A pilonidal sinus is a subcutaneous sinus. It may contain hair.
- It is generally believed to be an acquired condition.
- Pilonidal sinuses are lined by granulation tissue rather than epithelium. They are also seen in interdigital clefts, face and axilla.
- Inflamed hair follicles in the cleft result in abscess or sinus formation.
- Hair becomes trapped in cleft and enters sinuses.
- Results in a foreign body reaction and perpetuates sinus formation.
- Usually seen in young adults.
- Eighty percent present with recurrent pain.
- Eighty percent present with a purulent discharge.
- Rare after the age of 40 years.
- Male: female ratio is 4 : 1.

### Figure 8A, B

Karydakis procedure – primary closure with a lateral approach – appears to give the best results for surgical treatment of sacrococcygeal pilonidal sinus

### Figure 9A, B

Patient position for pilonidal sinus surgery

Figure 8A

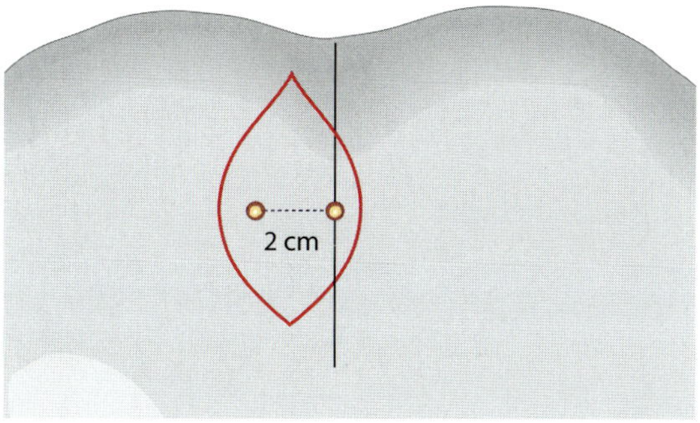


Figure 8B

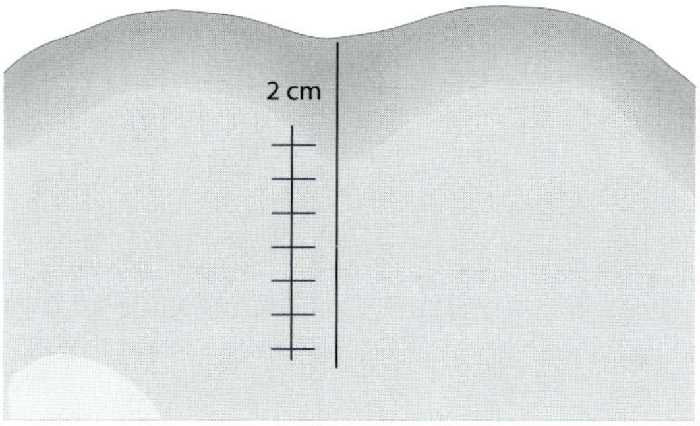


Figure 9A

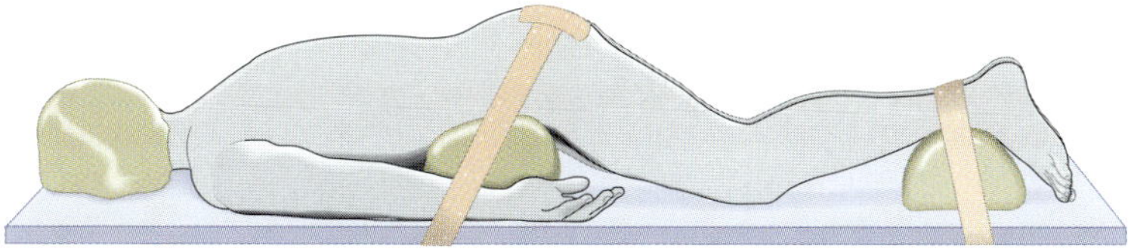

Figure 9B

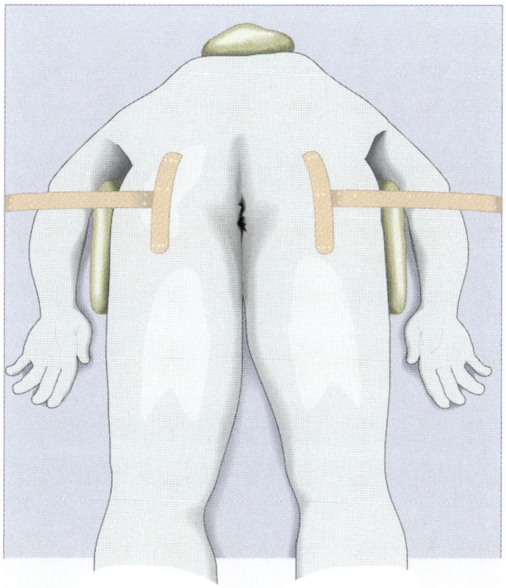

## Figure 10A: Exposure of the Sacral Area Using Tapes

## Figure 10B: Incision Over an Inserted Probe

Figure 10A

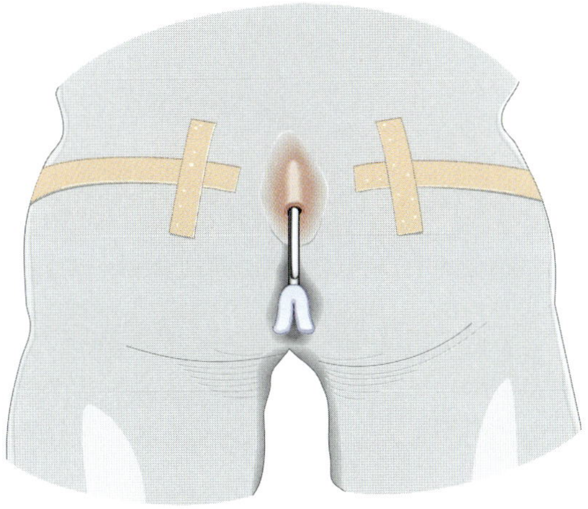

Figure 10B

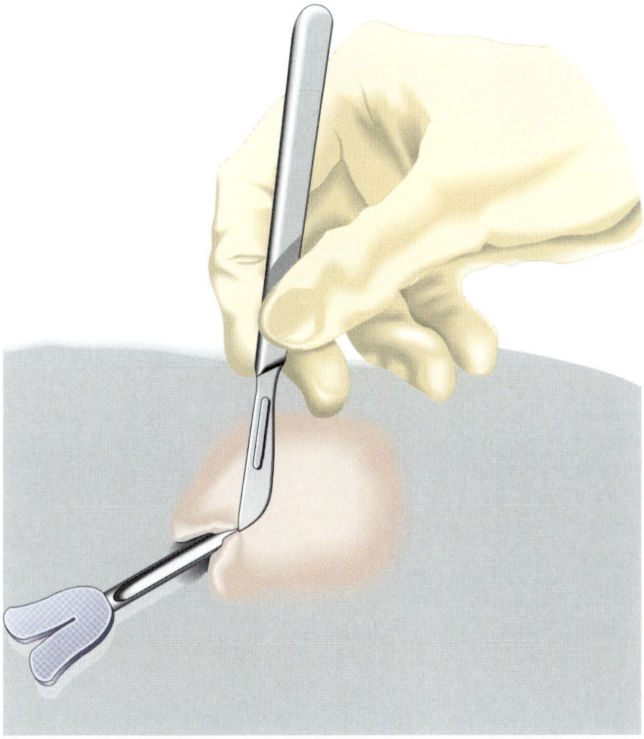

## Figure 11: Excision of a Pilonidal Sinus

Figure 11

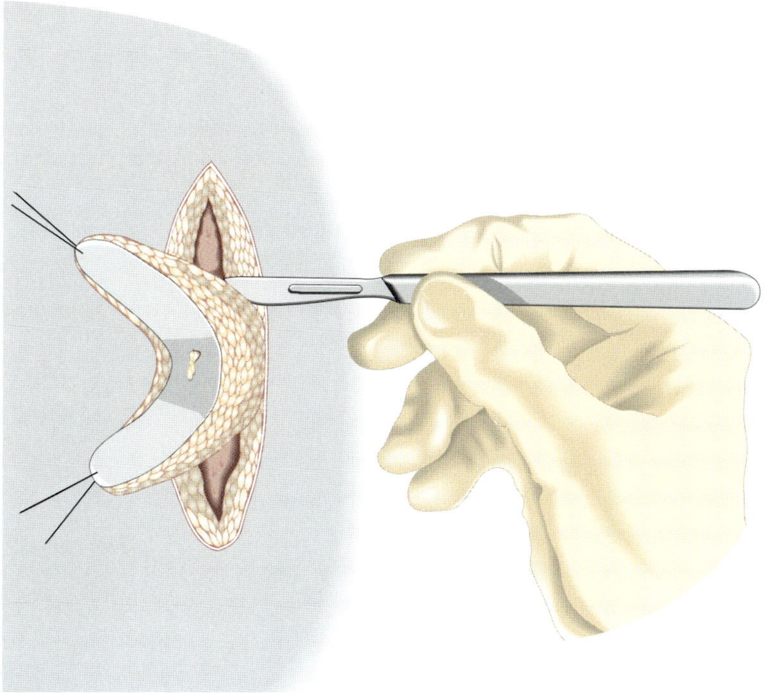

Table 2

| Procedure for pilonidal sinus | |
|---|---|
| Position | Laying face down |
| Preparation | Antibiotic prophylaxis may be of benefit |
| Anaesthesia | General or spinal |
| Procedure | 1. Fix extra large adhesive tape to both lower gluteal areas and perineum. Anchor the tape to the operating room table, separating the intergluteal fold (Fig. 9)<br>2. Probe the sinus gently, since occasionally it may travel laterally (Fig. 10). Consider methylene blue injection to identify all of the tracts. With an elliptical incision down to the fascia, remove the cyst and the sinuses en bloc and in toto, including subcutaneous tissue (Fig. 11)<br>3. After good haemostasis is established, pack the wound with iodoform gauze, or, if there is no infection, close the wound in one layer using 3–0 nylon with interrupted vertical mattress sutures, including the fascia<br>Excision and healing by secondary intention:<br>Requires regular wound dressing and shaving<br>Produces 70–90% healing at 70 days<br>Excision and primary closure:<br>Five to 15% recurrence rate after<br>Produces 70% healing at 2 weeks<br>Twenty percent develop wound infection<br>Skin flap procedures (e.g. Karydakis procedure; see Fig. 11) aim to flatten natal cleft and keep scar from midline. In expert hands this produces good results. Failure rates as low as 5% have been reported |

## SELECTED REFERENCES


Bascom JU (1994) Pilonidal sinus. Curr Pract Surg 6:175–180

Chintapatla S, Safarani N, Kumar S, Haboubi N (2003) Sacrococcygeal pilonidal sinus: historical review, pathological insight and surgical options. Tech Coloproctol 7(1):3–8

Duxbury MS, Blake SM, Dashfield A, Lambert AW (2003) A randomised trial of knife versus diathermy in pilonidal disease. Ann R Coll Surg Engl 85:405–407

Hughes F, Mehta S (2002) Anorectal sepsis. Hosp Med 63: 166–169

Khaira HS, Brown JH (1995) Excision and primary suture of pilonidal sinus. Ann R Coll Surg Eng 77:242–244

Kitchen PRB (1996) Pilonidal sinus: experience with the Karydakis flap. Br J Surg 83:1452–1455

McCourtney JS, Finlay IG (1995) Setons in the surgical management of fistula-in-ano. Br J Surg 82:448–452

Peterson S, Koch R, Stelzner S (2002) Primary closure techniques in chronic pilonidal sinus. A survey of the results of different surgical approaches. Dis Colon Rectum 45: 1458–1467

Senapati A, Cripps NPJ (2000) Pilonidal sinus. In: Johnson CD, Taylor I (eds) Recent advances in surgery, vol 23. Churchill Livingstone, Edinburgh, pp 33–42

Senapati A, Cripps NPJ, Thompson MR (2000) Bascom's operation in the day-surgical management of symptomatic pilonidal sinus. Br J Surg 87:1067–1070

Seow-Choen F, Nicholls RJ (1992) Anal fistula. Br J Surg 79: 197–205

Thomas P (1993) Decision making in surgery; acute anorectal sepsis. Br J Hosp Med 50:204–205

# Part V Urology

CHAPTER 16

# Vasectomy

**Vaithianathan Natarajan, Neil Oakley**

## INTRODUCTION

Bilateral scrotal vasectomy is a simple and effective operation to achieve permanent sterilisation in men. The operation is usually performed as a day case procedure under local anaesthesia.

Indications for formal exploration under general anaesthesia include:

- History of allergic reactions to local anaesthetic agents
- Anticipated difficulty at operation from factors such as obesity, previous scrotal surgery, or inability to palpate the vas preoperatively
- Patient preference

Pre-operative assessment of men requesting vasectomy should include:

1. Examination of the scrotum to determine that both vasa deferentia are palpable and no abnormality is evident in the testes.
2. Counselling to the effect that:
   - The procedure is intended to be permanent as although reversal is possible, its success is not certain.
   - Until informed otherwise by the surgeon, the patient should not assume the vasectomy has rendered him infertile and must continue to use alternate contraception. Confirmation that contraception may be discontinued requires the patient to provide a semen sample that is azoospermic. This is usually taken 16 weeks after surgery (and ideally after at least 24 ejaculations), and if viable sperm are still present is repeated at intervals.
   - There are two types of failure following vasectomy:
     Early – postsurgery semen analysis persistently fails to become azoospermic in 1:500 requiring a repeat vasectomy under GA.
     Late – despite azoospermia in postoperative semen analyses, in 1:2000 cases the man's partner will conceive. This results from late spontaneous recanalisation of the vas.
   - Besides immediate postoperative discomfort, chronic testicular or epididymal pain may complicate vasectomy in 1:4 patients. In the vast majority of patients, the pain is mild, transient and does not require intervention. In 2.2% of all vasectomy patients it may affect the quality of life sufficiently to warrant surgical intervention. The precise cause of such pain may be difficult to identify and the wide variety of operations employed (vasectomy reversal, excision of sperm granuloma, epididymectomy, denervation procedures and orchidectomy) indicate the surgical intervention is not always effective.
   - The overall immediate complication rate is low (5–8%), with haematoma (2%) and wound infection (3–12%) being the main complications in the early postoperative period.
   - Controversy surrounds the long term risk of prostate cancer, testicular cancer and cardiovascular disease following vasectomy but at present there is no conclusive evidence of substantially increased risk for any of these conditions following vasectomy.

Following counselling, a written, informed consent is taken documenting the above points.

■ **Technique.** The operation is performed with the patient in the supine position, in a theatre with warm ambient temperature to aid relaxation of the dartos muscle. Either a single midline incision or bilateral 1-cm transverse incisions in each hemiscrotum may be used. The scrotum, base of the penis and adjacent pubic hair should be shaved prior to the operation. Whether performed under local or general anaesthetic there is a small risk of bradycardia following a vasovagal reflex due to traction on the vas, and the resuscitation trolley must be available at all times.

## Figure 1

The key to successfully performing the operation is to locate the vas deferens on examination of the scrotum and to immobilise it between the forefinger and the middle finger of the surgeon's non-dominant hand over the pulp of the thumb. As the vas deferens lies posteriorly in the scrotum it is easier for a right-handed surgeon to stand at the right of the patient using the left hand to fix the vas. Once the vas deferens has been successfully palpated in the posterior scrotum it should be gently rolled round towards the anterior scrotal wall. The other cord structures will slip posteriorly leaving the vas isolated and fixed by the fingers superficially beneath the anterior scrotal wall.

The local anaesthetic is then infiltrated using 1% plain lignocaine. The first infiltration is a small skin bleb and through this the needle is inserted infiltrating local anaesthetic either side of the vas and then sliding the needle both proximally and distally alongside the vas keeping as close to it as possible to ensure instillation around the perivasal sheath.

## Figure 2

A 0.4-cm skin incision is then made with a number 15 blade at right angles to the vas deferens over the pulp of the operator's left thumb. The tips of small artery forceps are inserted through this and opened to develop access through the dartos muscle. The vas is then felt rolling under the tips of the forceps. These are inserted and opened on both sides of the vas along its length to create a small space.

## Figure 3

The vas ring is then inserted through the incision, the vas grasped and hinged upwards through the skin incision. The vas at this time cannot be pulled through the skin incision but can be tilted forward over the edge of the vas ring so that it appears as a small lump extending through the wound. An incision is made with a scalpel along the length of the vas as it arches over the edge of the vas ring. The incision should be a single incision through the perivasal facial layer. Multiple small incisions should be avoided as they cause false planes. The easiest way to avoid this is to make the first incision deep enough to incise the wall of the vas itself.

Figure 1

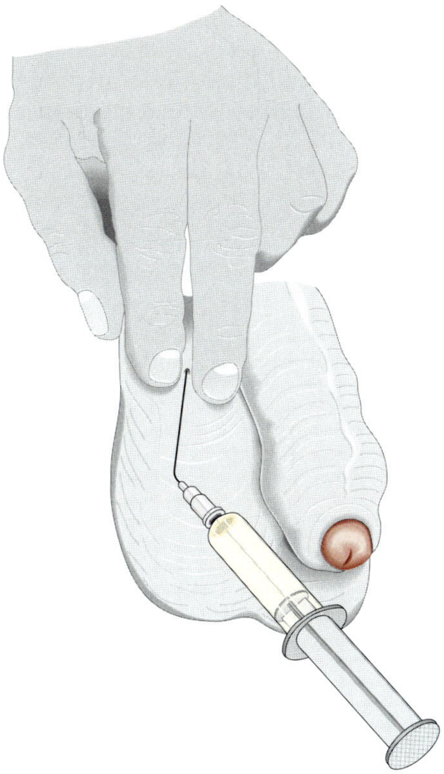

Figure 2

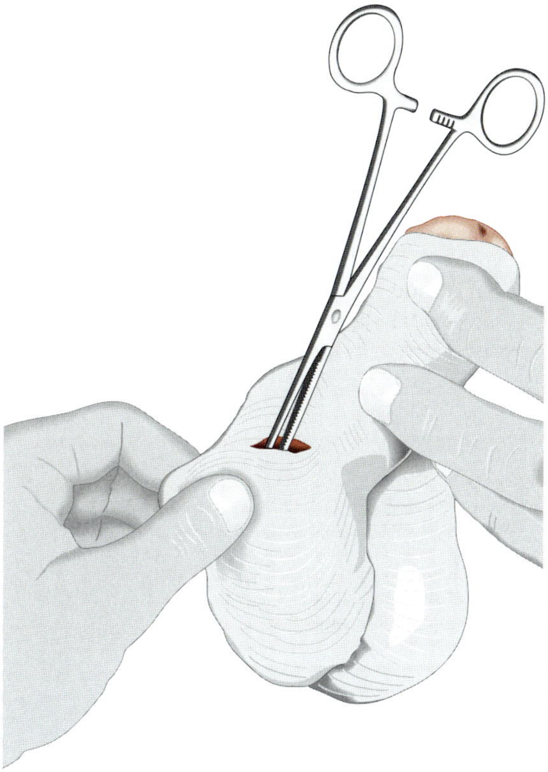

Figure 3

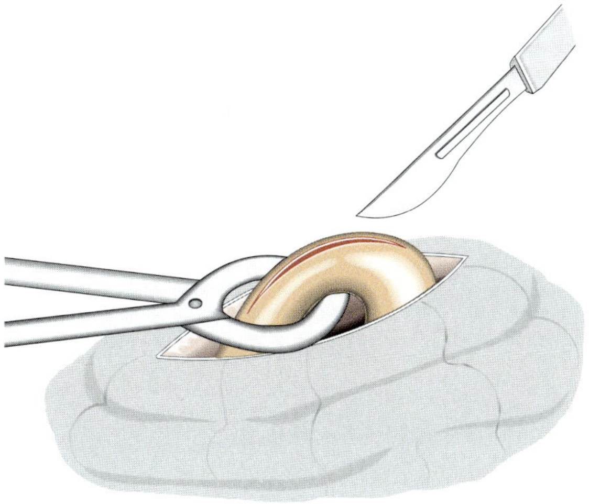

## Figure 4

The facial layers are then split apart with forceps and the tip of the artery forceps hooked between the facial layer and the vas in order to pull the vas up out of the wound in a loop. The apex of this loop is grasped with an artery clip and the fascia within the loop stripped down with forceps. Within this fascia is the artery to the vas and if the vas is properly exposed the artery will strip away without bleeding.

## Figure 5

The vas at the base of the now exposed loop is reclipped with artery forceps at the proximal and distal end and the intervening vas excised. Considerable debate exists over the treatment of the divided ends. Classically both ends have been ligated with absorbable suture and some have advocated then retying this suture proximally around the vas to essentially loop the vas. This can cause necrosis of the ends with a theoretical increased risk of early recanalisation. A recent change is to fulgurate the cut seminal end of the vas and to leave the testicular end open. The advantage of leaving this open is that a sperm granuloma will form which can lessen the risk of chronic pain syndrome; however, there is a potentially higher risk of failure of the vasectomy. If it is left open then the key manoeuvre is to release the vas whilst holding the facial sheath. The vas will retract into the scrotum and then the fascia sheath can be closed with an absorbable suture both for haemostatic purposes and to reduce the risk of re-canalisation. This skin is closed with a single mattress absorbable suture.

Figure 4

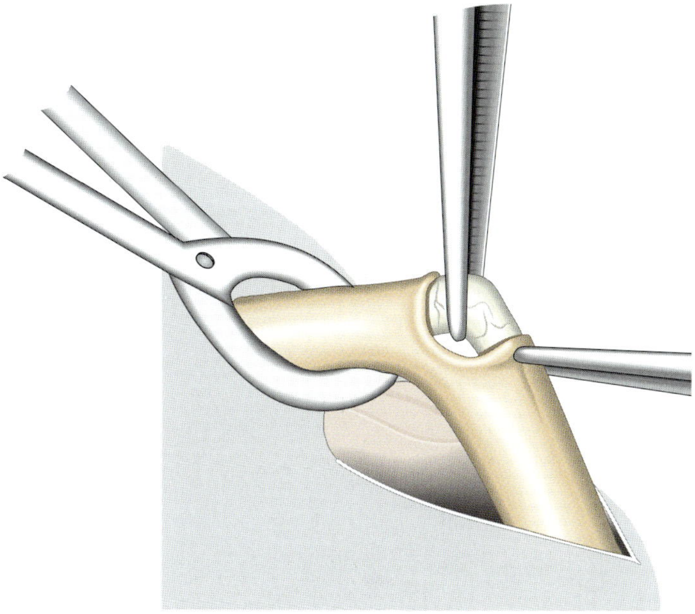

Figure 5

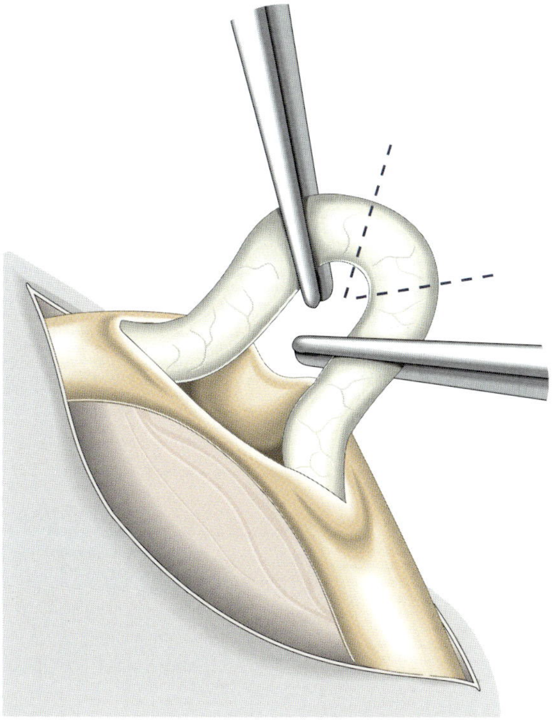

## SELECTED REFERENCES

Kendrick J, Gonzales B, Huber D et al. (1987) Complications of vasectomies in the United States. J Fam Pract 25:245–248
Labrecque M, Nazerali H, Mondor M, Fortin V, Nasution M (2002) Effectiveness and complications associated with 2 vasectomy occlusion techniques. J Urol 168(6):2495–2498
McConaghy P, Paxton LD, Loughlin V (1996) Chronic testicular pain following vasectomy. Br J Urol 77:328
McMahon AJ, Buckley J, Taylor A, Lloyd SN, Deane RF, Kirk D (1992) Chronic testicular pain following vasectomy. Br J Urol 69(2):188–191
Schwingl PJ, Guess HA (2000) Safety and effectiveness of vasectomy. Fertil Steril 73:923–936
Sokal D, McMullen S, Gates D, Dominik R (1999) The male sterilisation investigator team: A comparative study of the no scalpel and standard incision approaches to vasectomy in 5 countries. J Urol 162:1621–1625

CHAPTER 17

# Hydrocele

Vaithianathan Natarajan, Neil Oakley

## INTRODUCTION

A hydrocele is a collection of fluid in the tunica vaginalis of the testis and is one of the commonest scrotal pathologies. In its commonest form, a primary vaginal hydrocele is a cystic scrotal swelling, that is palpably inseparable from the testis and clearly transilluminates. It results from defective absorption of tunical fluid and therefore tends to be relatively large and tense. On the other hand, secondary hydroceles develop from excessive production of tunical fluid resulting from testicular pathology such as tumours, trauma and torsion. Since there is no defect in absorption of fluid from the tunical sac, these tend to be lax to palpate.

Non-surgical management of hydroceles by aspiration with or without sclerotherapy should only be attempted in patients unfit for anaesthesia, as this approach risks infection, recurrence and epididymal obstruction. The ideal management of symptomatic hydrocele in a fit patient is surgical. Whenever the underlying testis inside the hydrocele sac is clinically impalpable, ultrasonography is undertaken to rule out testicular pathology, especially tumours.

Surgical treatment of hydrocele is curative and recurrences are extremely uncommon. Wound infection and haematoma are rare complications preventable with careful haemostasis, wound drainage and scrotal support.

## Figure 1

A transverse scrotal skin incision is usually employed. The skin is prepared and towelled and the scrotum is grasped with the surgeon's non-dominant hand so that the hydrocele, testis and scrotum project from the fist, putting the scrotal skin under tension over the hydrocele. This compresses the small vessels in the scrotal skin and the subsequent incision is usually bloodless. The direction of the skin incision is made between and parallel to the visible vessels in the scrotal skin and is made 4–5 cm long in order to be able to deliver the testes. The incision is made through the skin, dartos muscle and areolar tissue initially with a knife and then with small curved scissors to avoid rupturing the tunica vaginalis.

Any bleeding from the wound edge or dartos muscle edge is controlled with bipolar diathermy.

## Figure 2

The tunica vaginalis is identified once the dartos fibres have been divided with scissors and at this point the dartos muscle is pushed gently off the tunica to expose it for a 5 cm length. A small incision is made in the tunica, which causes the hydrocele fluid under tension to squirt out and this is caught in a kidney dish. Once the hydrocele has been decompressed the edge of the small incision is grasped with artery forceps and a sucker inserted to aspirate the fluid to keep the operation site dry.

## Figure 3

The incision in the tunica is then enlarged to 5 cm and the testes squeezed from below, so this exteriorises through the defect of the tunica vaginalis and skin incision. This everts the sac (effectively turning the tunica sac inside out), leaving the superficial wall still attached to the dartos and fascia.

The testes is examined for signs of pathology.

The method of dealing with the tunica sac depends on the nature of the hydrocele.

Figure 1

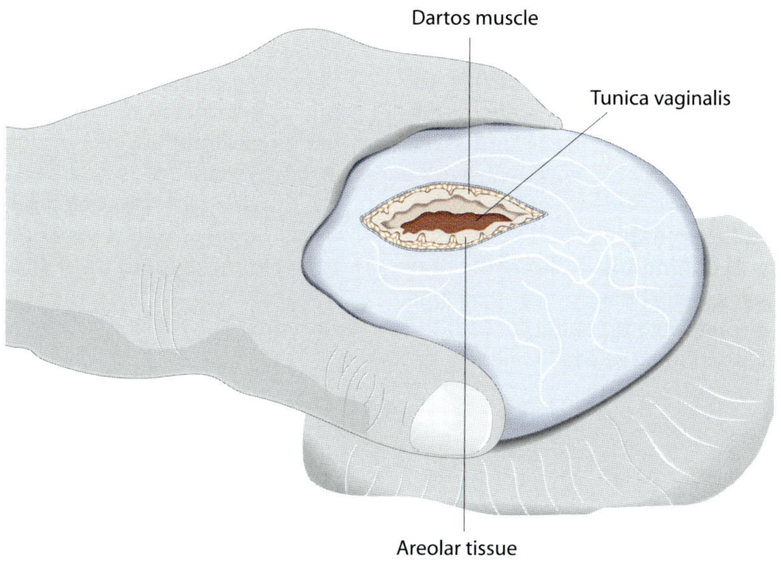


Figure 2

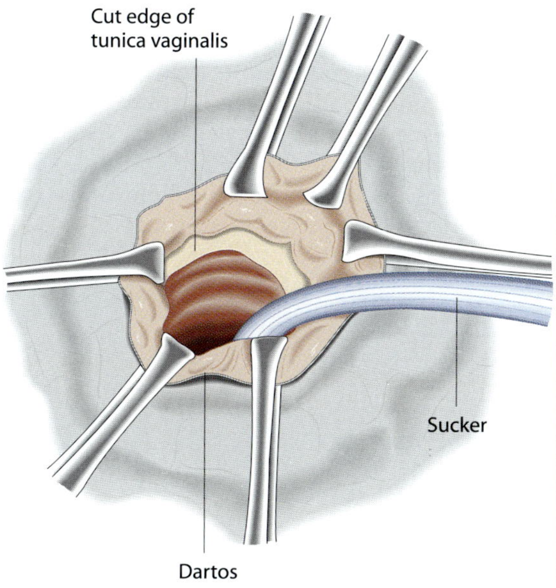


Figure 3

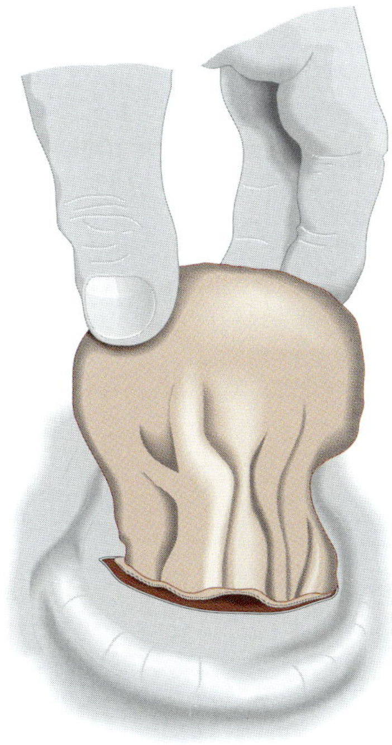

## Figure 4

1. Sac excision. In long-standing, thick walled or multiloculated sacs
   Once the hydrocele has been decompressed the cut edges are grasped by artery forceps. Using these as retractors the dartos muscle and fascia are stripped off the tunica by pushing away with a swab and sharp dissection. The sac is then excised to about 1 cm from the epididymis and a circumferential haemostatic running suture along the tunical cut margins using absorbable 3/0 suture is performed. Wound drainage would be required if this technique were applied to large hydroceles.

## Figure 5

2. Jaboulay procedure. If the sac is large but thin walled.
   Following eversion the testis is held in the air leaving a symmetrical curtain of tunica vaginalis hanging around it. This tunica vaginalis is not excised, but closure of the free margins behind the epididymis and the cord with 3/0 running haemostatic sutures is performed. Care should be taken to avoid strangulation of the cord by leaving an adequate gap between the tunical suture line and the cord.

## Figure 6

3. Lord's procedure. In moderate sized thin sacs.
   Radial plication of the opened sac wall achieves the same effect as the Jaboulay procedure without risking vascular compromise of the cord. As before the testes is held up leaving a curtain of tunica. This is gathered into a ruff by inserting a series of interrupted absorbable sutures picking up the tunica with 1-cm bites. These sutures are only tied once all are in place.

The advantage of the plication techniques over the excision technique is that they requires less dissection and hence less risk of haematoma. The disadvantage is that because the tunica is not freed from the dartos the plication effectively removes the scrotal cavity in which the testes was sitting.

Figure 4

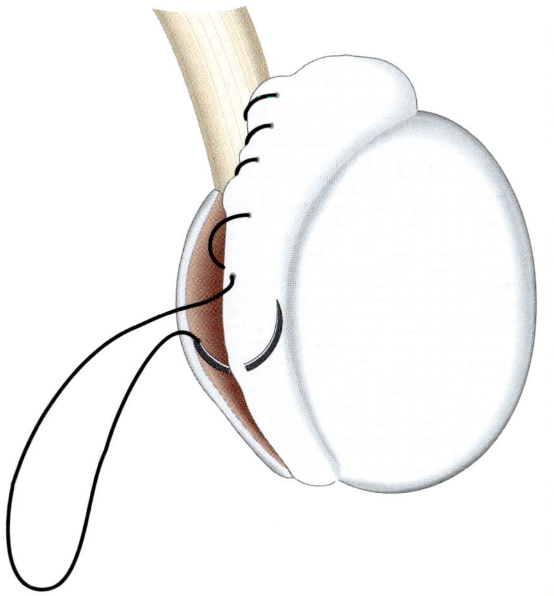

Figure 5

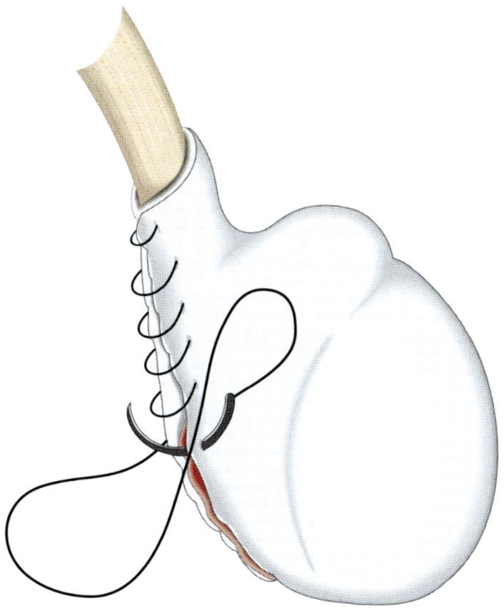

Figure 6

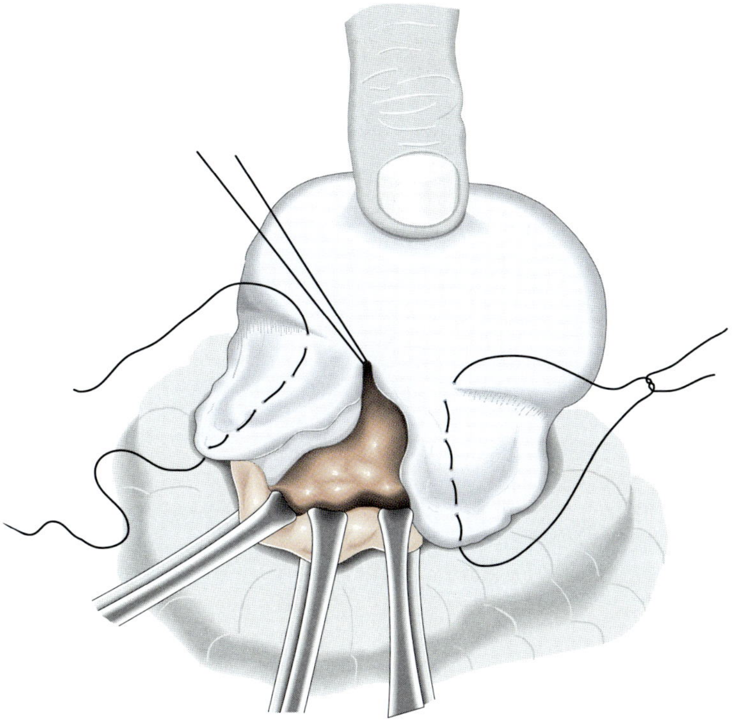

## Figure 7

Replacement of the testes within the scrotum can therefore be the most difficult part of the procedure. The key is to hold the edges of the dartos at the skin incision with four clips and to exert pressure on the dome of the testes, pushing it back into the scrotum so the dartos muscle then closes over the testes. The incision is then closed in two layers. Firstly the forceps are applied to either end of the incision and these stretch the incision line so that the testes cannot be seen but the dartos is easily opposed with a continuous 3/0 absorbable suture. The skin edges and subcutaneous tissue are then closed with a separate suture line picking up both skin edges and subcutaneous tissue with a continuous haemostatic over and over suture utilising undyed absorbable suture.

Figure 7

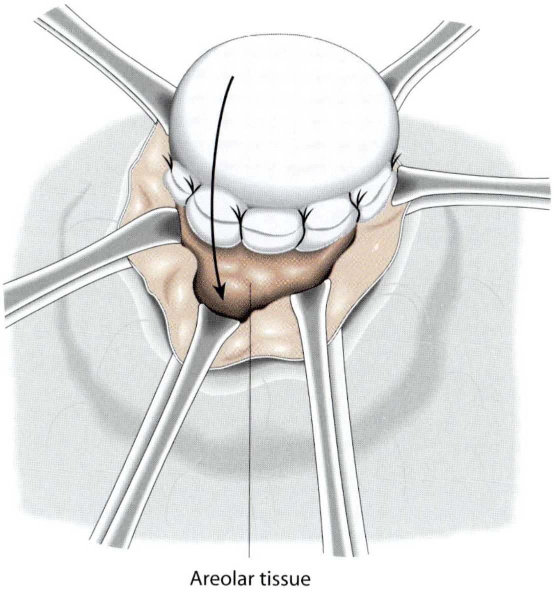

CHAPTER 18

# Epididymal Cyst/Epididymectomy

Vaithianathan Natarajan, Neil Oakley

## INTRODUCTION

### Epididymal Cysts

Epididymal cysts are the commonest intrascrotal cystic swellings and are invariably benign. The incidence increases with age and the commonest site is the caput epididymidis. The vast majority are asymptomatic and indications for surgery are uncommon but can include pain or cosmesis. Surgical extirpation of these cysts risks epididymal obstruction and should not be taken lightly in patients who may want to father children. Recurrence following cyst excision is very common due to the nature of the epididymis. Excision of the whole epididymal gland prevents this but with the consequence of causing irreversible unilateral testicular obstruction.

### Epididymal Cyst Excision

■ **Technique.** The cyst is usually a spermatocele arising as a tiny cyst at the head of the epididymis. As these gradually increase in size they carry their blood supply and push to one side the areolar tissues of the scrotum. This means there is usually a plane of cleavage between the wall of the cyst and the tissues of the scrotum.

The key to successful excision of the cyst is to try and remove the cyst as a whole so as not to leave residual wall behind. Therefore one must avoid incising the cyst wall unintentionally.

## Figure 1

The skin is incised over the cyst parallel to the skin vessels. The incision is deepened through the layer of the dartos using forceps and scissors. As the cyst is approached one can see a bluish hue over which will be very fine layers of fascia containing thin vessels. Each fine layer of fascia should be picked up with blunt forceps and incised with scissors so the epididymal cyst itself is exposed. The small bleeding vessels in each layer need to be coagulated with bipolar diathermy.

## Figure 2

As the incision between the facial layers is extended it is usually possible to gently manipulate the thin walled cyst out of the skin incision. The layers of fascia should be gently pushed away with a combination of fine sharp dissection and gentle stripping and this will leave the cyst attached at its base to the epididymis. If the cyst is inadvertently opened during the procedure it is best to put a small artery forceps across the opening to try and keep fluid within the cyst to aid the dissection.

Figure 1

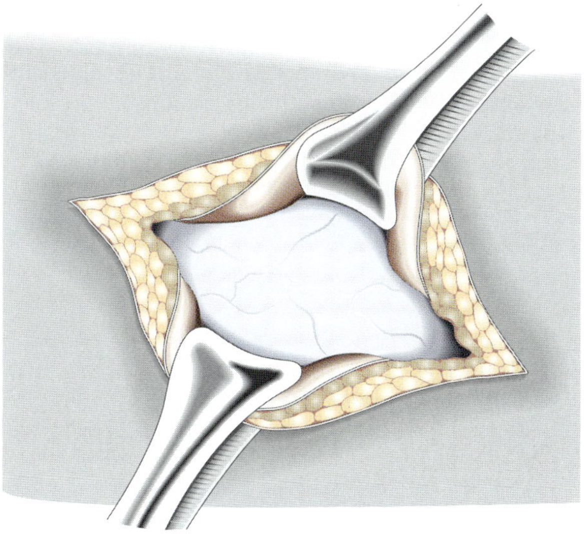

Figure 2

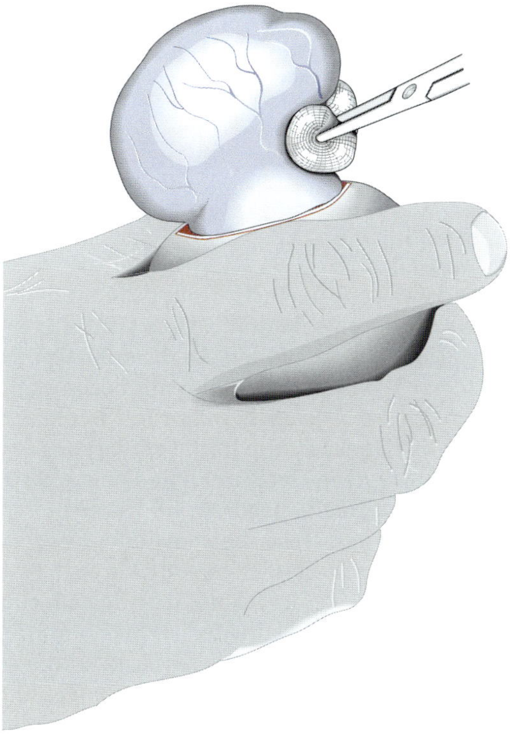

## Figure 3

Once the cyst is exposed, multiple small cysts will often be found around its base accompanied by fine vessels arising from the epididymis extending into the cyst. The pedicle needs to be cross-clamped and tied with an absorbable ligature. The wound is closed in layers as for hydrocele. As for all scrotal operations the patient should have a scrotal support applied postoperatively and be allowed to shower after 24 h and bathe after 3 days.

## Figure 4

## Epididymectomy

The scrotal skin, dartos and tunica vaginalis are incised as for a hydrocele repair. Care must be taken so as not to damage the testicle, which lies in close proximity to the tunica vaginalis as the hydrocele sac contains little fluid. The testis will be delivered through the incision in the tunica vaginalis and skin. The assistant holds the testis while artery forceps are applied to the head of the epididymis. The tail and body of the epididymis are closely applied to the testis but the head can be gently retracted away from the testis leaving an obvious plane of cleavage. This plane of cleavage contains the rete testis surrounded by tunica. This layer of tunica is incised close to the epididymis and with traction between the testis and the epididymis the fibrous bands between epididymis and testis are divided with fine scissors and any bleeding controlled with bipolar cautery. It is important that the incision of the tunica stays close to the epididymis at all times so as not to cause damage to the testicular artery. Any epididymal cyst is excised from the areolar tissue as previously described but without freeing it from the epididymis. The dissection of the epididymis from the testis proceeds towards the body and tail. As the tail is approached (particularly where the epididymis becomes the convoluted vas) it is especially important to make sure that dissection keeps close to the epididymis as the cord structures lie in close proximity. The reflection of the tunica vaginalis needs to be incised to trace the convoluted vas. Once the convoluted vas has been reached, this will be the final attachment of the epididymis and therefore it should be ligated with 3/0 absorbable suture and divided at this point.

The testis is replaced within the scrotum by clipping and lifting the cut edges of the tunica vaginalis with artery forceps reducing the testis into this sac. Care must be taken to ensure the cord is not twisted in order to prevent torsion. The tunica vaginalis is closed with continuous absorbable sutures.

Closure of the dartos and skin is as described previously.

Figure 3

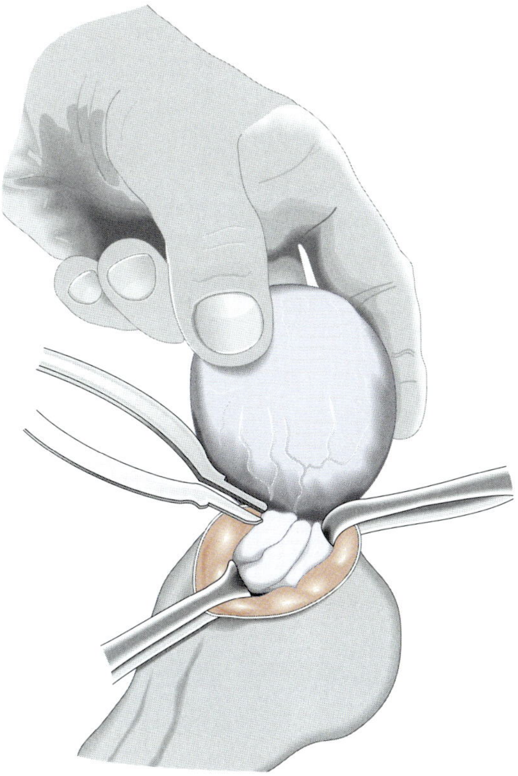

Figure 4

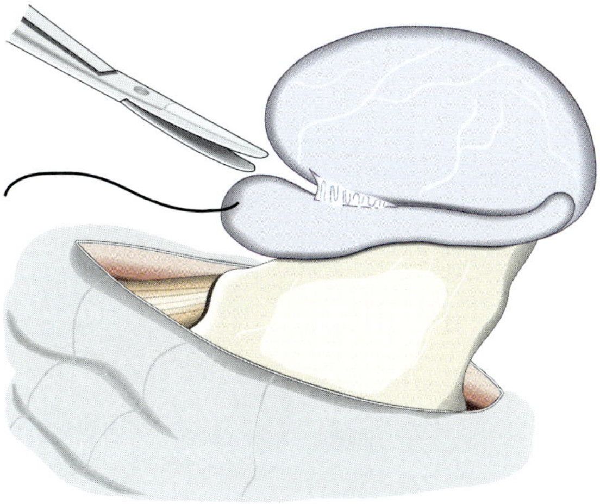

# CHAPTER 19 Varicocelectomy

Vaithianathan Natarajan, Neil Oakley

## INTRODUCTION

Varicoceles are present in approximately 15% of the population and are left sided in 90%. The indications for surgical intervention for varicoceles in the adult include pain and infertility whilst in the adolescent the role of intervention is to prevent testicular atrophy and non-development. Subclinical varicoceles detected on colour Doppler alone do not merit treatment.

Treatment options include vascular embolisation or surgical division. Embolisation has a success rate in the order of 80% but requires radiological expense and expertise.

Conventional open surgical options include a high retroperitoneal approach in which all the testicular vessels are ligated en masse or a lower selective approach (inguinal or subinguinal) which is used to spare the testicular arteries and lymphatics. The high approach is easier as there are fewer veins and it does not run the risk of testicular atrophy by damaging vasal collateral arteries. The low approaches involve ligation of multiple veins encountered at this level and, particularly in the subinguinal approach, carries a risk of damage to the testicular arterial supply (multiple branches of the testicular artery are intertwined with veins of the pampiniform plexus). These approaches involve exposure of the spermatic cord through the inguinal canal or just distal to the external inguinal ring. The subinguinal approach, which is technically more difficult, is preferred in those with prior inguinal surgery and in obese patients and should be performed with the aid of an operating microscope.

## RETROPERITONEAL APPROACH: PALOMO PROCEDURE

This involves ligation of the testicular veins just above the deep inguinal ring. At this level there are two to three veins and the testicular artery may be separable from the veins even though this is not routinely attempted because of the potential distal collateral supply from the cremasteric and vasal arteries.

## Figure 1

A 5–6 cm skin crease incision is made 3 cm medial to the anterior superior iliac spine. The external oblique aponeurosis is divided along the line of its fibres and the deeper muscles are then split. Sweeping the peritoneum medially exposes the retroperitoneal space just above and lateral to the deep inguinal ring. The inferior epigastric vessels are identified deep to the transversalis fascia. The spermatic vessels can be seen running laterally and superiorly from the deep inguinal ring whilst the vas can be seen running medially and inferiorly.

## Figure 2

The vas and its surrounding vessels are not exposed but the testicular vessels are exposed as high as possible and the internal testicular veins and lymphatics are ligated en masse and divided. There is sufficient blood supply via the artery to the vas to maintain the viability of the testes as long as the surrounding tissue is not dissected. After ensuring haemostasis, the aponeurosis is closed with a 2–0 absorbable suture and the skin with subcuticular monofilament suture material.

Figure 1

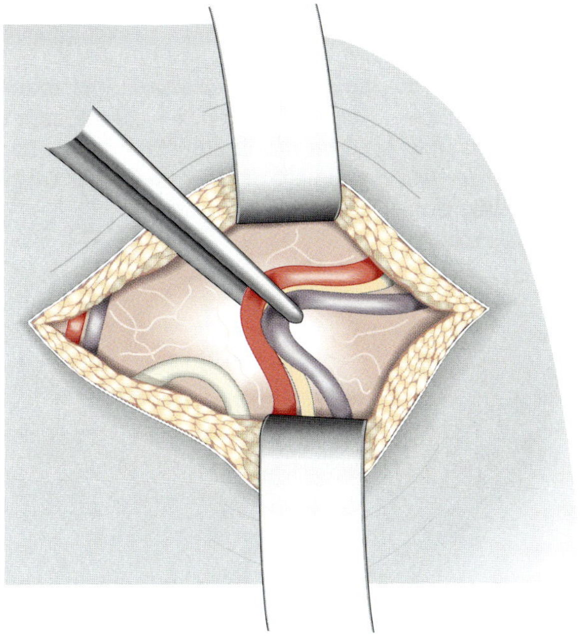

Figure 2

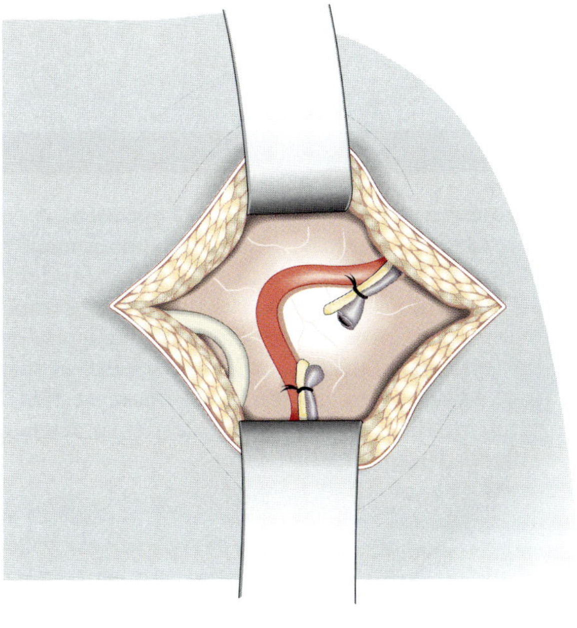

## INGUINAL APPROACH

### Figure 3

A 5–10 cm skin crease incision is made, 1.5–2 cm above and parallel to the inguinal ligament. The incision is deepened through Camper's and Scarpa's fascia, controlling the larger subcutaneous veins with fine ligatures. The inguinal canal is opened by division of the external oblique aponeurosis along the direction of its fibres, taking care to identify and preserve the ilioinguinal nerve. The cord is mobilised and held in a hernia ring or surgical tape to allow retraction.

### Figure 4

The table is tilted with the head raised 5–10 degrees to fill the spermatic veins. The cremasteric fascia is divided and the cord contents exposed. Veins of the pampiniform plexus are gently dissected free from the vas and individually ligated and divided. An attempt is made to identify and preserve the testicular artery and, if possible, the lymphatics. Any additional veins running parallel to the cord or piercing the posterior wall of inguinal canal are similarly dealt with. At the end of the procedure, only the vas with its blood supply, testicular artery and lymphatics should remain in the inguinal canal. After ensuring haemostasis, the wound is closed in layers using absorbable suture material.

■ **Subinguinal Approach.** A 3–4 cm oblique or transverse skin incision is made below and medial to the external inguinal ring and the cord structures are delivered after division of Camper's and Scarpa's fasciae. The remaining steps are essentially similar to the inguinal approach except that the number of testicular veins are more at this level and the finer branches of the testicular artery are more difficult to identify.

Figure 3

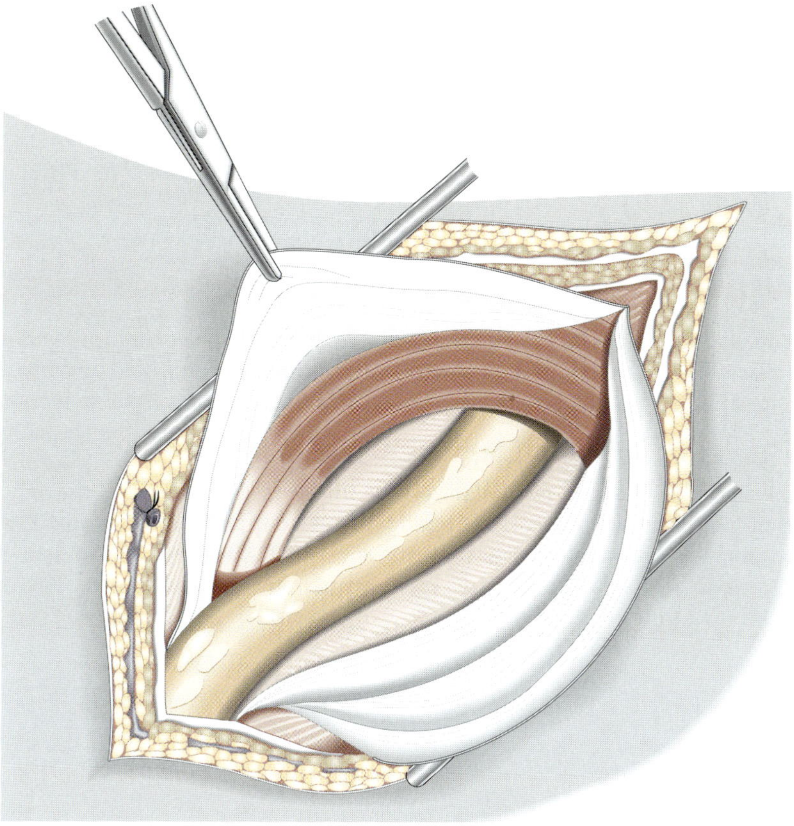

Figure 4

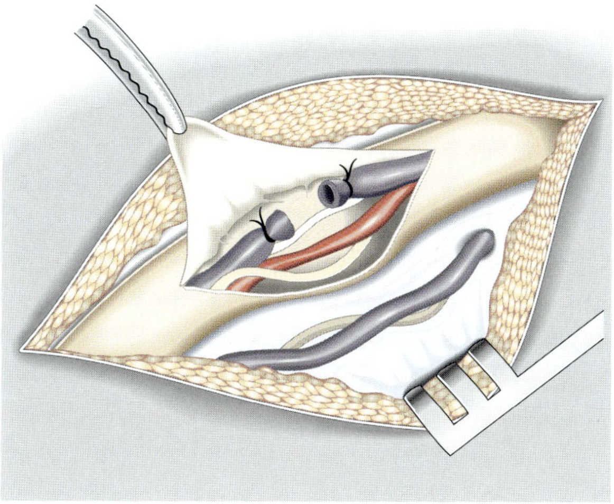

## LAPAROSCOPIC APPROACH

The patient's bladder is emptied and he is positioned supine with a 20-degree left lateral tilt side. The surgeon stands at the right side of the patient with the monitor at the patient's feet.

Three laparoscopic ports are inserted, one 10 mm at the umbilicus for the laparoscope, a 10-mm port in the midline halfway between the pubis and umbilicus and one 5 mm at the left side of the rectus sheath lateral to the umbilicus. Adhesions between the sigmoid colon and the lateral pelvic wall are taken down with sharp dissection until the vas and testicular vessels are seen entering the deep inguinal ring.

## Figure 5

Knowledge of the anatomy is important as the testicular vessels form one side of the 'triangle of doom' along with the ureter and vas, which contains the external iliac vessels.

In the original descriptions a 'T'-shaped incision was made in the peritoneum over the testicular vessels. These were then mobilised and the veins clipped but the artery left intact. The vas deferential vessels were then exposed and divided as were any veins visible at the medial end of the inguinal ligament. However, this is time consuming and due to spasm the artery was only identified and protected in 60–80% of patients. A more simple is to reproduce the Palomo approach and divide the testicular vessels en masse. After the 'T' incision is made the testicular vessel bundle is grasped with the left hand grasper and double clipped with a 10-mm applicator via the midline port. Care must be taken to avoid the nerve which lies on the psoas. The vessels are divided between the clips but the vas is left undisturbed.

Figure 5

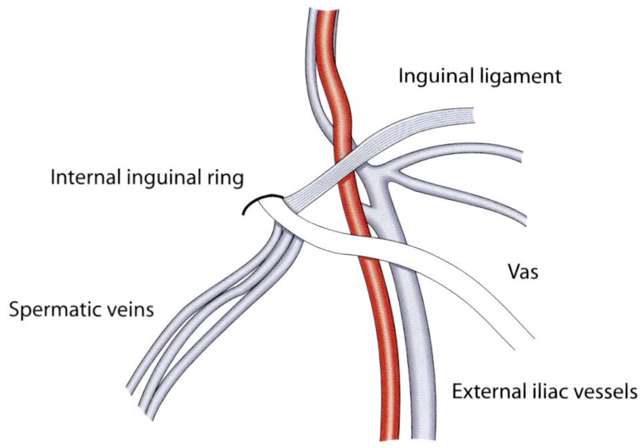
Inguinal ligament
Internal inguinal ring
Vas
Spermatic veins
External iliac vessels

## CONCLUSION

In experienced hands there is a low chance of recurrence but the retroperitoneal approach, when compared to the low approach, has a reputation for having a higher risk of hydrocele formation (up to 10% vs 5%) but lower recurrence rate (<10% vs 15%). The incidence of testicular arterial injury with the low approach is 14% except when microsurgical dissection techniques are used with the subinguinal approach.

The laparoscopic approach was developed initially to utilise the advantages of a high approach with a lower morbidity as well as offering the advantage of magnification to aid testicular artery preservation. Wound complications from the laparoscopic approach are seen in <1% of cases.

The need for preservation of the testicular artery in the high approach is debatable. In adult series in which comparisons were made between a laparoscopic artery-sparing approach or en masse division, no difference in semen parameters or Doppler resistive index was seen. In one series the selective approach had a failure rate on venography of 39% vs 6% if the testicular vessels were divide en masse. In the paediatric population there seems to be little difference in the chance of atrophy if the testicular artery is divided or not; however, division of all the vessels en masse has a lower incidence of recurrence (2–8%).

The effect on fertility from varicocele ligation is debatable. In infertile men the prevalence increases to up to 40% and clinically evident varicocele is associated with alterations in sperm density, motility and morphology. Varicocelectomy is known to improve these semen parameters in up to 50%, but studies comparing fertility in men with treated and untreated varicoceles, however, have shown that improvement in fertility with varicocelectomy is not evident.

## SELECTED REFERENCES

Esposito C, Monguzzi G, Gonzalez-Sabin MA, Rubino R, Montinaro L, Papparella A, Esposito G, Settimi A, Mastroianni L, Zamparelli M, Sacco R, Amici G, Damiano R, Innaro N (2001) Results and complications of laparoscopic surgery for pediatric varicocele. J Pediatr Surg 36(5):767–769

Fisch H (1991) The surety of surgical repair of varicocoeles. Contemp Urol 3:69–74

Jarow JP, Assimos DG, Pittaway DE (1993) Effectiveness of laparoscopic varicocelectomy. Urology 42(5):544–547

Kass EJ, Marcol B (1992) Results of varicocele surgery in adolescents: a comparison of techniques. J Urol 148(2):694–696

Kattan S (2001) The impact of internal spermatic artery ligation during laparoscopic varicocelectomy on recurrence rate and short post operative outcome. Scand J Urol Nephrol 35(3):218–221

Lenk S, Fahlenkamp D, Gliech V, Lindeke A (1994) Comparison of different methods of treating varicocele. J Androl 15 Suppl:34S–37S

Podkamenev VV, Stalmakhovich VN, Urkov PS, Solovjev AA, Iljin VP (2002) Laparoscopic surgery for pediatric varicoceles: Randomized controlled trial. J Pediatr Surg 37(5):727–729

Student V, Zatura F, Scheinar J, Vrtal R, Vrana J (1998) Testicle hemodynamics in patients after laparoscopic varicocelectomy evaluated using color Doppler sonography. Eur Urol 33(1):91–93

Varlet F, Becmeur F (2001) Laparoscopic treatment of varicoceles in children. Multicentric prospective study of 90 cases. Eur J Pediatr Surg 11(6):399–403

CHAPTER 20

# Circumcision and Frenuloplasty

Vaithianathan Natarajan, Neil Oakley

## CIRCUMCISION: INTRODUCTION

Circumcision is one of the oldest surgical operations, dating back to the Egyptian Pharaohs, and probably initially performed to prevent irritative balanitis in a hot, sandy environment. Religious circumcision performed neonatally or in infancy, as practiced by Jews, Muslims, Coptic Christians of Ethiopia, Bushmen of the Kalahari and Australian Aborigines, reflects similar geoclimatic origins of their forebears.

"Routine" circumcision, mainly practiced in the North American continent, aims to prevent urinary infections and its consequences in male infants and penile carcinoma. The role of circumcision in prevention of HIV transmission is controversial.

The vast majority of circumcisions performed on adults in the Western world, however, are for established medical conditions such as symptomatic phimosis, recurrent paraphimosis and recurrent balanoposthitis as well as for carcinoma of the penis confined to the preputial skin.

Care should be exercised before making the clinical diagnosis of phimosis in children, as physiological non-retractile foreskin with an adherent prepuce can mimic true phimosis [fibrotic constriction of the preputial orifice, usually by balanitis xerotica obliterans (BXO)]. BXO is rarely seen in preschool children but a non-retractile foreskin is present in 95% of term babies. This can cause ballooning of the foreskin during micturition or balanoposthitis. Neither of these is an indication for circumcision in a child, for if left untreated, over 95% become retractile by adolescence.

Devices such as the Plastibell and Gemco clamp are employed exclusively for neonatal circumcision. In older boys and adults, the technique of sleeve resection or freehand circumcision is most commonly used.

The operation of frenuloplasty is only indicated for a tight frenulum that results in recurrent tears, pain, and fibrosis, associated with sexual intercourse. Frenuloplasty is only effective in about 50% of these men; the remainder are best served by circumcision to produce lasting symptom relief.

Contraindications to circumcision include hypospadias, ammonia dermatitis in infants and buried penis.

■ **Technique.** Although circumcision is possible under local anaesthetic penile block, this can be incomplete and general or spinal anaesthesia is preferred:

There are many techniques of circumcision but the key to a successful outcome is to ensure:

1. Sufficient preputial skin is removed to prevent future adhesions
2. Care is taken not to remove too much skin
3. Sufficient inner preputial mucosa is left attached to the corona for cosmesis and sensation
4. The anastomosis is symmetrical
5. The frenulum is not shortened

The simplest and most accurate way to ensure this is to perform incisions with a scalpel at the correct level on both the inner preputial mucosa and the outer preputial skin and to join these by dividing through.

## Figure 1

The penis is thoroughly prepared with aqueous antiseptic. In order to get the correct level of incision for the circumcision the glans must first of all be fully freed from the foreskin since often, especially in cases of chronic phimosis, there will be multiple adhesions between the foreskin and the glans.

The foreskin is retracted over the glans and any adhesions between the two are broken down with a combination of sharp dissection and pushing the foreskin back off the glans with a swab so that eventually the subcoronal sulcus can be fully exposed.

## Figure 2

If retracting the foreskin proves difficult due to the phimosis, this can be ruptured by carefully inserting haemostats between the glans and foreskin through the preputial meatus and forcibly opening them. Once the glans has been fully exposed it is re-prepped with the aqueous solution.

**Figure 1**

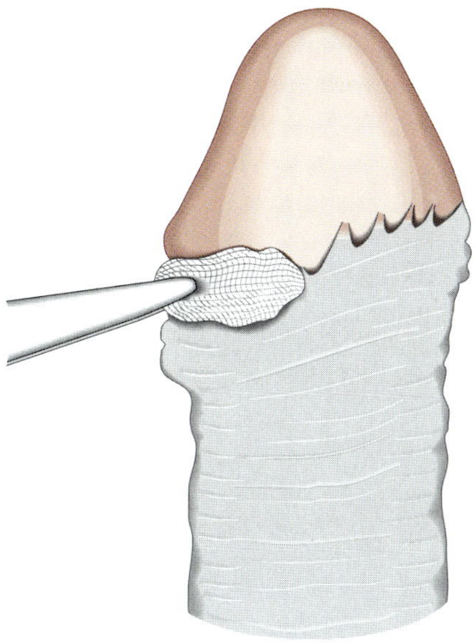

**Figure 2**

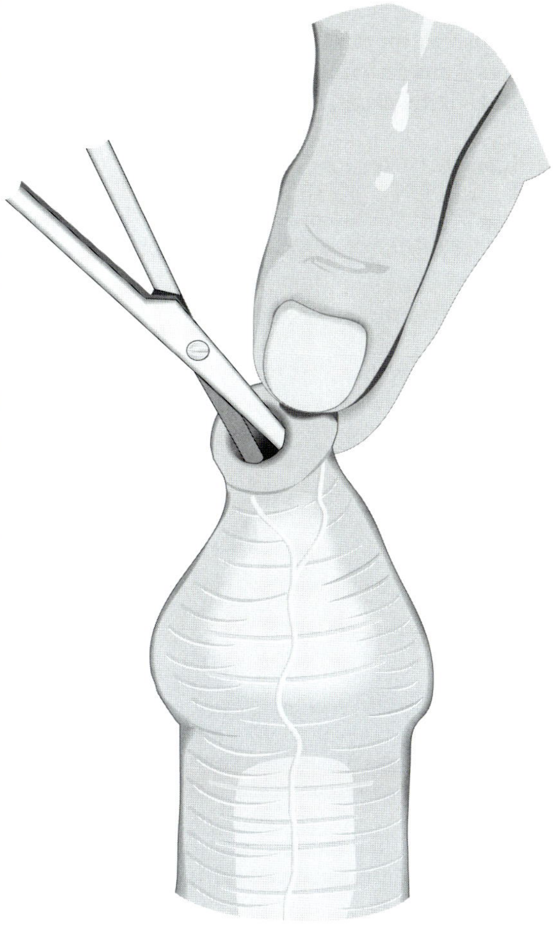

## Figure 3A, B

The shaft of the penis is gripped and proximal traction is placed on the skin. A circumferential scalpel incision is made though the preputial mucosa 1 cm proximal to the glans. The edges of the incised mucosa will spring apart when the correct plane is reached. The frenular artery may bleed and requires suture ligation with 4/0 absorbable suture.

## Figure 4A, B

The foreskin is then reduced over the glans. The shaft of the penis is lightly gripped, which causes the glans to advance slightly. A circumferential scalpel incision is then made through the skin at the level of the glans corona.

Figure 3A

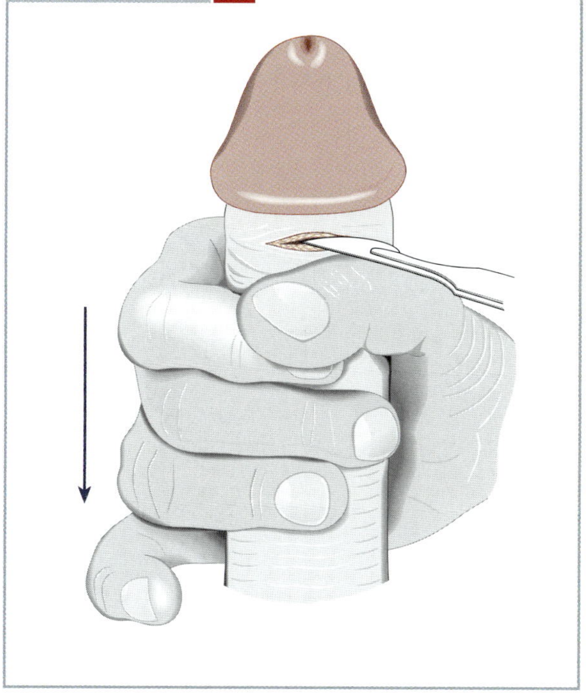

Figure 3B

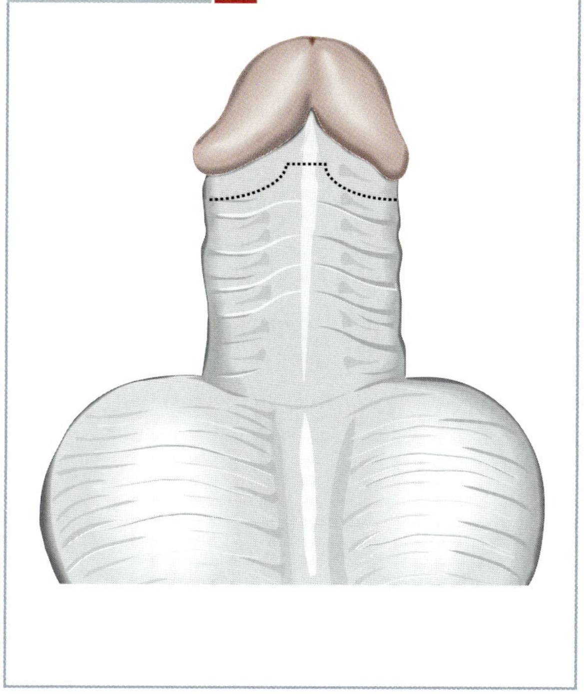

Figure 4A

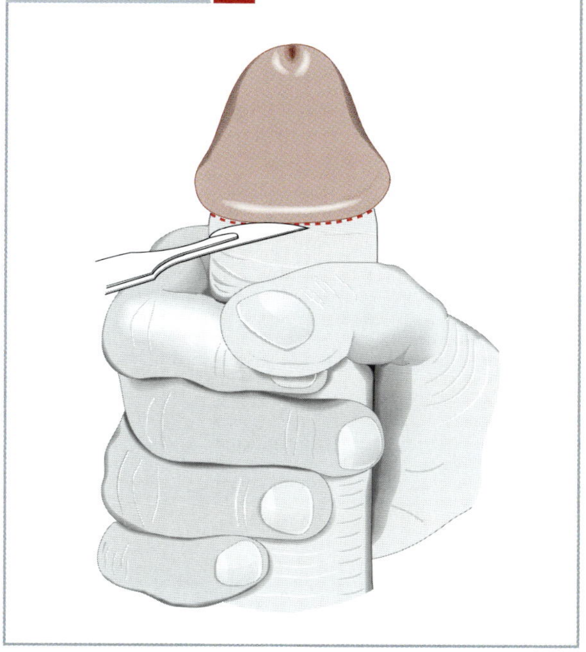

Figure 4B

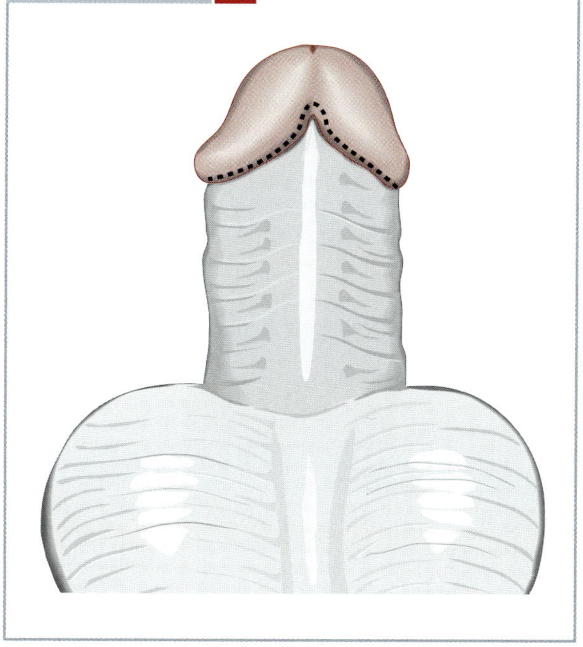

## Figure 5A, B

Haemostat clips are placed on the edges of the preputial meatus and traction is applied. The skin is cut with scissors on the ventral and dorsal aspect until both circumferential incisions are reached. This leaves two 'wings', which are excised by either scissors or scalpel along the inner and outer incision line.

## Figure 6A, B

The penile skin is then retracted and haemostasis is controlled by a combination of absorbable ligature and bipolar diathermy. The anastomosis is performed with interrupted undyed absorbable sutures. The first two are placed at the opposite dorsal and ventral aspects of the anastomosis line and held up for retraction. This brings the anastomosis together correctly to be completed by a series of interrupted sutures. A Vaseline gauze dressing over the suture line, while notoriously difficult to retain, helps the patient to direct the stream of urine in the initial postoperative period. It is our practice to routinely send the preputial skin for histology, both to confirm BXO and to rule out any unsuspected malignancy.

Figure 5A

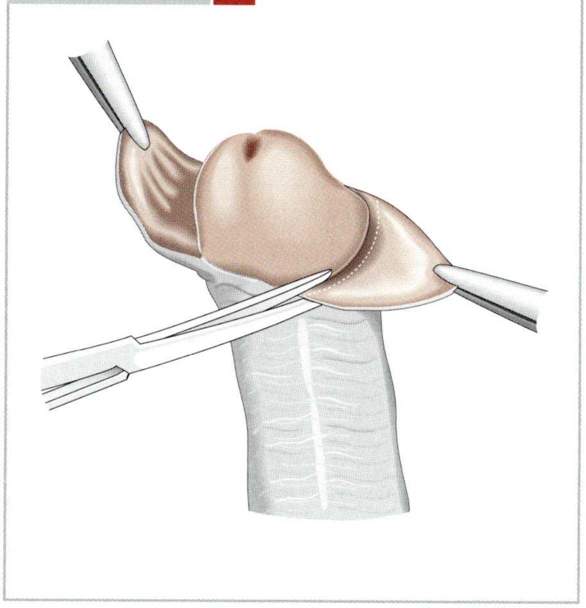

Figure 5B

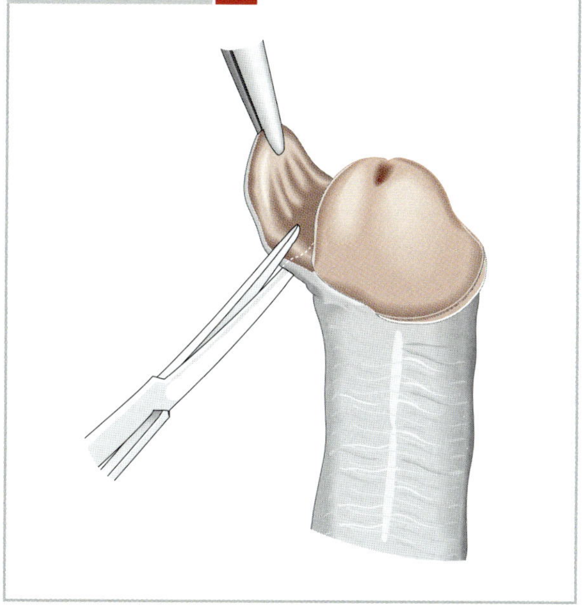

Figure 6A

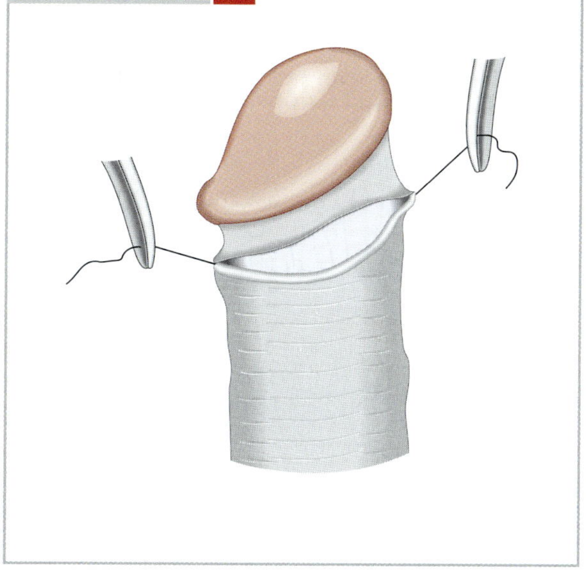

Figure 6B

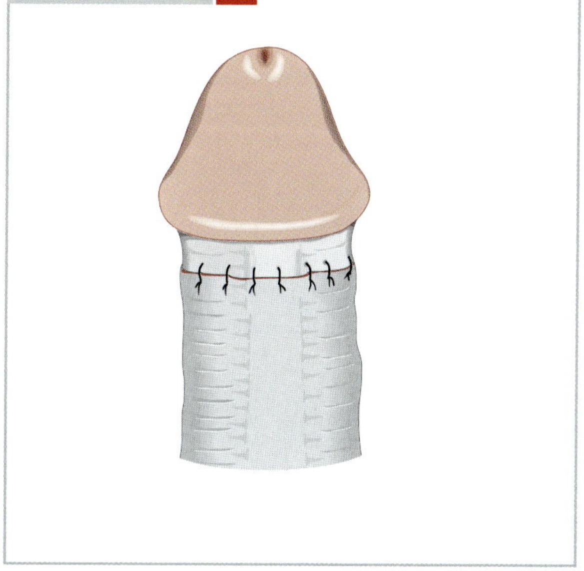

## FRENULOPLASTY

### Figure 7

Retracting the foreskin should not reveal adhesions or preputial stenosis but will cause a chordee due to the tight frenulum. Whilst proximal traction on the shaft skin is maintained by lightly gripping the penis, a transverse incision is made across the frenulum. Often this will not bleed due to repeated trauma and fibrosis, but if it does it is usually minimal and can be treated with bipolar diathermy.

### Figure 8

The incision is carefully deepened until satisfactory release is achieved. Care must be taken not to cause urethral injury. The incision will now lie vertically and may be closed with interrupted absorbable sutures before covering with lignocaine jelly and the foreskin reduced.

Figure 7

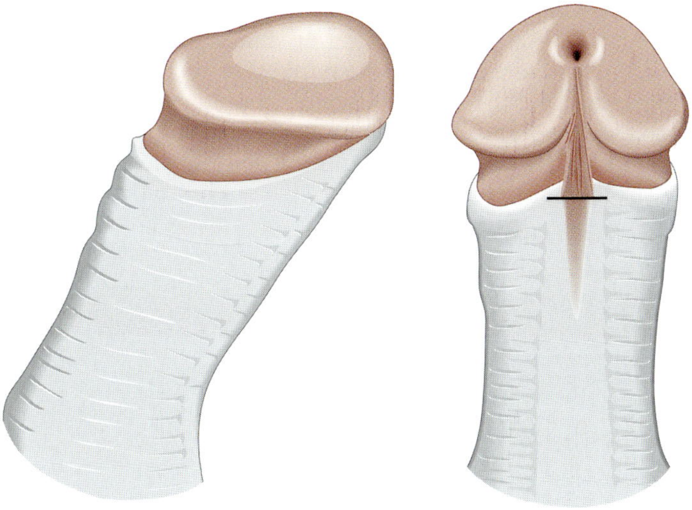

Figure 8

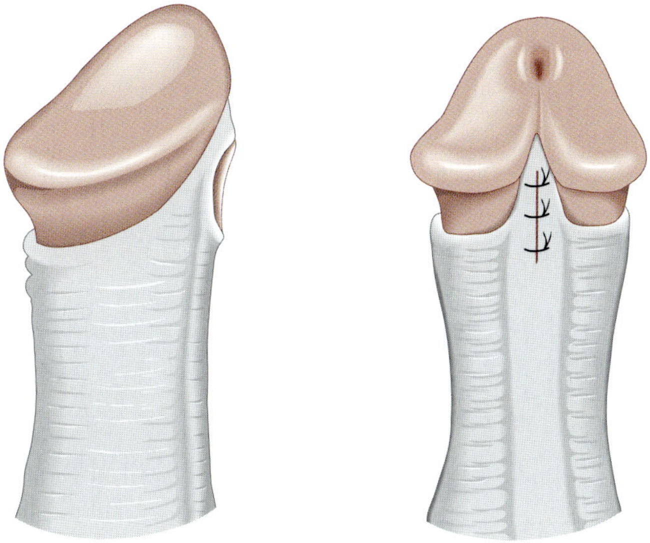

## CONCLUSION

Circumcision is complicated by bleeding and sepsis in 2–10% of cases. The cause of late meatal stenosis, occurring in 8% of boys undergoing circumcision, is unclear. Meatitis/meatal ischaemia, resulting from frenular artery ligation, is a possible mechanism. Patients should be warned of glandular hypersensitivity, which may take several weeks to improve. A poor cosmetic result usually results from over-/underexcision of skin or dense adhesions between the inner preputial skin and the glans. Laceration of the glans, usually caused by insertion of one blade of the scissors, is a surgical misadventure caused by inadequate exposure of the glans/breakdown of adhesions rather than a true complication.

## SELECTED REFERENCE

Rickwood AMK, Cornford P (1998) Male circumcision. Br J Urol (Eur Urol Update Series) 7:29–38

# Part VI Vascular Surgery

CHAPTER 21

# Operations for Varicose Veins

Matthias H. Seelig, Friedrich W. Pelster

## INTRODUCTION

Venous diseases of the lower extremities are of paramount medical importance due to their frequency and their potential long-term complications such as venous ulcers and post-thrombotic syndrome. This is mirrored by the prevalence of varicose veins in the Western world of 30% in women and about 15% in men. The vast majority of this population suffers from the stem-type insufficiency with an incompetent channel consisting of either the long or short saphenous vein. Subsequently the tributary veins dilate and form the typical varicosities.

Secondary varicose veins may also result as a consequence of venous outflow obstruction and valve destruction following deep vein thrombosis or extraluminal compression. The pattern of post-thrombotic secondary varicose veins is mostly determined by the site and extent of the original thrombosis and the relative predominance of valve incompetence and obstruction. The clinical picture is characterized by deep vein reflux, incompetent perforators and typical skin changes such as hyperpigmentation and lipodermatosclerosis. In contrast, patients suffering from primary varicose veins progress to chronic venous insufficiency only on rare occasions.

Chronic venous insufficiency is a clinical syndrome caused by continuous venous hypertension in the erect posture that is not reduced by exercise and activation of the calf muscle pump. It relates to all subsequent changes resulting from primary varicosities or phlebothrombosis. It can result in discomfort while standing, leg-swelling, development of varicose veins and pathological changes in the skin and subcutaneous tissues such as hyperpigmentation, induration, inflammation, eczema and ulceration. A clinically oriented system of classification has been provided by the CEAP classification (Consensus Group 1996).

## LONG SAPHENOUS VEIN STRIPPING

Preoperative evaluation is performed with the patient in the upright position. A careful physical examination is a sine qua non for assessing the distribution and for determining the severity of the diseased venous system. The state of competency or incompetency of the saphenofemoral and saphenopopliteal junctions is investigated by using continuous wave Doppler scanning while color-flow duplex scanning should be performed to evaluate the haemodynamic and anatomical status of the saphenous trunks. The information obtained will help to determine whether stripping of the long or short saphenous veins needs to be performed and will assist the surgeon in tailoring the operation to the patient's haemodynamic findings. All varicose trunks and incompetent perforators are carefully marked with a permanent marker.

A phlebogram should be obtained in equivocal cases and always when the patient has a history of deep vein thrombosis.

## Figure 1: Position

The operation is performed with the patient under spinal, epidural or general anesthesia. The patient is placed supine and in the Trendelenburg position. The contralateral leg may be lowered to facilitate access to the perforators on the medial thigh and the calf. The knee is slightly flexed by means of a roll and rotated externally. Skin preparation includes the leg from the inguinal region to the foot.

## Figure 2: Incision

The surface marking of the saphenofemoral junction is approximately 3–4 cm below and lateral to the pubic tubercle. The incision is centered on this point and is made parallel to the inguinal ligament. A length of 3–4 cm usually guarantees comfortable exploration. The incision should allow an adequate exposure of the saphenofemoral junction with all its tributaries.

The incision is deepened by blunt dissection through the superficial fascia, until the long saphenous vein is identified. Exposure is maintained by means of a self-retaining retractor or Langenbeck hooks.

## Figure 3: Identification of the Long Saphenous Vein

Division of the long saphenous vein should be postponed until the saphenofemoral junction, the femoral vein and the femoral artery have been unequivocally identified together with the network of small tributaries that join the saphenous vein at the hiatus saphenus.

## Figure 4: Ligation and Division of Tributaries

All these tributaries should be isolated and divided after ligation with 3/0 absorbable sutures (polyglactin, Vicryl). If the division is performed incompletely or if these veins are simply ligated, recurrence of varices occurs by a persisting network of superficial veins communicating with the perineum, lower abdominal wall and iliac region. Therefore every effort should be made to expose and divide each of the saphenous tributaries within the groin incision.

Figure 1

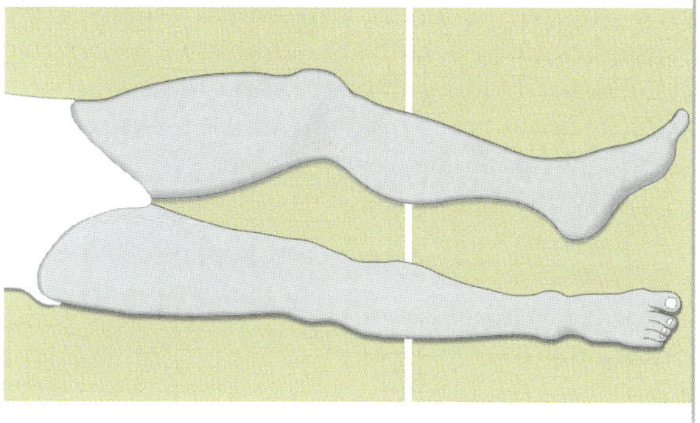

Figure 2

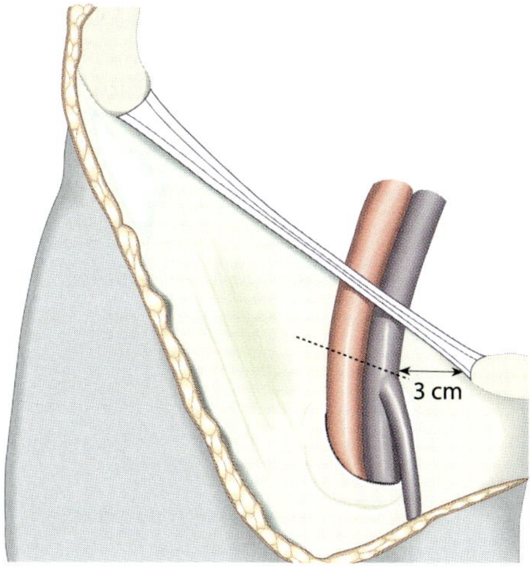


Figure 3

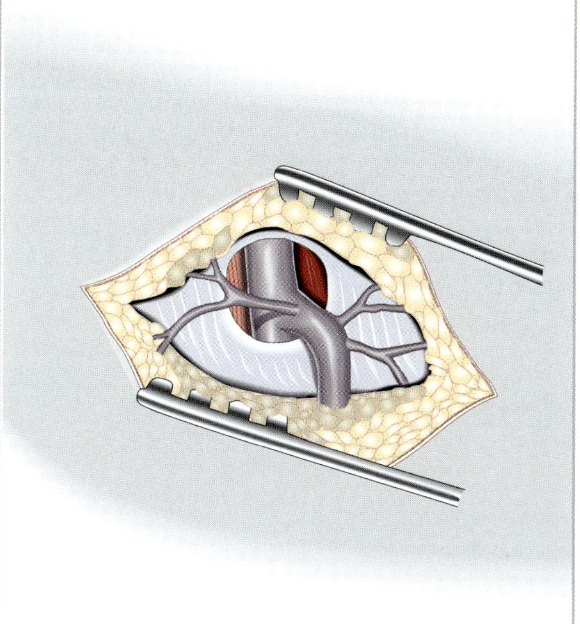

Figure 4

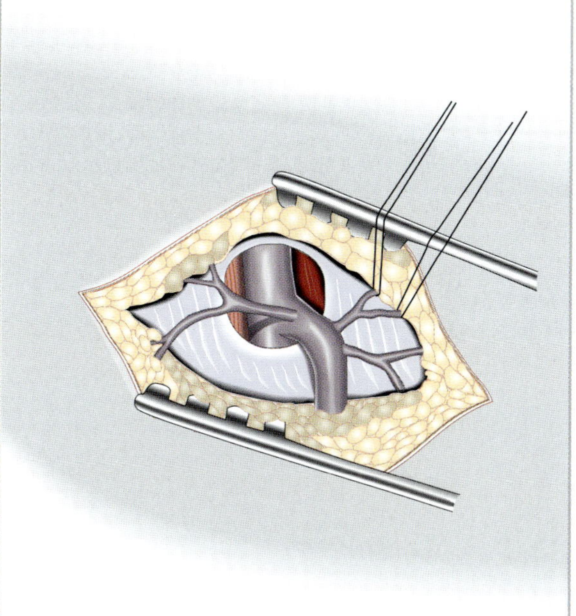

## Figure 5: Dissection of Saphenofemoral Junction

When all subdivisions have been divided the long saphenous vein should be encircled by a Vicryl ligature and divided between two Overholt clamps. The mobile upper end of the vein facilitates the mobilization of the remaining tributaries and allows exact identification of the saphenofemoral junction. The deep external pudendal vein, which usually enters the saphenous vein at the junction, must be carefully divided. By dividing the upper and lower border of the cribriform fascia over the foramen ovale, the femoral vein should be clearly visible.

Figure 5

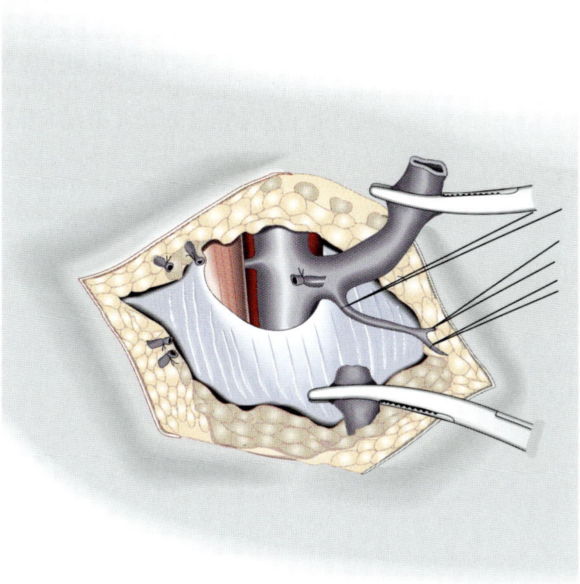

## Figure 6A, B: Dissection of Distal Saphenous Vein

In most instances the long saphenous vein is removed from the groin to the main trifurcation 3-4 cm below the knee joint. Stripping of the complete vein from the ankle to the groin has been abandoned due to the potential for saphenous nerve damage and the fact that a clear benefit of stripping the calf portion has not been proven. However, in the presence of complete insufficiency at the level of the ankle (Hach IV), complete stripping may be indicated.

When retrograde insertion of the stripper into the long saphenous vein proves to be impossible, the vein is identified through a small incision in the upper medial calf or just anterior to the medial malleolus. The vein is then encircled proximally and distally with an absorbable ligature. Following a distal ligation, a venotomy is performed and the stripper is introduced into the lumen of the vein and gently advanced until the tip of the stripper reaches the groin. At the malleolus or just distal the knee joint, the vein is divided completely. In the groin the tip is exteriorized via a small venotomy and the vein is ligated distally. A cap is applied to the end of the vein stripper and the vein is ligated behind the cap (Fig. 6A).

If the vein cannot be stripped away completely, several incisions are performed over the largest varicosities and the vein is stripped away in small segments (Fig. 6B).

**Figure 6A, B**

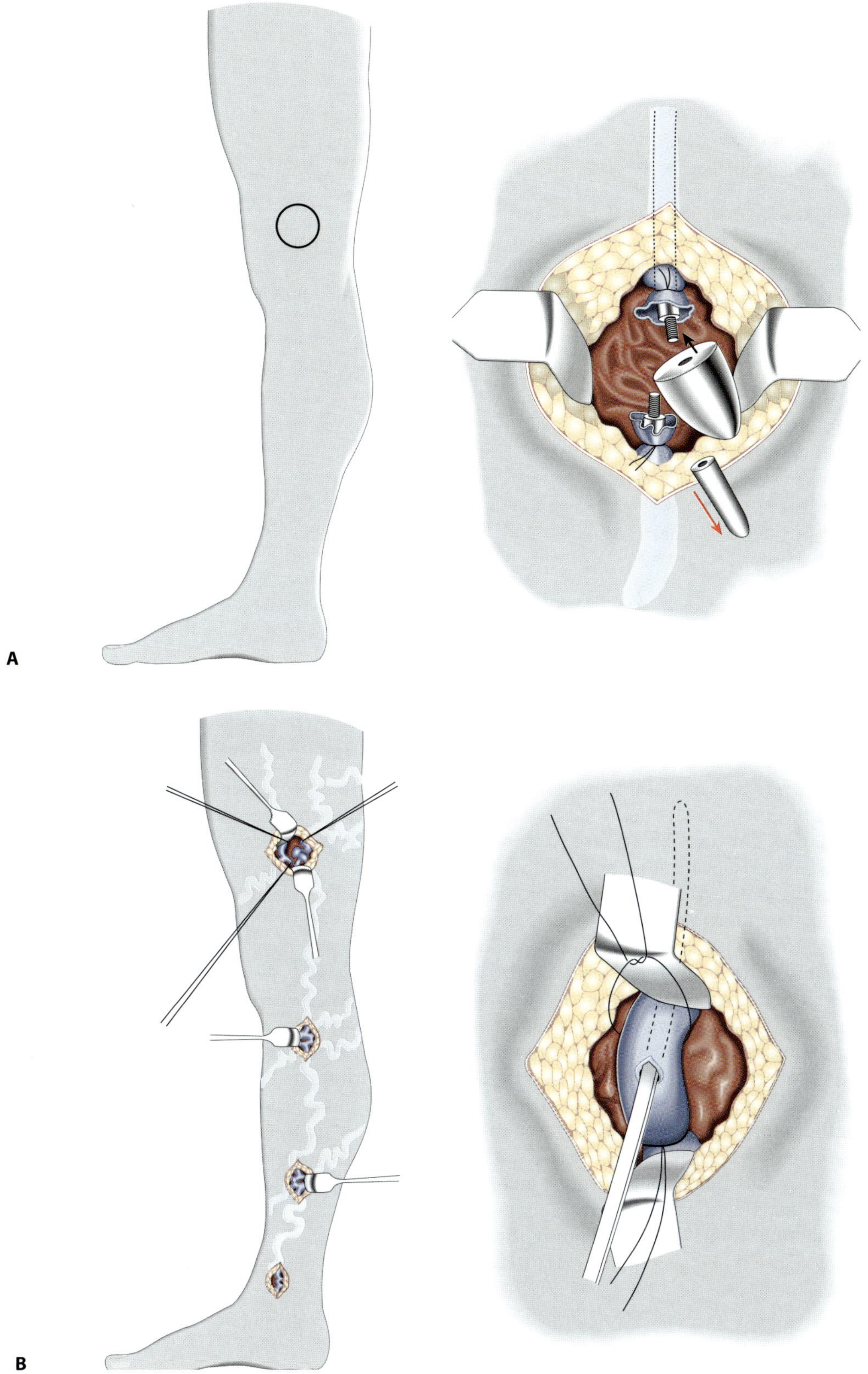

## Figure 7: Ligation of the Long Saphenous Vein at the Saphenofemoral Junction

The long saphenous vein is then transected and transfixed with a 3/0 polyglactin suture. Care should be taken neither to leave a blind sac nor to place the suture too close to the femoral vein, resulting in stenosis of the vein.

## Figure 8, 9: Phlebectomy and Ligation of Perforators

This part of the operation is preferably performed using controlled ischaemia, which allows for operating in a bloodless field. This may be achieved by using a tourniquet. The leg is elevated and exsanguinated by tightly wrapping an Esmarch bandage from the foot to the level of the tourniquet. Subsequently a Löfqvist rolling tourniquet is applied around the mid-thigh and kept in place by means of a small rubber wedge (Fig. 8). It remains in place for the remainder of the operation and is only removed after the final elastic compression bandage has been applied.

The varicosities are removed through small 5-mm incisions. These are placed at intervals of 5–10 cm along the line of the veins, the aim being total removal of the underlying varices. In the case of significant clusters of dilated varicosities, slightly larger incisions (2–3 cm ) will be required. The preferred direction of incisions is longitudinal except for over the ankle and the knee, since the best cosmetic results are obtained with vertical incisions throughout the leg and thigh, which also allow preservation of lymphatics. At each incision the vein is mobilized with a combination of fine instruments including a small phlebectomy hook and mosquito forceps and brought to the surface, freed from subcutaneous tissues and avulsed.

A medial ankle venous flare or lipodermatosclerosis in the classical gaiter distribution are two signs indicating the presence of incompetent venae perforantes (perforator veins), which should be identified.

The perforators should be approached through an incision allowing the tip of the finger to palpate the facial gap where the vein leaves the subfacial area. The perforators are ligated with absorbable sutures (Fig. 9).

Figure 7

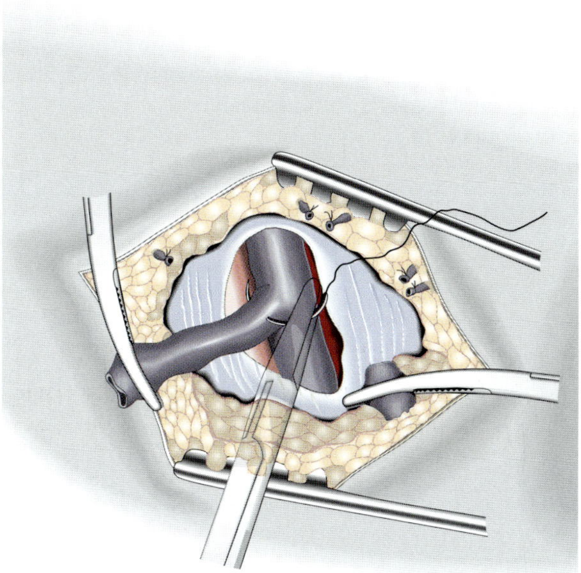

Figure 8

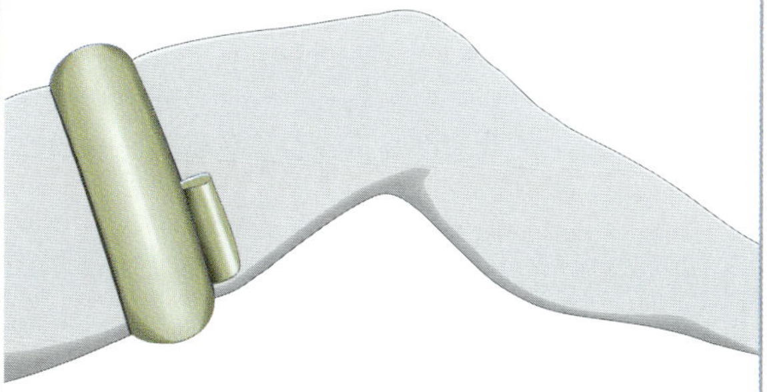

Figure 9

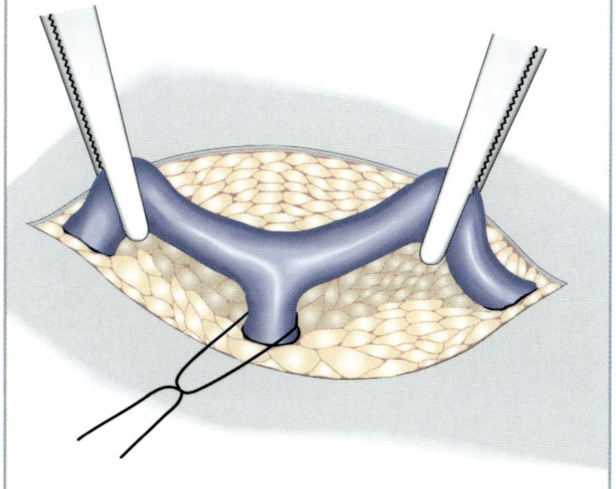

## Figure 10: Stripping of Long Saphenous Vein

The long saphenous vein is stripped from distal to proximal. At the same time the wounds are closed using absorbable 4/0 intracutaneous sutures. When indicated, stripping is performed while the tourniquet remains in situ. The entire extremity is bandaged with a cohesive elastic bandage. The tourniquet is removed or deflated and the return of colour and peripheral pulses is carefully verified. A drain may be placed in the proximal bed of the vein. The groin is closed with absorbable subcutaneous 4/0 synthetic suture material.

Figure 10

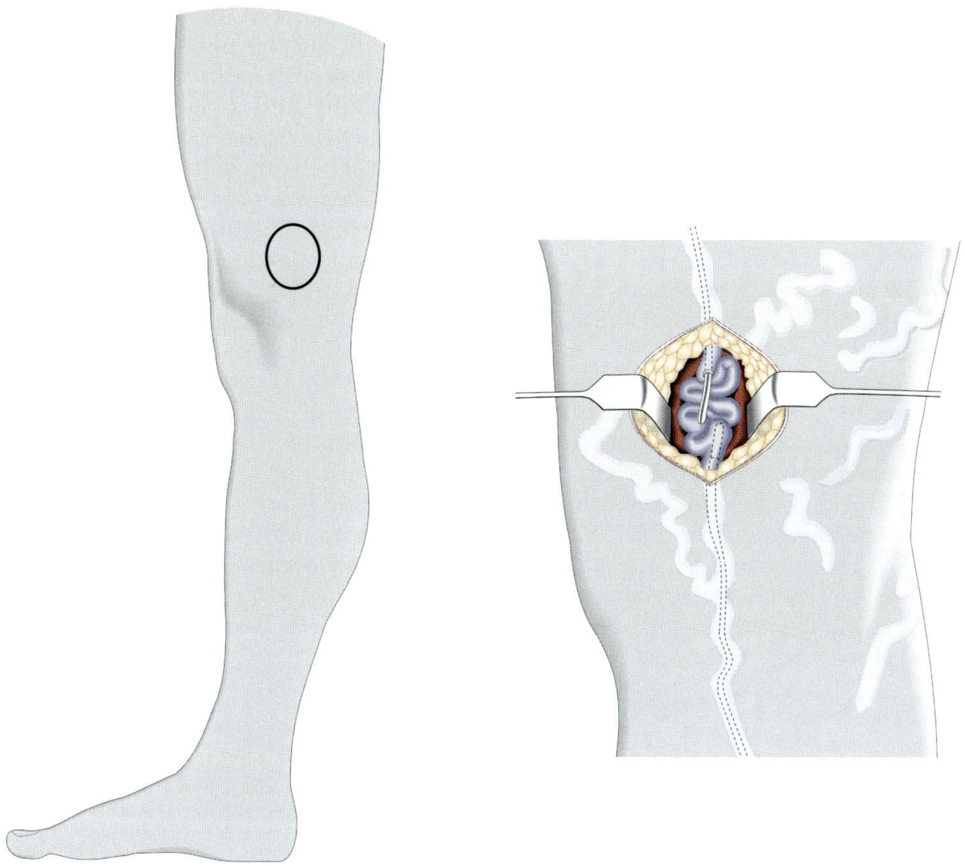

## Figure 11A, B: Subfascial Endoscopic Perforator Surgery

Endoscopic ablation of perforating veins may be performed using a single scope to both view and work within a created subfascial channel. To achieve a bloodless field a Löfqvist tourniquet is applied. Using a 2–3 cm incision dorsal to the line of Linton, the skin, subcutaneous tissue and fascia are incised. The subfascial compartment is explored digitally and the scope is gently introduced. Insufflation of air or $CO_2$ is not necessary since a subfascial space can be created by elevation of the scope. The perforators are identified and are dissected by either using bipolar coagulation or vascular clips.

An alternative involves instrumentation from laparoscopic surgery. After the thigh is exsanguinated by using an Esmarch bandage, a thigh tourniquet is applied and inflated to 300 mmHg. A longitudinal incision is made in the proximal calf approximately 2 cm dorsomedial to the medial edge of the tibia. The fascia is opened and the tube is introduced. Alternatively two 10-mm endoscopic ports are introduced into the subfascial space with the help of a blunt obturator and positioned 6–10 cm apart from each other proximal to the diseased skin of the calf. The skin incision should be small to allow an air seal around the port. Carbon dioxide is insufflated into the subfascial pace, and pressure is maintained around 30 - mmHg to improve access to the perforators. The connective tissue can be bluntly divided by moving the camera. The subfascial space is widely explored from the medial border of the tibia to the posterior midline and down to the level of the ankle. All perforators encountered which have preoperatively been identified with duplex scanning are divided by either using the harmonic scalpel or clips. In addition, a paratibial fasciotomy is performed by incising the fascia of the posterior deep compartment.

At the completion of the endoscopic portion of the procedure, the instruments and ports are removed, the carbon dioxide is manually expressed from the limb and the tourniquet is deflated.

If concomitant superficial reflux is present, high ligation and stripping of the greater saphenous vein from the groin to below the knee is performed.

Figure 11A

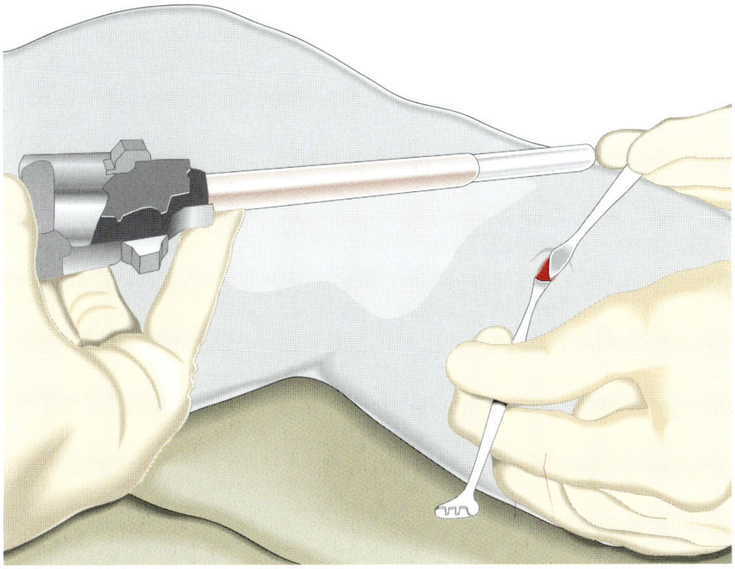

Figure 11B

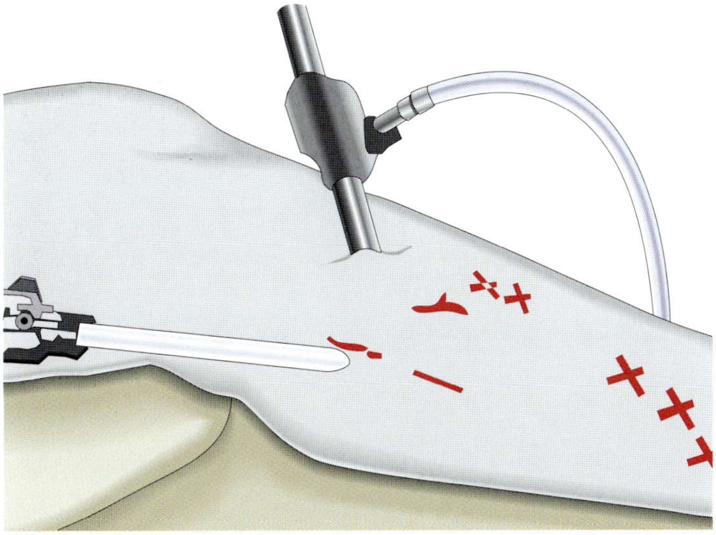

## Figure 11C, D: Subfascial Endoscopic Perforator Surgery

The subcutaneous junction between perforating vein and saphenous vein is seen trough the endoscpe. The dotted lines indicate the levels of occlusion by e.g. clips prior to surgical seperation of the veins.

Figure 11C

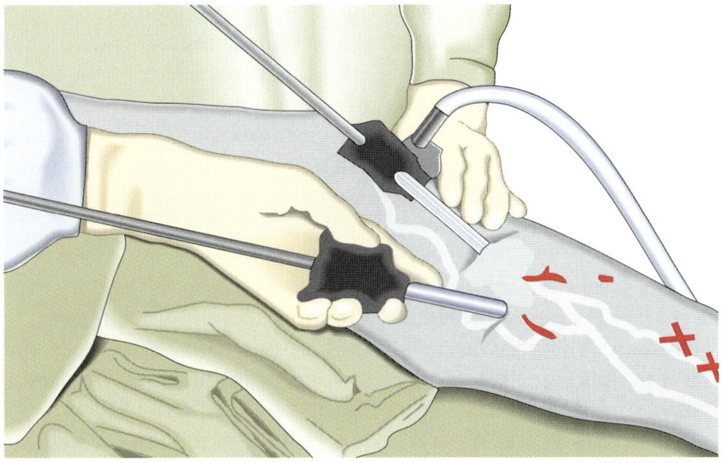

Figure 11D

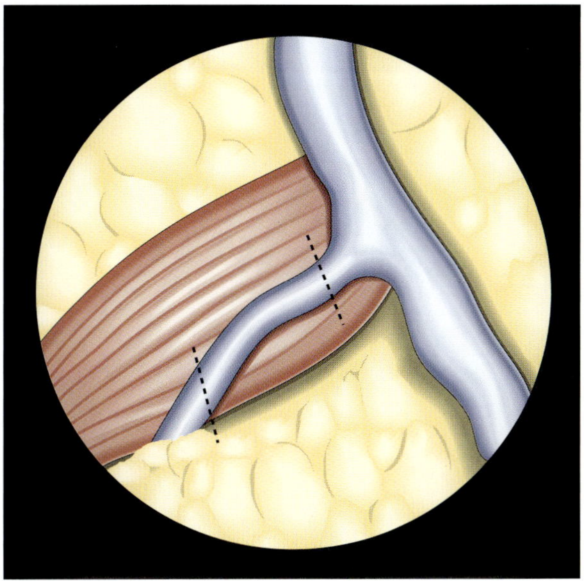

## Figure 12: Short Saphenous Vein Ligation

If no surgery of the long saphenous vein is required, the patient is positioned prone after a tourniquet has been applied to the thigh. If short saphenous vein ligation is part of a more complex vein operation which started with the patient in the supine position, the tourniquet is kept in place. The patient is turned and redraped.

The saphenopopliteal junction should have been accurately mapped prior to the operation. In the vast majority of cases the junction can be found 2–3 cm above the transverse skin crease. Therefore the incision should be placed in the crease. The deep fascia is opened vertically, which allows the dissection of the vein in either direction should it be required. The short saphenous vein is identified and carefully mobilized. The vein is freed by blunt dissection from the sural nerve and popliteal fat. Once it has been identified with certainty, it is divided between haemostats and the proximal end is mobilized. Mobilization must be done with care since nerve damage is not uncommon in short saphenous vein surgery. The saphenopopliteal junction is less distinct than the saphenofemoral junction, and the popliteal vein may be quite mobile.

The short saphenous vein is transsected and ligated with 3/0 Vicryl. It is only rarely required to strip the short saphenous vein down to the ankle, particularly as this is liable to cause sural nerve damage. A stripper may, however, be useful as a guide, as it is much more difficult to feel the short saphenous vein through the skin than the long saphenous vein.

Figure 12

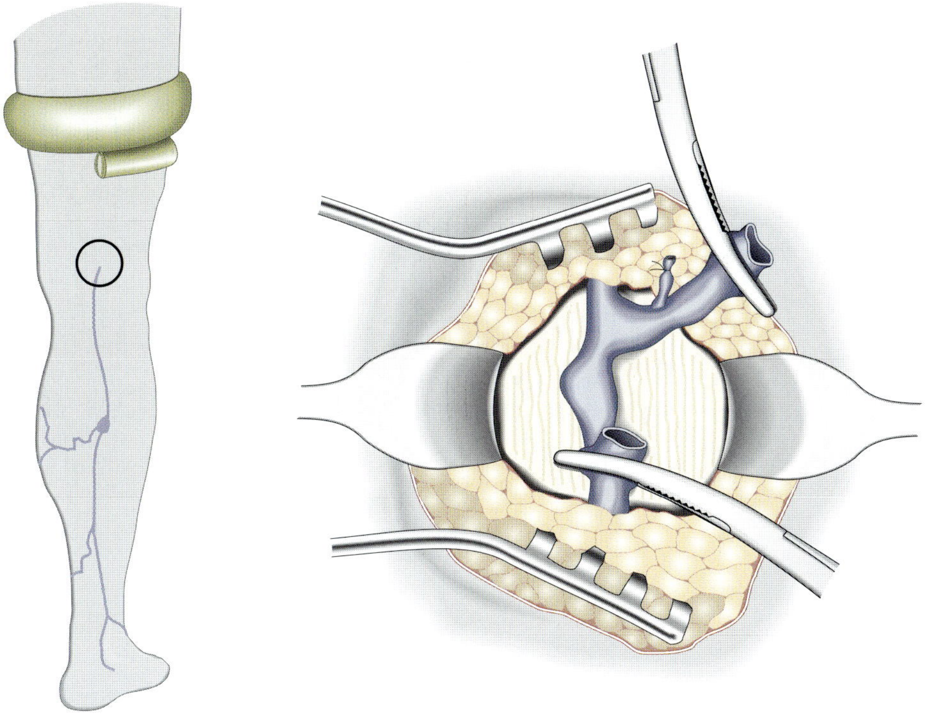

## CONCLUSION

Operative treatment of primary varicose veins is aimed at complete removal of the diseased venous segment, prevention of venous hypertension in the superficial venous system, prophylaxis against secondary insufficiency of the large veins and prevention of further complications such as dermatoliposclerosis or venous ulcer. In addition thrombophlebitis and bleeding should be prevented. These aims should be achieved with minimal complication and optimal cosmetic results. The sine qua non to achieving optimal results is an adequate clinical diagnosis of the morphological abnormalities and their haemodynamic consequences, a carefully planned operative procedure based on a clear understanding of the state of the venous system, and an accurate surgical technique.

## SELECTED REFERENCES


1. Löfqvist J (1998) Chirurgie in Blutleere mit Rollmanschetten. Chirurg 59:853--854
2. Raivio P, Perhoniemi V, Lehtola A (2002) Long-term results of vein sparing varicose vein surgery. World J Surg 26:1507–1511
3. Villavicencio JL, Gillespie DL, Kreishman P (2001) Controlled ischemia for complex venous surgery: The technique of choice. J Vasc Surg 34:947–951

CHAPTER 22

# Vascular Access

Friedrich W. Pelster, Matthias H. Seelig

## INTRODUCTION

Up until 60 years ago central venous catheterization was not even possible or could only be performed using a metal cannula for short periods of time. With the development of plastic catheters long-term medical treatment via the central venous system evolved rapidly. Meyers and Zimmermann were the first to publish the value of plastic catheters for long-term central venous infusion in 1945.

The leading cause of failure of the first clinically used catheter systems was due to a lack of biocompatibility, lack of flexibility of the material, and recurrent severe infections at the exit site.

Following 25 years of experiments with various materials, Broviac and Hickman achieved significant progress by using a cuff of polyester Dacron at the exit site. The fibrosis resulting between cuff and skin provided a significant mechanical barrier for microorganisms, leading to a dramatic decrease of infections of implanted systems.

Although the infection rate of central venous catheters can be reduced significantly by using cuffs at the exit of the skin surface (infection rate of 4–13 per 1000 treatment days), the problem of secondary infection with invasive microorganisms still remains. The primary source of infections is the skin flora of the patients themselves or the hand flora of the medical staff.

Large bore central venous access catheters for temporary use are percutaneously implanted Hickman or Broviac catheters. In contrast, small diameter catheters such as intraport catheters can remain in place for unlimited use. These systems are completely covered and protected and access is obtained via a temporary transcutaneous puncture.

## Figure 1, 2: The Hickman Catheter

Hickman or Broviac catheters are single-lumen catheters made of silicone and used for chemotherapy or parenteral nutrition. Proximal to the exit site these catheters have a Dacon cuff to prevent bacterial contamination. The catheters are visible under X-ray, permitting an exact localization of the tip of the catheter.

After obtaining informed consent, the subclavian vein of both sides is identified using Doppler sonography. With the patient positioned supine and the head inclined to the contralateral side, the operative field is disinfected. The infraclavicular area and the periosteum of the clavicle are injected with local anaesthetic (lidocaine 2%). The subclavian vein is punctured using Seldinger's technique and the wire is advanced into the right atrium under X-ray control. The introducer is inserted over the wire and the wire is extracted. Using a second incision below the clavicle, the catheter is advanced to the first incision and inserted through the introducer. The correct position is verified using X-rays and subsequently the introducer is removed. The cuff is fixed with the surrounding tissue using 4–0 absorbable monofilament suture material and a sterile dressing is applied.

The implanted catheter is flushed with heparinized saline and can be used without delay.

### Figure 1

Hickmann-catheter with infection barrier and security clamp

### Figure 2

Catherization of the cephalic vein or V. suclavia using Seldingers technique to introduce the catheter

Figure 1

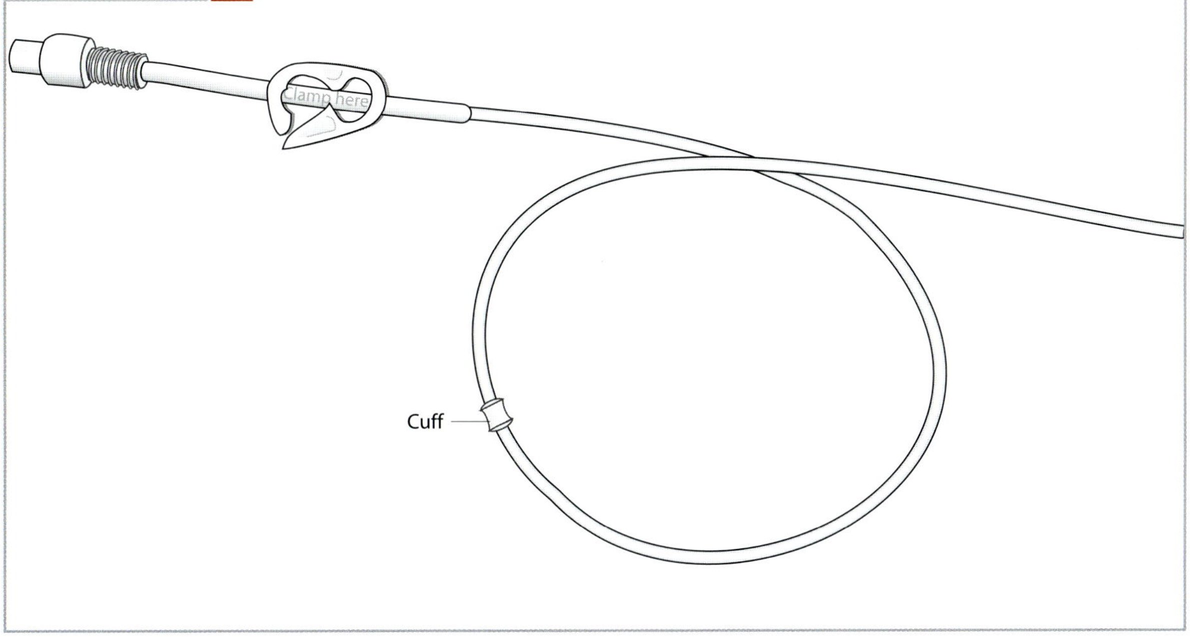


Figure 2

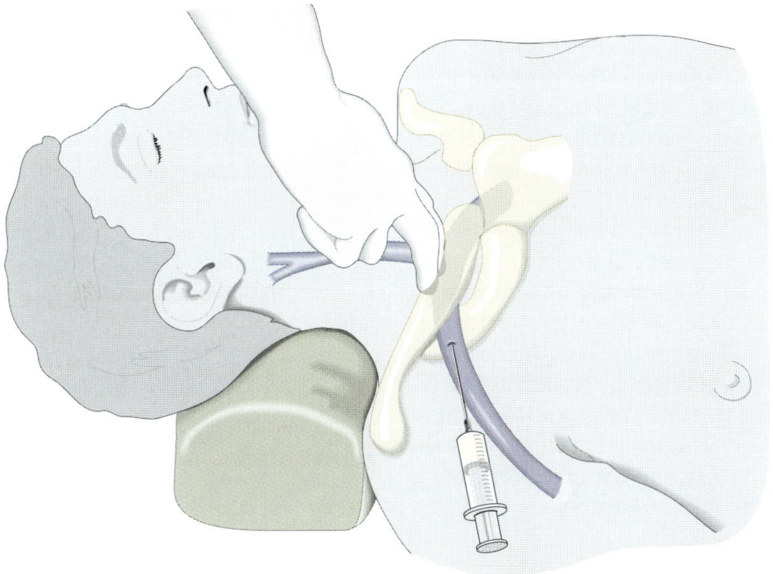

## Figure 3: Vascular Systems

Central venous port systems are a further development of implantable pumps which have been developed for regular bolus administration of medications. However, these pumps do not allow for any modification or change of medication after implantation. A reservoir has been developed, which allows for transcutaneous puncture through a specialized membrane and injection of various medications. This reservoir (the port chamber) is positioned completely beneath the skin. Connected to the reservoir is a silicone catheter 15–20 cm in length which is localized with its tip in the superior vena cava. Due to the large volume vessel, local irritation of the vessel wall, a common problem when small peripheral veins are used for infusions of irritant agents, is significantly reduced.

The port chamber itself is made of plastic or titanium, and modern systems are made of ceramics. Both materials are visible under X-ray and do not interfere when magnetic resonance imaging is performed. Different sizes of systems are available and can be chosen according to patient size and therapy requirements.

The port chamber is cylindrical and can be palpated easily through the overlying tissue. The ventral side bears the silicone membrane, and the base of the system is usually larger and has holes for fixation on the fascia. The chamber and the catheter can be connected securely after cutting for the required length.

Port systems can be used about 3–6 days after the operation. Puncture of the port should only be performed with a specially designed needle and under sterile conditions. After use the system must be flushed with heparinized saline. Bleeding should be prevented due to the increased risk of thrombosis of the system.

### Figure 3

Port system (with injection chamber) and "Huber"-injection needle

## Figure 4–9: Venous Port Systems

Venous port systems can be inserted into any vein. Usual implantation sites include the cephalic vein, the subclavian vein and the internal jugular vein. The cephalic vein can be easily accessed but the lumen is often small and sometimes valves may inhibit the insertion of the catheter.

Insertion via the subclavian vein carries the advantage of a larger lumen, but due to its close proximity to the thorax, haemothorax and pneumothorax are potential risks. In order to place the port reservoir a second incision is sometimes required. Access via the internal jugular vein seems to be more difficult when undertaken beneath the sternocleidomastoid muscle. However, after a steep learning curve the operation is relatively easy, the complication rate is low and a second incision is not necessary.

After informed consent the patient is examined clinically and duplex sonography of both sites of the neck is performed. The operation is performed with the patient supine and the head turned to the opposite site. The skin is disinfected from the neck to the thorax. A single shot of antibiotic prophylaxis is given and local anaesthetic is injected. A 3-cm skin incision is performed at the upper border of the medial part of the clavicle. After incision of the platysma the pars clavicularis of the sternocleidomastoid muscle is retracted medially and the jugular vein can be isolated.

### Figure 4

Site of insertion of the catheter in the jugular vein on the right side between clavicle and M. sternocleidomastoideus

Figure 3

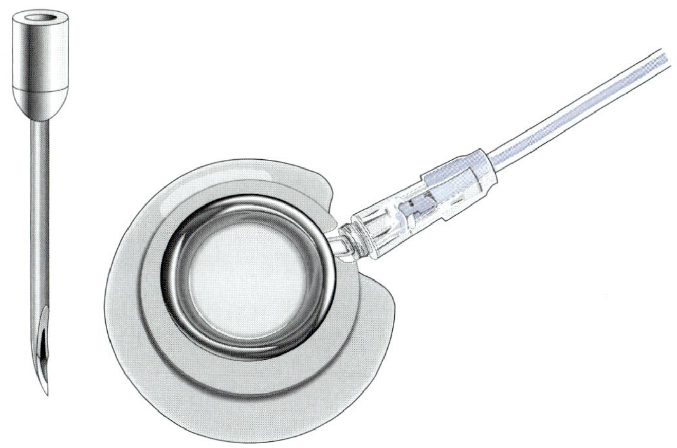

Figure 4

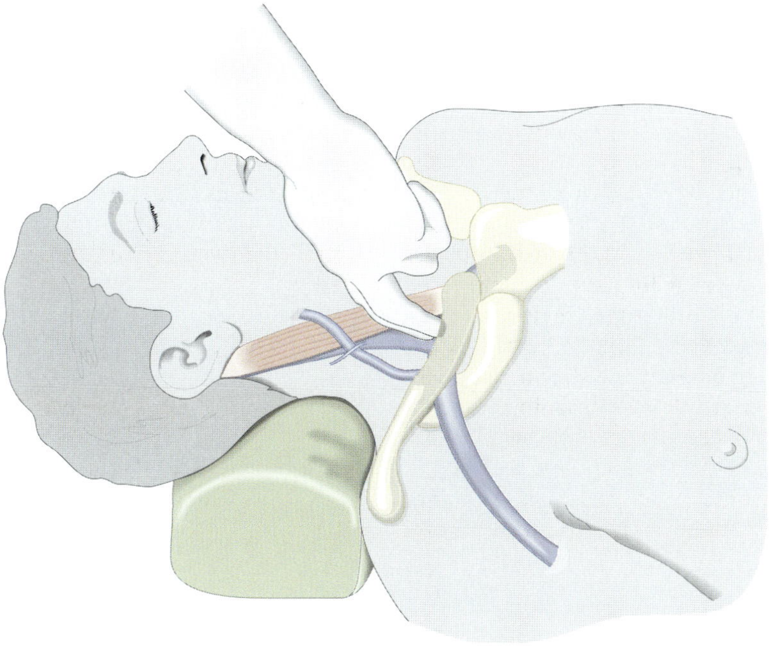

## Figure 4–9: Venous Port Systems

The vein is punctured using Seldinger's technique and the tip of the catheter is placed approximately 2–3 cm above the right atrium. The correct position is verified using X-rays. The catheter is fixed to the vein using an absorbable suture.

From the skin incision, the subcutaneous tissue over the second rib lateral to the sternum is dissected to create a tunnel for the port. The correct length of the catheter is determined and the catheter and the port are connected. The port is inserted into the tunnel. Usually, any additional fixation is not required, and a small drain can be placed. The skin is closed in layers. Finally, the port is punctured transcutaneously, filled with heparinized saline and a dressing is applied.

The operation can be performed with the patient ambulatory. If a drain is placed, it can be removed on the first postoperative day. The port can be used on the third postoperative day. The system must be flushed with heparinized saline after each application to prevent thrombosis, although the risk of thrombosis can not be completely eliminated.

### Figure 5

3 cm skin insertion and preparation of the internal jugular vein underneath the M. sternocleidomastoideus

### Figure 6

Catherization of the right jugular vein

Figure 5

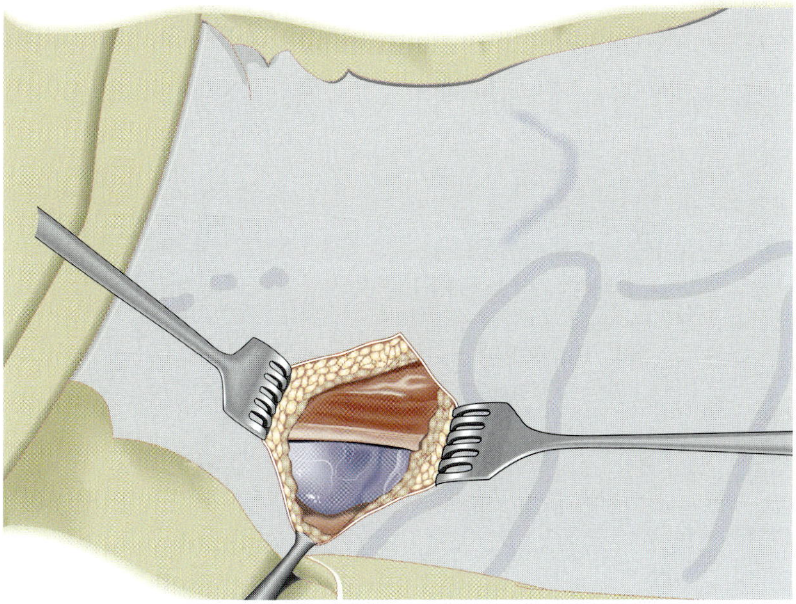

Figure 6

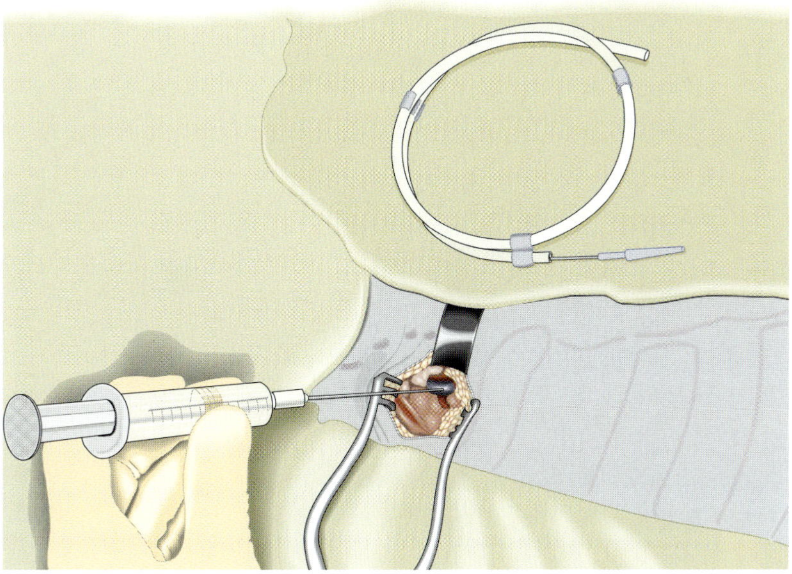

## Figure 4–9: Venous Port Systems

### Figure 7

Introduction of the port system using a split introduction catheter

### Figure 8

Shortening of the catheter and conncetion with the injection reservoir

Figure 7

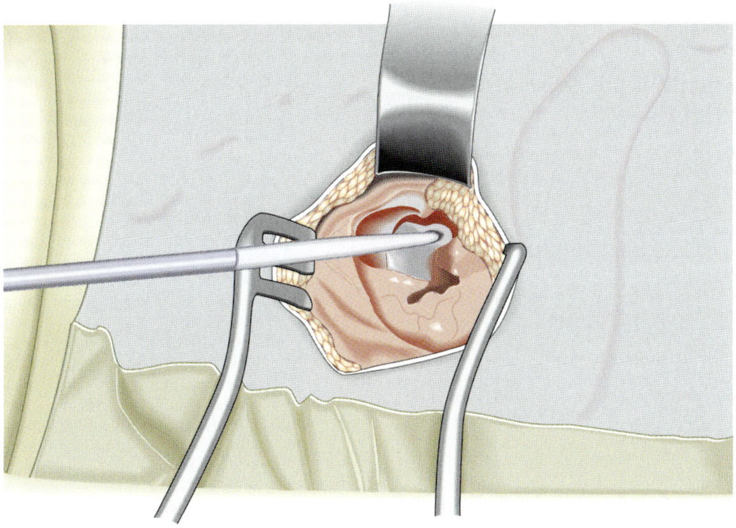

Figure 8

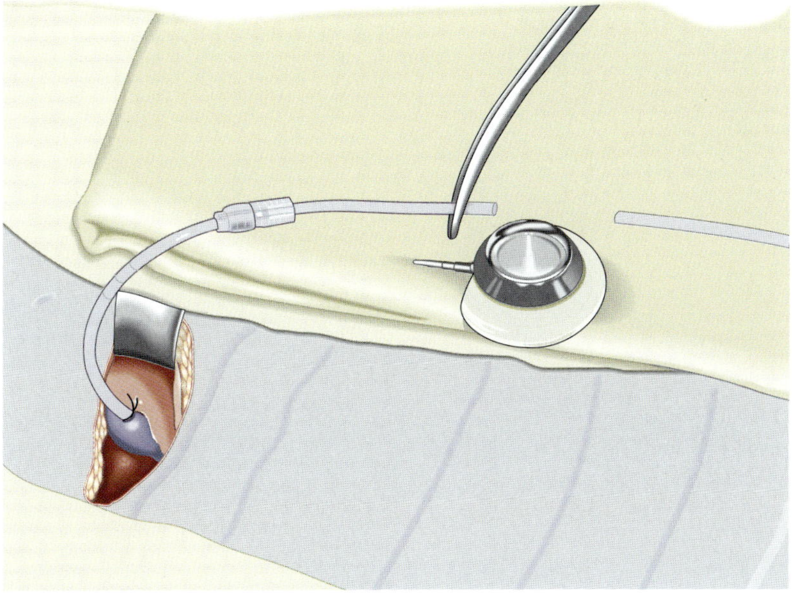

## Figure 4–9: Venous Port Systems

### Figure 9

Correct and solid placement of the reservoir alining with the 2nd rib on the right side

Figure 9

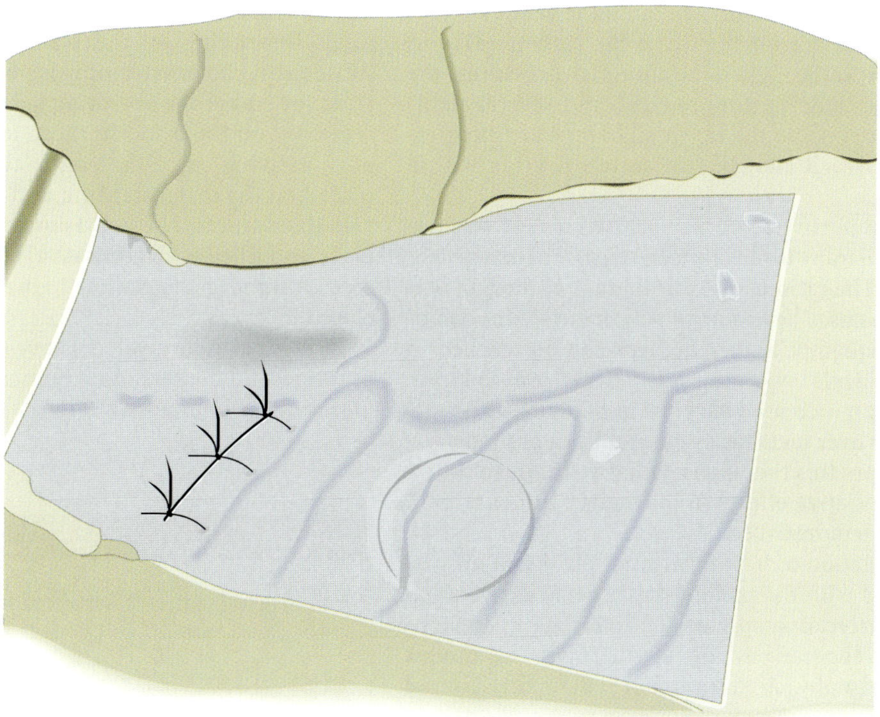

## Figure 10, 11: Arterial Port Systems

Arterial port systems are similar to the venous catheter system except for the tip of the catheter. Due to the significantly higher intraluminal pressures, the wall of the catheter is more rigid, and several centimetres proximal to the tip small humps are integrated into the wall allowing for secure fixation within the vessel.

Arterial port systems may be used for locoregional chemotherapy for liver metastases or primary liver tumours. The rationale of this therapy is the fact that liver metastases have a primarily arterial blood supply. Subsequently, higher dosages can be reached in the liver while systemic side effects are reduced. However, an increased survival in patients with non-resectable liver metastases has not been demonstrated; therefore this therapy is palliative in the majority of cases. Positive effects in other liver tumours have not been demonstrated.

Implantation of hepatic arterial ports can only be performed with the patient under general anaesthesia. The arterial supply of the liver has to be confirmed preoperatively by angiography or duplex ultrasonography. A tumour burden in the liver of more than 70%, liver cirrhosis or extrahepatic metastases are a contraindication for arterial port implantation.

Using a right subcostal incision the gastroduodenal artery is identified and distally ligated. Via a small arteriotomy the catheter is advanced into the common hepatic artery. The catheter is fixed to the gastroduodenal artery using three non-absorbable sutures. Depending on the planned chemotherapy a subsequent cholecystectomy is performed.

At the end of the operation a subcutaneous tunnel is created on the distal sternum for placement of the port. Leaving enough length the port system is placed on the distal sternum and fixed with non-absorbable sutures. The port is punctured transcutaneously and filled with contrast agent to verify the correct location of the catheter. Finally the abdomen is closed in layers.

Arterial catheter systems have a high endoluminal pressure, and the risk of thrombosis according to the literature is about 40–60%.

### Figure 10

Tip of arterial catheter with fixation sleeve

### Figure 11

Arterial port system for therapy of liver disorders, transabdominal approach and placement of the catheter tip in the gastroduodenal artery, placement of the reservoir extraabdominally (presternal placement)

Figure 10

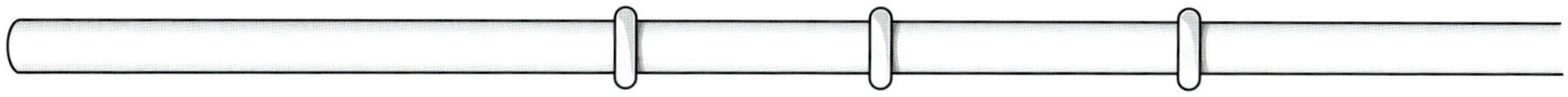

Figure 11

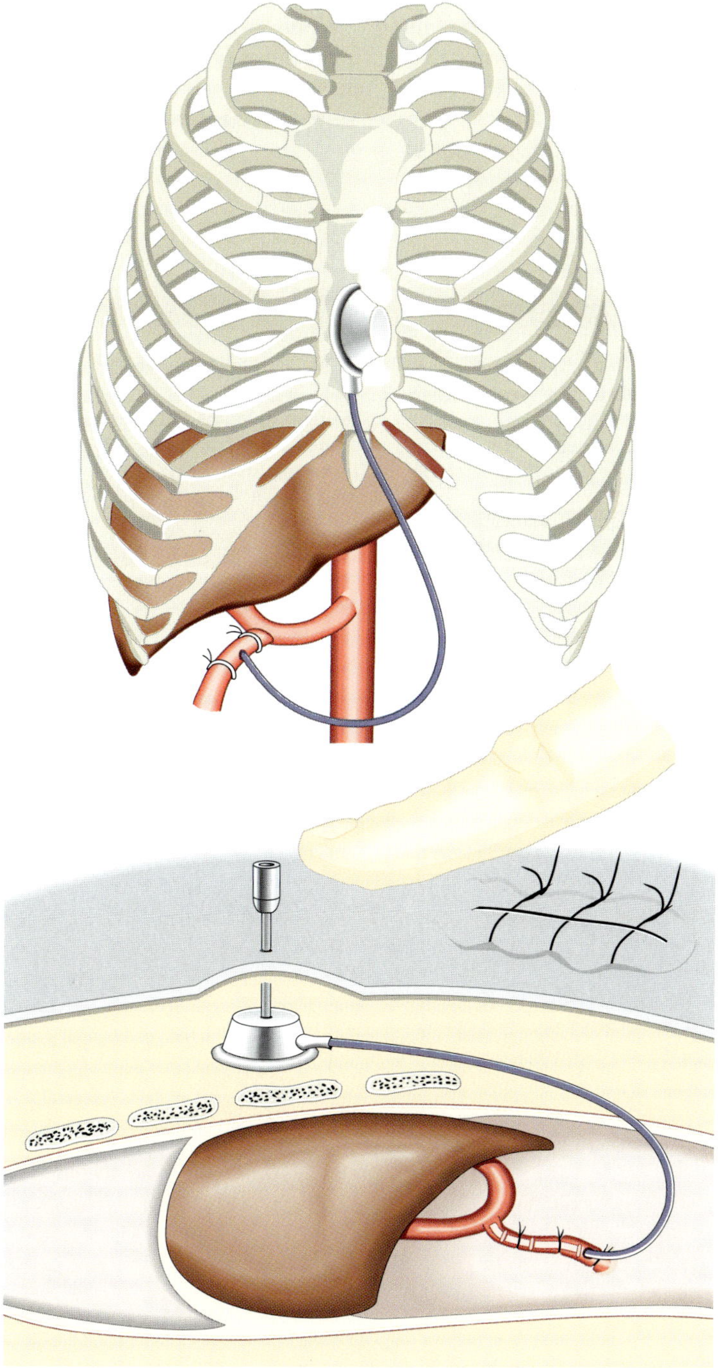

## CONCLUSIONS

Central venous catheter systems can be categorized into large bore percutaneous systems and subcutaneous port systems. Percutaneously implanted Hickman and Broviac catheters are the first choice for temporary systems for intravenous chemotherapy and also allow for withdrawal of central venous blood. Due to the exit site, infections and septic complications are potential drawbacks. Recent studies demonstrate that up to 70% of nosocomial infections occur in patients with central venous catheters.

Subcutaneously implantable port catheter systems have a much lower infection rate; however, since regular transcutaneous punctures are required infection may not be completely preventable.

The second main complication is thrombosis of the catheter tip. Correct siting in the superior vena cava and regular flushing with heparinized saline may reduce this risk significantly. New generation systems have a mechanism at the tip of the catheter to prevent venous backflow into the lumen.

Besides infection and thrombosis the third most important complication is dislocation of the port reservoir. Therefore the port should always be placed on the bony structures of the thorax. Fixation using sutures may not be required under these circumstances.

When implanted correctly and regular care is provided, these systems can be used to an unlimited extent and have significant advantages for the patient compared to other systems.

## SELECTED REFERENCES

Beckmann MW, Lorenz C, Dall P (2000) Platzierung und Pflege von venösen Verweilkathetern und Portsystemen. Gynakologe 33: 255–260

Broviac JW (1973) A silicone rubber arterial catheter for prolonged parenteral alimentation. Surg Gynecol Obstet 136: 602–606

Hickman RO et al (1979) A modified right arterial catheter for access to the venous system in marrow transplant recipients. Surg Gynecol Obstet 148: 871–875

Meyers L (1945) Intravenous catheterization. Am J Nurs 45: 930–931

Seldinger SI (1953) Catheter replacement of needle in percutaneous arteriography. Acta Radiol 39: 368–371

Zimmermann B (1945) Intravenous tubing for parenteral therapy. Science 101: 567–568

# Part VII Endoscopy

CHAPTER 23

# Surgical Endoscopy

Dirk Tübergen, Emile Rijcken

## INTRODUCTION

Surgical endoscopy provides a paradigm for short stay surgery, since operative access by the natural orifices is minimally invasive, which guarantees a short recovery phase for the patient. However, one should not be deceived in that complex operative procedures can be performed endoscopically that require special postoperative surveillance. Such patients are perfectly well looked after in existing surgical environments, with access to operating rooms, intensive care units and close cooperation with anaesthetists. Furthermore the possible complications and the corresponding complication management are familiar to surgeons from their routine training.

This chapter deals with interventional endoscopy that can be performed during a short hospital stay. In this context we are not specifically concerned with diagnostic endoscopic examinations or with intra- or postoperative endoscopy. We also will not consider emergency endoscopy such as gastrointestinal bleeding situations or foreign body extractions, since the subsequent course and the hospital stay cannot be planned in advance.

Like all operative disciplines, surgical endoscopy requires appropriate facilities, technical expertise, and experienced personnel to provide a friction-free and low-risk procedure.

The spatial requirements comprise one or more specially equipped examination rooms and a separate room for the preparation and cleaning of instruments with special attention to standards of hygiene and health and safety requirements. Also a changing room for staff and a recovery room are needed.

The technical requirements include appropriate modern videoendoscopes and an X-ray unit. Such a unit with digital imaging and the latest features in terms of radiation protection are preferred. This unit should be run in cooperation with radiologists. Furthermore an electronic image processing unit is desirable, which enables the endoscopist to document interesting and pathological findings during the endoscopic, ultrasound, and X-ray examinations and allows word processing at the same time. Ideally, a computer based documentation system can also produce statistics for audit, assessment and material requirements and can make scientific evaluations easier.

Special examination tables are required and suitable instruments for patient monitoring (e.g. pulse oximeter, blood pressure and ECG) are mandatory. It is important to maintain a set of emergency equipment with intubation and mechanical ventilation facilities within reach. Drugs for sedation and analgesia as well as their antidotes should be available.

The staff team should contain at least one fully trained and responsible endoscopist and the nurses should also be specially trained in the field of endoscopy. Particularly important is a close cooperation with the anaesthetist when caring for co-morbid patients and for cases of long and complex endoscopic procedures (e.g. airway maintenance during endoscopy with the patient in the supine position).

## UPPER GASTROINTESTINAL TRACT

## Figure 1A–C: Endoscopic Diverticulotomy of Zenker's Diverticulum

■ **Indications.** Symptomatic diverticula with dysphagia, regurgitation and repeated aspiration should be treated. In contrast to the open surgical procedure, the endoscopic diverticulotomy does not resect the diverticulum. Furthermore the cricopharyngeal muscle is not incised; merely the septum between the diverticulum and the oesophageal wall is divided in order to promote the emptying of the diverticulum.

■ **Special Conditions and Instruments.** A gastroscope with a protection cap, gastric tube, high-frequency instruments, needle knife or argon plasmacoagulation probe or laser probe (Nd-YAG) are required. If applicable an oblique suction cap as used in endoscopic mucosa resection (EMR) is also used.

■ **Technique.** Initially an oesophago-gastro-duodenoscopy is undertaken in the left lateral position in order to exclude secondary pathological findings. When withdrawing the endoscope, a flexible wire is positioned in the stomach and subsequently a gastric tube is inserted over the wire. After this, the diverticulum is visualised and the septum is divided in a stepwise manner.

■ **Pitfalls.** Bleeding can occur when the ratio between cutting and coagulating current is inappropriate. In most cases this bleeding can be stopped by endoscopic coagulation. Perforations can occur especially when the diverticulotomy is performed too fast. For this reason it is better to undertake multiple sessions and to retain a small part of the septum at the bottom of the diverticulum.

**Figure 1A–C**

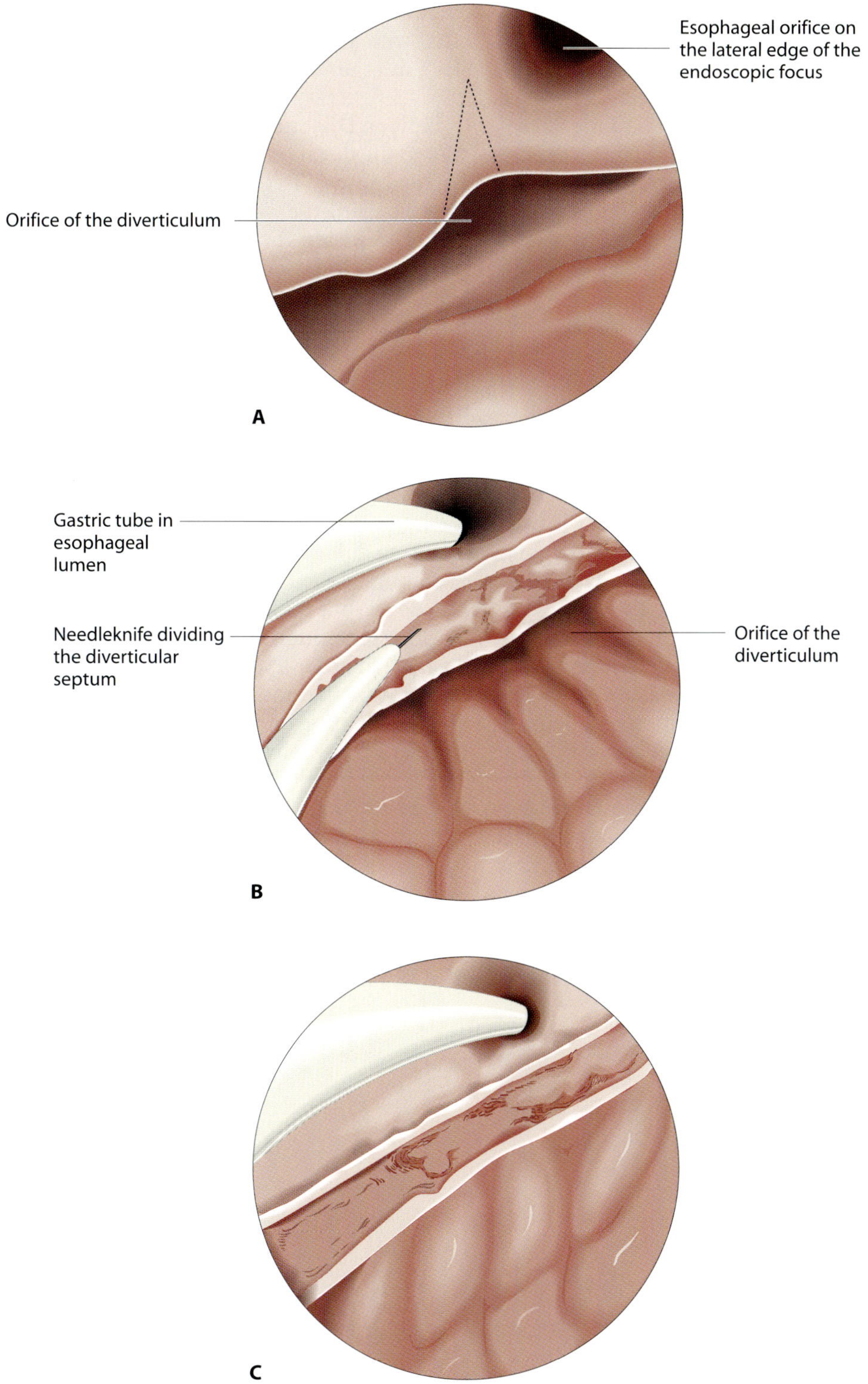


After diverticulotomy esophageal orifice and the bottom of the diverticulum are at the same level

## Figure 2A–D: Treatment of Stenoses

■ **Indications.** Before a stenosis in the upper or lower gastrointestinal tract can be treated effectively, malignancy must be excluded and the underlying pathological process should be clarified. The choice of both the endoscopic management and the subsequent therapy are directed at this issue. In cases of benign stenoses, dilatation or bougienage is sufficient, whereas in cases of malignant stenoses palliative maintenance of the lumen is achieved by a durable tube (metal or plastic stents).

■ **Special Conditions and Instruments.** Requirements are a gastroscope, possibly a small paediatric gastroscope or bronchoscope, guidewires of different grades of stiffness, catheters for administration of contrast medium, bougies of different diameters (Savary bougies) or dilatation-balloon catheters [guided by wire, OTW (over the wire), or guided by sight, TTS (through the scope)], possibly high frequency instruments with a needle-knife or argon plasma-coagulation probe or papillotomy instruments, and X-ray unit.

■ **Technique.** Before treatment, knowledge of the exact nature of the stenosis is mandatory. When the stenosis cannot be passed by an endoscope, adequate X-ray assessment with contrast medium can help. Malignancies must be excluded by biopsy and histological examination before any further intervention is performed. Furthermore the surrounding tissues should be evaluated prior to intervention by means of CT scanning and endoultrasonography.

■ **Incision of the Stenosis.** Short sail-like cicatricial stenoses are most likely to be anastomotic stenoses. After adequate assessment, these stenoses can be incised with a needle knife in the shape of a Mercedes star until the original organ wall is reached.

■ **Balloon Dilatation.** When the length of the stenosis and the distal course of the lumen can be seen endoscopically, a TTS dilatation balloon catheter can be inserted using the working channel of the endoscope and sited within the stenosis. Then the stenosis can be dilated under endoscopic vision. By pulling the pellucid balloon close to the endoscope's optic the success of the dilatation can be assessed but possible complications can also be dealt with endoscopically. Particularly useful are newly developed dilatation balloons with pressure-variable diameters.

If the length of the stenosis and the course of the distal lumen remain unclear, the situation can be clarified by contrast medium examination using image intensification. Thereafter a guidewire can be inserted, to guide the balloon through the stenosis. The dilatation is then performed analogous to the TTS procedure, but under X-ray control. Immediately after the intervention one should perform a further endoscopy in order to check the postinterventional situation. A further radiological contrast medium swallow examination on the following morning is recommended. Close clinical surveillance is mandatory. These examinations can reveal perforation, which is the most serious complication at this early stage .

### Figure 2A–D

Incision of anastomotic stenosis after oesophagojejunostomy

**Figure 2A**

Esophageal lumen

Sail-like stenosis
consisting of scar tissue

**Figure 2B**

Incision with a needleknife

**Figure 2C**

Balloon dilatation through the scope

**Figure 2D**

Final result after incision and dilatation

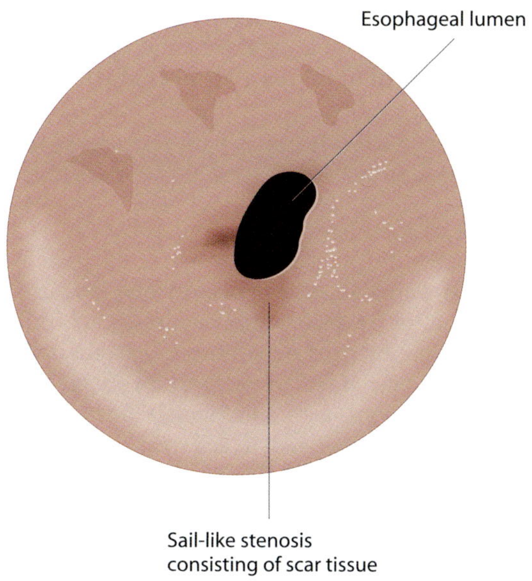

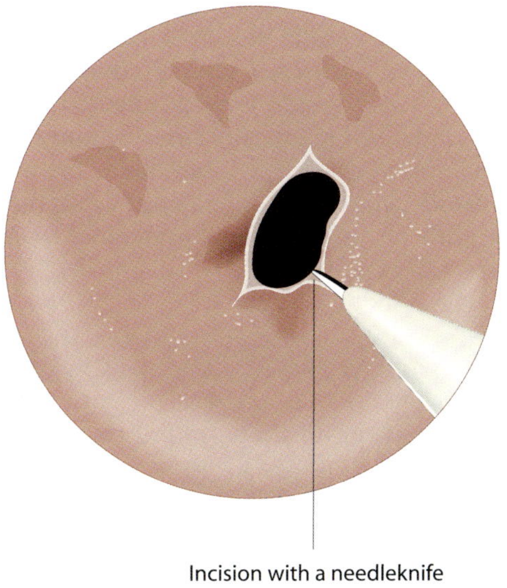

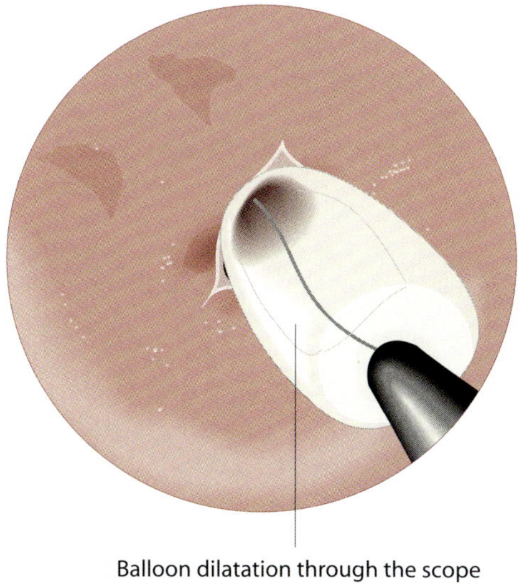

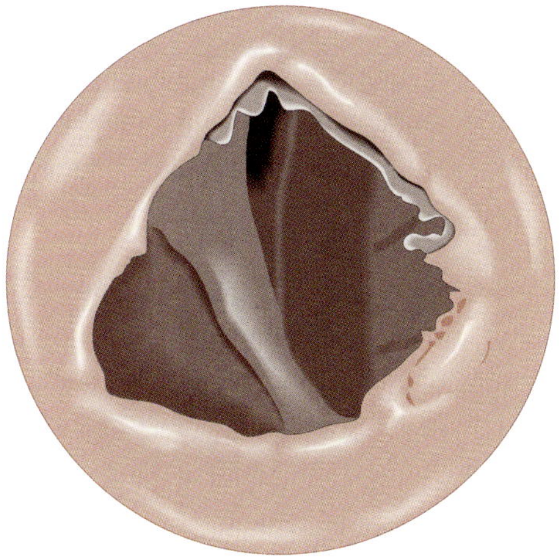

## Figure 2E–G: Treatment of Stenoses

**Bougienage.** Bougienage is especially applicable for the treatment of long distant stenoses (e.g. in the oesophagus) and stenoses with a straight course. Once again a stiff guide wire is inserted into the stomach under X-ray control. After removal of the endoscope, bougies of ascending diameters are applied over the wire. This is monitored using the centimetre scale on the bougie or preferably under X-ray control (Fig. 2E).

### Figure 2E

Principle of tumour dilatation by means of bougies

**Stent Insertion.** Because of the difficult removal of stents and the uncertain long term behaviour of these stents, stent insertion is restricted in general to malignant stenoses. Prior to stent insertion, the passage through the stenosis should be clarified by means of a small-bore endoscope or, if passage of the endoscope is not possible, by a contrast medium study and insertion of a guidewire which allows dilatation until the lumen is secured. Thereafter the tumour borders are measured and marked either endoluminally by injection of dye or alternatively by placing opaque markers externally on the skin. Then a stiff guidewire is inserted using the working channel of the endoscope. Thereafter the endoscope is removed and in most cases a covered metal stent is put in place. The stent should bridge the tumour completely. Usually one can dispense with dilatation of the stent, because most stents expand spontaneously due to their own flexibility (Fig. 2F and G).

### Figure 2F and G

Principle of stent insertion

**Pitfalls.** Perforations can occur when dilatation or bougienage is performed too aggressively. Inflammatory, neoplastic, or neoadjuvantly irradiated stenoses are at special risk of perforation. In such cases, a stepwise dilatation or bougienage during several sessions is recommended. In contrast to the implantation of plastic tubes, the risk of perforation is low when using self-expandable metal stents, and small tears of the mucosa during implantation are sealed when the covered metal stent is expanded. Stent dislocation occurs mostly when insertion has been performed too early in the disease process and the lumen is still too wide. In these cases, one should wait until the lumen is narrow enough that the stenosis fixes the stent securely. Stenoses of the cardia are especially at risk of stent dislocation, since the stent is only secured by the proximal border of the tumour while the distal end of the tube terminates freely in the stomach. To avoid a false positioning of the stent, the exact expansion properties of the stent type used should be known and the patient must be sedated adequately during stent implantation.

Figure 2E

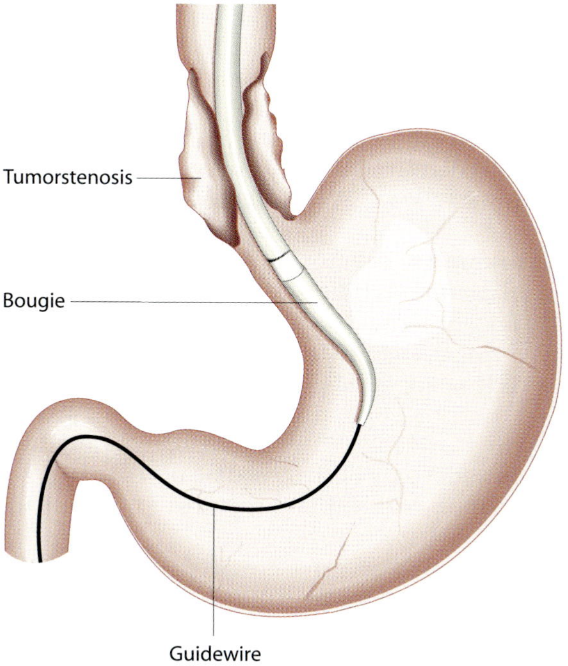


Figure 2F

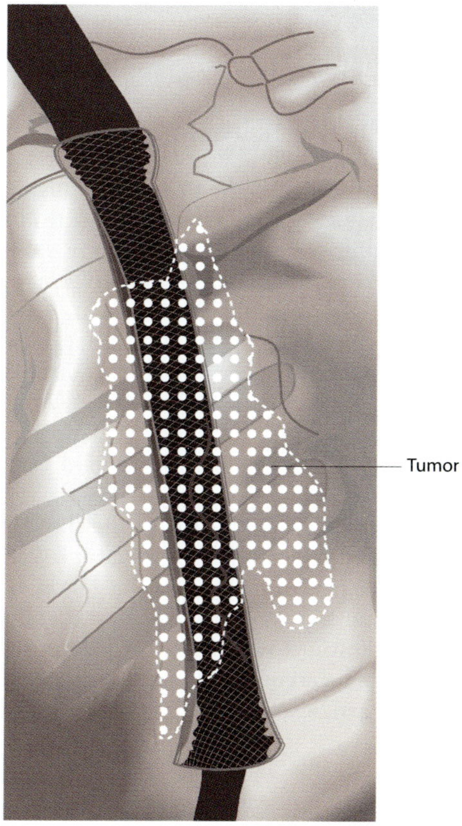


Contrast dye flowing unimpeded through the lumen of the stent

Figure 2G

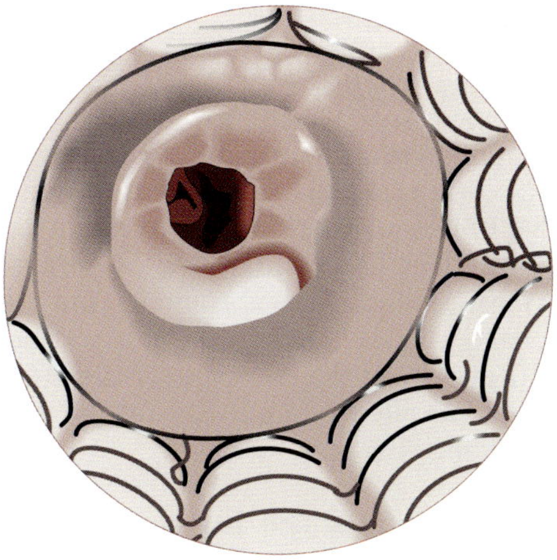

Endoscopic view through the stent on to healthy esophageal tissue

## Figure 3A, B: Ligature of Varices

■ **Indications.** All varices which are associated with current or former bleeding events should be treated. Apart from this, prophylactic treatment of varices is indicated in those case of varices at risk of bleeding, for example if full varices show "cherry red spots" or the patient has Child C liver cirrhosis (Fig. 3A).

■ **Special Conditions and Instruments.** Requirements are a gastroscope, a variceal ligature set (this is in general an industry provided set which contains a suction cap with multiple rubber rings), and instruments for blood-staunching (sclerosing needles, ethoxysclerol 5%, Histoacryl).

■ **Technique.** A quick orientation endoscopy of the oesophagus, stomach and duodenum is required to exclude further sources of bleeding, e.g. hypertensive gastropathy, or relevant fundus varices. After connecting the ligature set to the tip of the endoscope, one should proceed to the gastro-oesophageal junction. From this point one proceeds from distal to proximal. The variceal cord moves into the cap by suction and a rubber ring is applied to the base of the varix (Fig. 3B).

■ **Pitfalls.** Bleeding during the treatment session is a rare event but should be taken into account, and one should be able to treat bleeding at any time. Any coagulation defect must be corrected and one should utilise large-diameter venous lines and have blood transfusion and vasoactive substances at one's disposal. The endoscopist should be familiar with the technique of emergency variceal sclerosis with ethoxysclerol. In the case of bleeding, once a varix is sucked into the cap, one should always complete the suction procedure and fire the rubber ring. This procedure should never be interrupted because the treatment of ruptured varices is always more difficult.

### Figure 3A, B

Ligation of esophageal varices

## Figure 4A–F: Percutaneous Endoscopic Gastrostomy or Jejunostomy

■ **Indications.** The indication for placement of a percutaneous endoscopic gastrostomy or jejunostomy (PEG/PEJ) is malnutrition due to eating or swallowing disorders. This disorder can be for anatomical reasons, e.g. oesophageal tumours, but also for functional or central nervous reasons, e.g. stroke. Before PEG placement the rationale for the procedure should be critically reviewed with special regard to the underlying disease.

■ **Special Conditions and Instruments.** Requirements are a gastroscope, possibly a small paediatric gastroscope or bronchoscope in cases of stenosis in the upper gastrointestinal tract, disinfectants, sterile covering sheets, sterile gowns, face masks and sterile gloves for the assistant, a single-shot antibiotic with broad spectrum cephalosporin, loop or grasping forceps, and a PEG set containing all the necessary instruments such as syringes, scalpels, and sutures.

■ **Technique.** Pull through procedure: An orientating endoscopy is performed to exclude relevant unexpected pathological findings in the upper gastrointestinal tract. The next steps are illumination of the distal gastric corpus and the antrum on the anterior wall and observation from the outside for transillumination in order to identify a suitable position for the PEG. At the site of the brightest transillumination, local anaesthetic is injected with a thin needle and an exploratory puncture into the stomach can be made. Then a small incision is performed and the cannula is inserted into the stomach, which is used to insert a thread. The cannula is grasped by the endoscopist endoluminally with some forceps or preferably by a loop to avoid its dislocation with consequent pneumoperitoneum. After grasping the thread with the loop the thread is pulled through perorally.

The PEG cannula is connected to the thread and pulled through into the stomach and out through the abdominal wall, just until the internal plate of the cannula fixes the stomach with sufficient pressure to the internal abdominal wall. In this position the external fixation plate is connected to the probe and the closing system can be applied (Fig.4A).

### Figure 4A

Pull through technique of PEG

Figure 3A

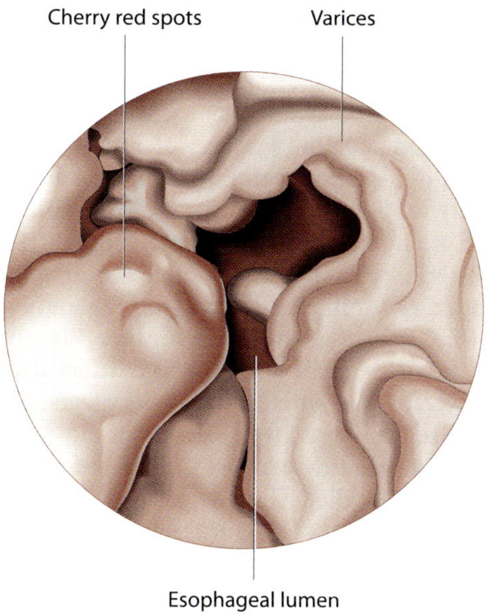


Figure 3B

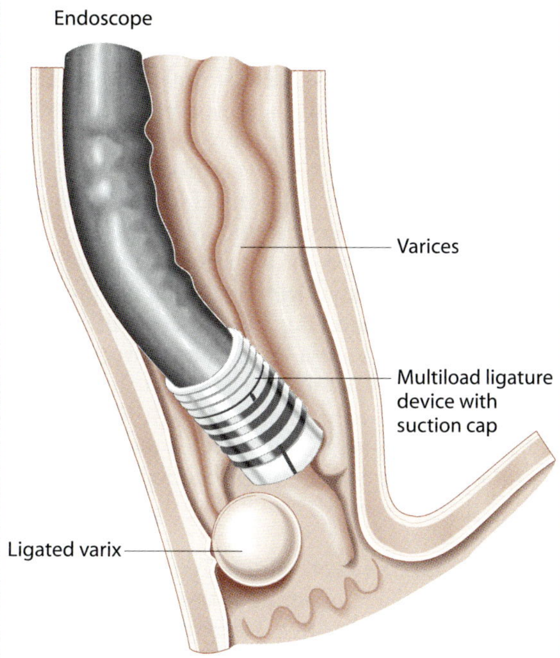


Figure 4A

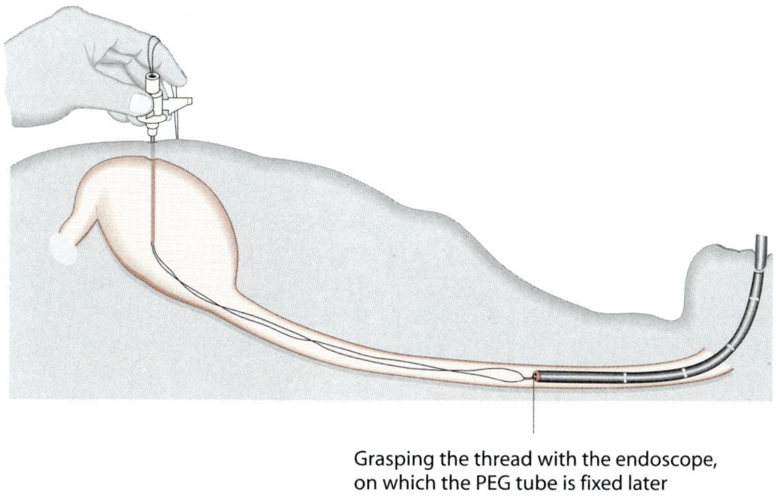

## Figure 4A–F: Percutaneous Endoscopic Gastrostomy or Jejunostomy

■ **Percutaneous Endoscopic Jejunostomy.** This consists of insertion of the jejunal nutrition cannula over the already existing gastric PEG. The proximal end of the jejunal cannula is grasped with endoscopic forceps, leaving the gastric probe in place. Under endoscopic and radiological control the tip of the jejunal probe is placed as far distal in the duodenum as possible or in the first jejunal loop.

In rare cases, such as a tumour-occupying the stomach or after gastric surgery, it may become necessary to avoid puncturing the stomach, but rather to puncture the duodenum or jejunum directly under transillumination control and to insert the PEJ cannula directly into the bowel. Although the risks are higher and the lumen is narrower, the technique used is similar to that for the implantation of a gastric PEG.

■ **Direct Puncture Proceedings.** In the case of direct puncture, the place of optimal transillumination is localized endoscopically similarly to the pull-through method. After local anaesthesia infiltration, a channel is dilated through which a balloon-tipped PEG cannual is advanced into the stomach. The balloon is secured by two previously placed sutures, which can be applied with endoscopic assistance using a specially prepared set (Fig. 4B–F).

■ **Pitfalls.** The most serious complication is a missed puncture and especially a puncture of interpositioned bowel, especially the colon. This complication can only be avoided by secure transillumination. Bleeding from the well-vascularised gastric wall at the site of puncture is not unusual but can be controlled by moderate tension on the PEG disk. In the early phase, infection of the puncture site is the most common problem. Bacteria usually originate from the upper gastrointestinal tract of the patient. To avoid this complication, we discontinue any proton pump inhibitors, since gastric acid is bactericidal. In addition a single shot of antibiotic is given immediately before the procedure. Patients should also practice adequate oral hygiene. A typical late complication is the so-called "buried bumper syndrome", caused by too high a pressure between the internal plate of the cannula and the gastric wall, which leads to necrosis and penetration of the plate through the mucosa and finally through the entire gastric wall. Therefore it is important to take care that a loose fit of the PEG plate is achieved, once the adherence between the stomach and the abdominal wall is stable, usually after 2 weeks.

### Figure 4B–F

Direct puncture of PEG

**Figure 4B–F**

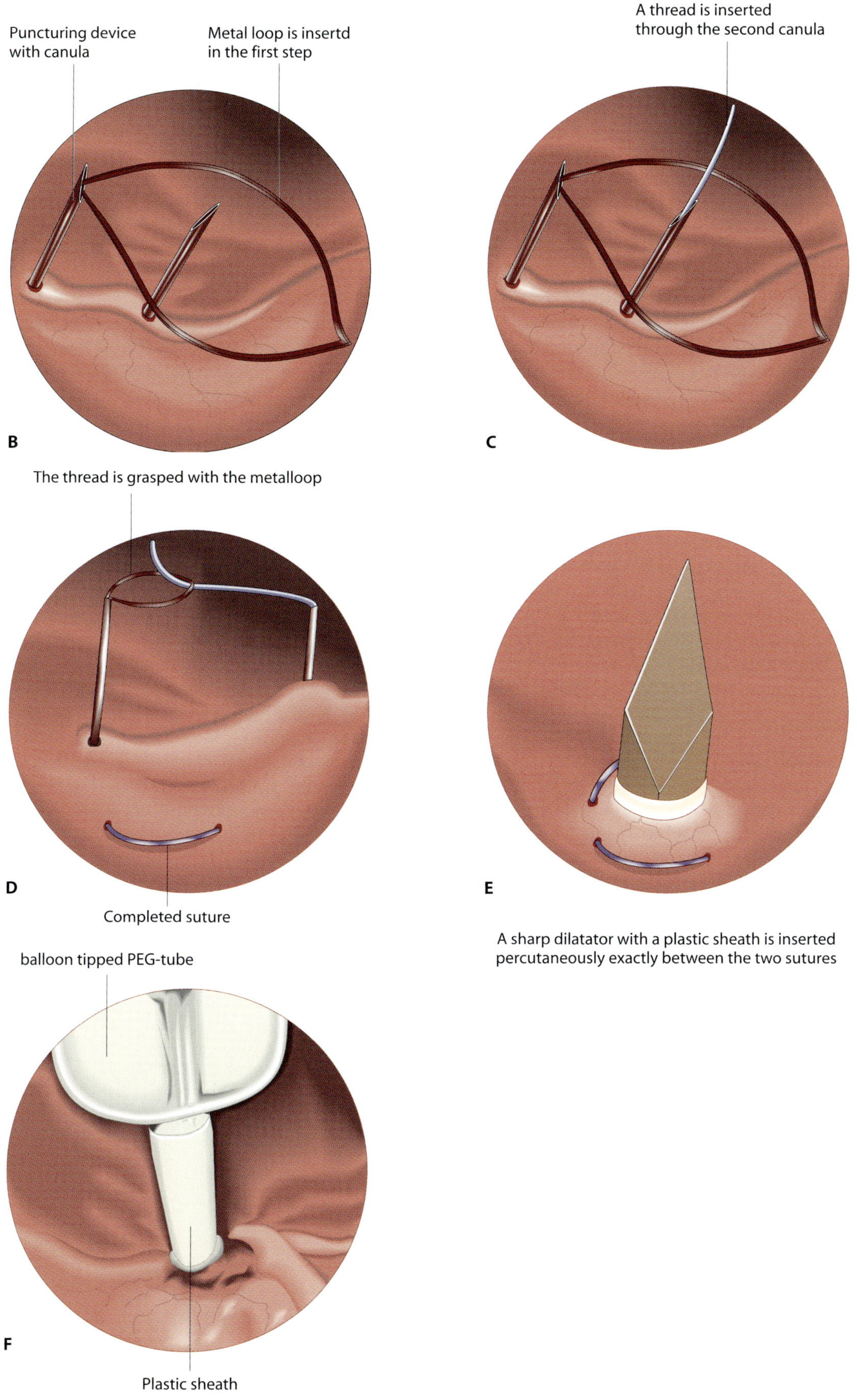
Puncturing device with canula
Metal loop is insertd in the first step
A thread is inserted through the second canula
B
C
The thread is grasped with the metalloop
D
Completed suture
E
A sharp dilatator with a plastic sheath is inserted percutaneously exactly between the two sutures
balloon tipped PEG-tube
F
Plastic sheath

## Figure 5A, B: Tumour Excision

■ **Indications.** Because of the possibility of malignant transformation there is nearly always an indication to remove all epithelial lesions/neoplasms from the upper gastrointestinal tract. The precondition for a local endoscopic procedure is an exact knowledge of the size and site of the lesion. Furthermore the type of growth, e.g. polyp, superficial, submucosal spreading, or infiltrating lesions must be assessed as well as the exact localisation. If possible, the endosonographic T and N stage should be recorded. This is crucial because although all benign neoplasms can potentially be removed endoscopically, only stage T1 malignant mucosal lesions may be removed in this manner. It is also important that such malignant lesions are well or moderately well differentiated and no lymph node metastases or lymphangitis carcinomatosa is apparent.

■ **Special Conditions and Instruments.** A therapeutic endoscope, preferably one with two working channels, is required. The instrument requirements depend on the technique of tumour removal. Different types of loops, caps, suction caps with rubber rings, and a sclerosing needle with a 1:100,000 adrenaline solution for injection of sessile polyps are required. In addition, instruments for controlling any bleeding should be available (1:10,000 adrenaline solution, fibrin glue, a double lumen needle and metal clips).

■ **Technique.** *Polypectomy:* In the case of pedunculated polyps a simple diathermy snare is sufficient in most cases. However, for better exposure of the polyp, prophylactic bleeding control, and to avoid damaging the organ wall, a submucosal injection of diluted adrenaline/saline solution is helpful. For polypectomy a mix of cutting and coagulation current is applied to the snare (e.g. Endocut function).

*EMR (endoscopic mucosa resection):* This is a technique especially developed for endoscopic removal of broad based sessile lesions. In these cases the lesion is elevated by a submucous injection with an adrenaline solution and is then drawn into a specially constructed suction cap mounted on the tip of the endoscope. This cap contains an electrical snare, which enables endoscopic removal of the tissue. Alternatively, the tumour can be drawn into the suction cap and then ligated by a rubber ring. The removal is then performed in a similar manner to pedunculated polyps. Other techniques utilise a double lumen endoscope, which allows the tumour to be lifted with some grasping forceps inserted down one channel and removed by snare excision using the second channel. However, the technically easiest method is the submucosal injection of the tumour and removal with a snare, e.g. a feather snare (Fig. 5A and B).

*Papillectomy:* The endoscopic excision of a lesion of the papilla of Vater is a very specialised form of tumour excision. The removal is analogous to an EMR utilising a submucosal injection of the papillary lesion followed by removal by snare excision. To avoid postinterventional pancreatitis, many endoscopists recommend short term use of a stent in the pancreatic duct.

■ **Pitfalls.** The risk of bleeding is significant in this procedure. Therefore one should keep instruments for bleeding control readily at hand at all times during the procedure (sclerosing needle with adrenaline solution, double lumen needle with fibrin glue, clip applicator, etc.). The most important precautionary measure for avoiding perforation is to adhere to clear guidelines and protocols with regard to the indications for the endoscopic procedure. Sessile tumours should be significantly elevated by submucosal injection before the tumour is removed by snare excision.

### Figure 5A and B

EMR with a suction cap

**Figure 5A, B**

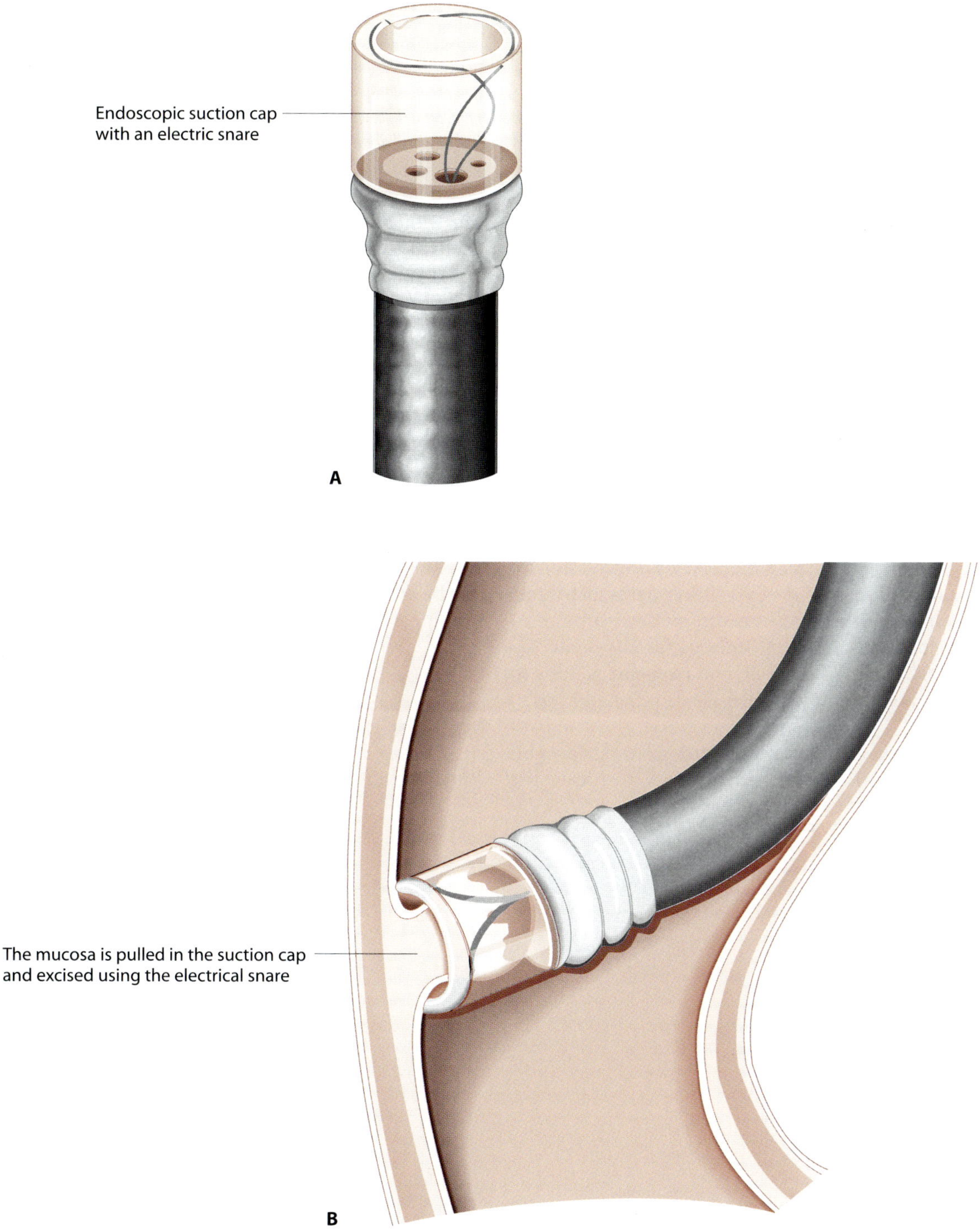
Endoscopic suction cap
with an electric snare
A
The mucosa is pulled in the suction cap
and excised using the electrical snare
B

## Figure 6A–D: Puncture and Drainage of Pancreatic Pseudocysts

■ **Indications.** The main indication to puncture a pancreatic pseudocyst is for a large symptomatic pseudocyst, which is causing pain and/or compression syndromes of the stomach or biliary and pancreatic ducts. In contrast to a simple peripancreatic fluid collection, the cyst should have a visible wall and be immediately adjacent to the stomach or duodenum. A fistula between the cyst and the pancreatic duct should be excluded by endoscopic retrograde pancreaticography (ERP) before the intervention. In the case of a proven fistula, the drainage of the pseudocyst should be undertaken via a transpapillary approach, or drainage should be improved by the use of a stent in the pancreatic duct.

■ **Special Conditions and Instruments.** A therapeutic duodenoscope or gastroscope is required. Also necessary is a longitudinal ultrasound scanner with Doppler function to locate the best puncture site and to exclude the presence of intramural vessels in the line of puncture. An X-ray unit is also needed to confirm correct puncture of the cyst by installation of contrast medium into the cyst. Other necessary items are an appropriate hollow needle, guidewire, papillotome or balloon catheter to enlarge the cystoenterostomy, double pigtail catheter, and nasogastric tube to initiate lavage therapy in the case of infected cysts.

■ **Technique.** Initially a standard gastroscopy and duodenoscopy is performed in order to locate the site of maximal gastric or duodenal impression by the pseudocyst. Ideally this region is examined by linear scanner in order to verify the direct contact of the cyst to the organ wall and to exclude intramural vessels. Thereafter the cyst is punctured using the hollow needle and the guidewire can be pushed forward through the needle into the cyst. Confirmation of its intracystic position is established by installation of contrast medium. After that the puncture channel is dilated by a guidewire papillotome or by an OTW (over the wire) balloon catheter. The double pigtail catheter is then inserted into the pseudocyst.

■ **Pitfalls.** Pseudocyst infection due to insufficient drainage of the secretion and bacterial colonisation after endoluminal puncture is a frequent problem. This is avoided by the use of sufficiently wide catheters. The pigtail catheters should be changed regularly in case they become obstructed. In the case of established infection of the cyst or when the secretion is very glutinous, one should carry out additional irrigation therapy using a nasocystic tube. Bleeding can be avoided in most cases by prior Doppler sonographic examination of the gastric wall (Fig. 6A–D).

### Figure 6A–D

Puncture and drainage of a pancreatic pseudocyst

**Figure 6A**

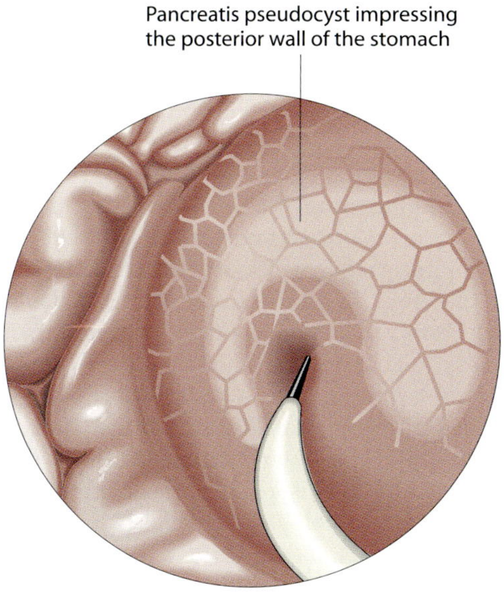


The wall of the pancreatis pseudocyst
is punctured using the needle knife

**Figure 6B**

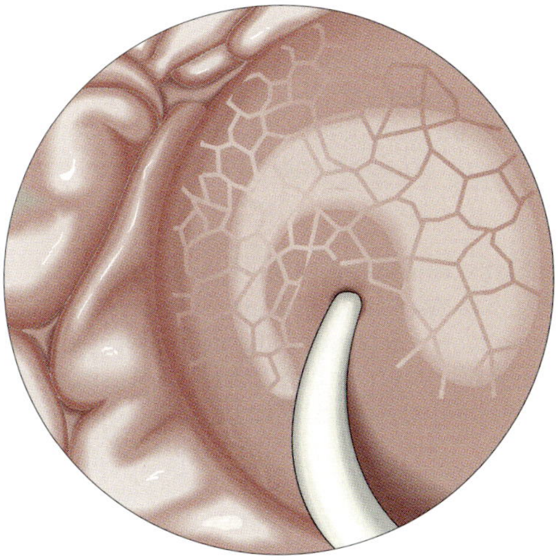

A guide wire is inserted into the pseudocyst through a catheter

**Figure 6C**

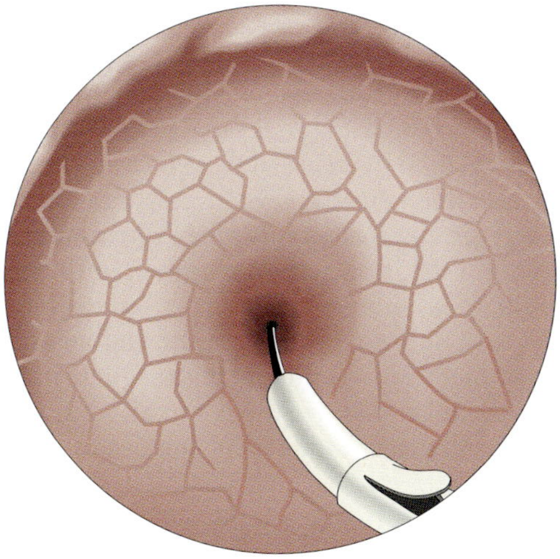

A pigtail prothesis is pushed over the guide wire

**Figure 6D**

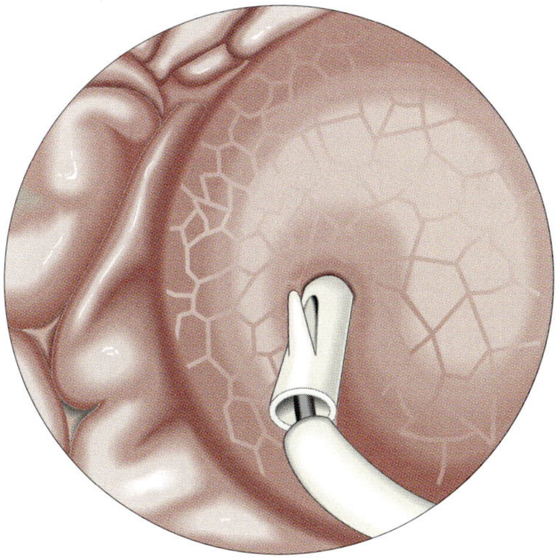

A pigtail prothesis disposes flaps to avoid
migration of the plastic stent

## Figure 7A–C: Tumour Recanalisation

**Indications.** Malignant obstructions of the lower gastrointestinal tract should be treated in the first instance by surgical resection, even when there is a palliative intention. Only in the case of very advanced tumours with extensive metastatic spread, when the patient's general condition is very poor, or in the rare cases of technically irresectable tumours of the rectum is there an indication for an endoscopic approach.

**Special Conditions and Instruments.** A laser (mostly Nd-YAG laser), argon plasma-coagulation equipment, stents, therapeutic colonoscope with a (-heat resistant) ceramic cap, a variety of wires and dilatation balloons, and an X-ray unit are required.

**Technique.**

A. Laser vaporisation: Laser therapy leads to the best possible elimination of endoluminal elements of a tumour by vaporisation of tumour tissue. Due to the high energy density there is always a significant risk of iatrogenic complications. Therefore the application of lasers must always be performed under direct visual control. Preferably the tumour is first passed endoscopically, possibly after gentle dilatation, and then the endoluminal parts of the tumour are treated symmetrically on retreat.

B. Argon plasma coagulation (APC): Argon plasma coagulation merely leads to carbonisation of the tissue, but the technique possesses a definite depth of penetration and is therefore easier to control. Because of this, argon plasma coagulation can be applied with a lower risk of complications. Other advantages are the lack of laser regulations, relatively inexpensive and transportable equipment, and the possibility of lateral treatment, since argon gas not only flows forward, but also sideways. The more shallow depth of penetration of APC necessitates repeated treatment in certain cases before final recanalisation is achieved. A further disadvantage is a delayed effect of recanalisation, since the necrotic tissue must separate from the tumour first. Also repeated treatment is often necessary in the case of further tumour growth while other side effects of tumour growth such as pain and development of a fistula are also not affected by APC. Finally, repeated hospitalisation of the patient in their final days is frequently required when choosing APC therapy (Fig. 7A).

C. Stent implantation: Based on long-term experience with endoprostheses in the vascular system and upper gastrointestinal tract, nowadays stents for the lower gastrointestinal tract are also available. However, technical and clinical success is not as easy to achieve as in the upper gastrointestinal tract. Reasons for this phenomenon are the increased motility and elasticity of the colon, leading to a higher vulnerability and higher rates of dislocation. The insertion is performed in most cases under radiological control using an endoscopically inserted guidewire. If the stenosis is not passable with the endoscope initially, either a balloon dilatation is performed or the passage to the proximal side of the stenosis may be explored using a flexible guide wire in a contrast medium catheter under X-ray control. Thereafter, following radiological confirmation of a satisfactory endoluminal position, one can exchange the flexible wire for a stiff guidewire, over which the stent is finally inserted. For better fixation of the stent, most models are not covered, but this can lead to later tumour ingrowth into the stent and to failure (Fig. 7B and C).

**Pitfalls.** The most frequent complication of endoscopic tumour destruction is bowel perforation. This can be prevented by gentle and well controlled techniques, possibly during several sessions. Increased caution is required especially when the tumour is located within the intraperitoneal colon. In the case of stent implantation a degree of experience is required to ensure an optimal position of the endoprosthesis. In this connection, not only is the adequate bridging of the tumour stenosis required, but also optimal adaptation of the stent to the local anatomical configuration.

**Figure 7A**

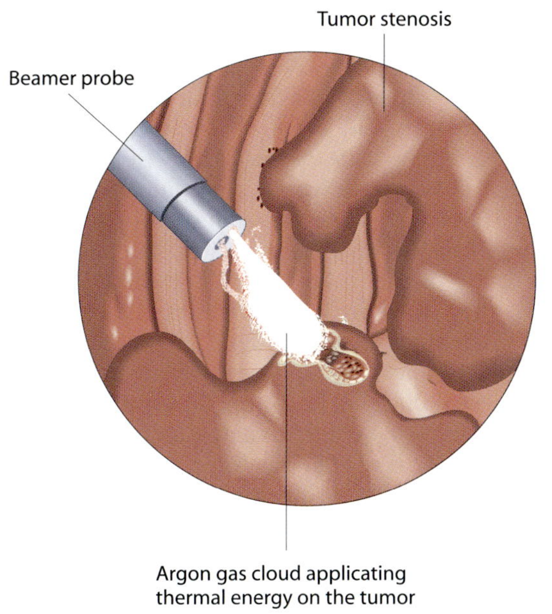


**Figure 7B**

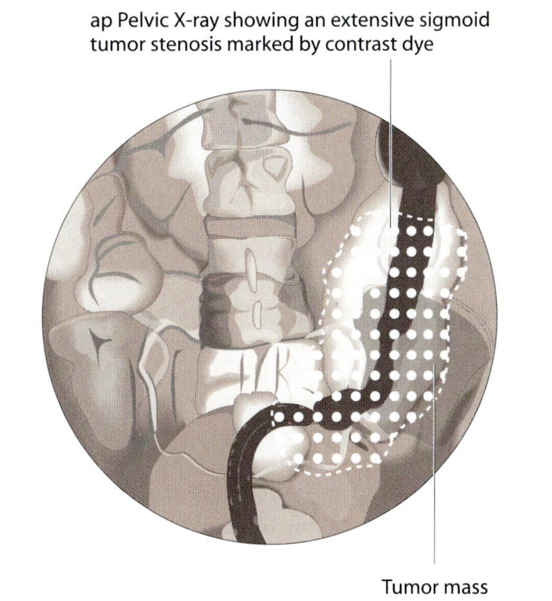


**Figure 7C**

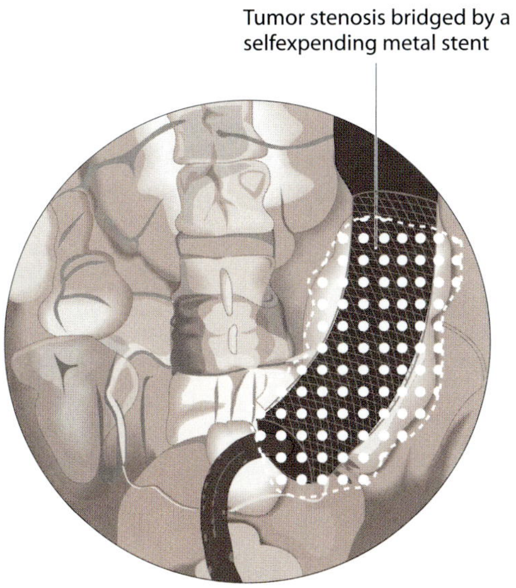

## ERCP

### Figure 8A, B: Stone Extraction

■ **Indications.** One should differentiate between stone extraction from the bile duct and that from the pancreatic duct. Bile duct stones are certainly more frequent. The indication for stone extraction depends simply on the detection of concrements (stones) in the bile duct as there is a high risk of possible complications, independent to the presence or absence of symptoms. In general a joint therapeutic approach is utilised in the case of simultaneous choledocholithiasis and cholecystolithiasis. This concept consists of endoscopic extraction of bile duct stones, followed by laparoscopic cholecystectomy. In cases of very large stones, a large number of concrements, or when stones are located intrahepatically and further pathologies such as stenoses and strictures are present, the chances of success and the expenditure of various lithotripsy techniques must be compared to open cholecystectomy with operative exploration of the bile duct.

The indication for extraction of stones from the pancreatic duct depends on symptoms such as pain and chronic pancreatitis.

■ **Special Conditions and Instruments.** Requirements include a sideviewing endoscope, contrast medium catheters, a variety of guidewires, papillotomes, precut papillotomes, needle knife papillotomes, Dormia baskets, balloon catheters, and a mechanical lithotripsy set.

■ **Technique.** The papilla of Vater is identified using the sideviewing endoscope. An oedematous papilla without any signs of bile flow indicates an impacted intrapapillary stone. Usually the bile duct is entered using an appropriate cannula followed by cautious instillation of diluted contrast medium. In the presence of bile duct stones, a papillotomy is performed using a guidewire papillotome, and a left laterocranial cutting direction (11 o'clock) should be chosen. The extent of the incision should be adjusted to the size of the stone, but only after careful consideration of the anatomical limitations, which are usually indicated by the diagonal fold immediately above the papilla. In cases where an initial cannulation with a flexible ERCP wire is not possible, e.g. due to an impacted intrapapillary stone, a so-called precut is performed using a precut papillotome or a needle knife papillotome. Following this, attempted cannulation of the precut papilla is again undertaken using a flexible Terumo wire. Once the correct position in the bile duct is confirmed radiologically, the papillotomy can be completed with a guidewire papillotome. Any ductal stone can be caught using a Dormia basket or a balloon catheter and the stone extraction can be completed (Fig. 8A and B). In case of multiple stones, each should be extracted separately. When the size of the stone and the width of the opening after papillotomy do not correspond, a variety of lithotripsy techniques can be applied (see below).

After successful extraction of any stones, unhindered drainage of the contrast medium should be documented by repeated filling of the bile duct with contrast.

Figure 8A

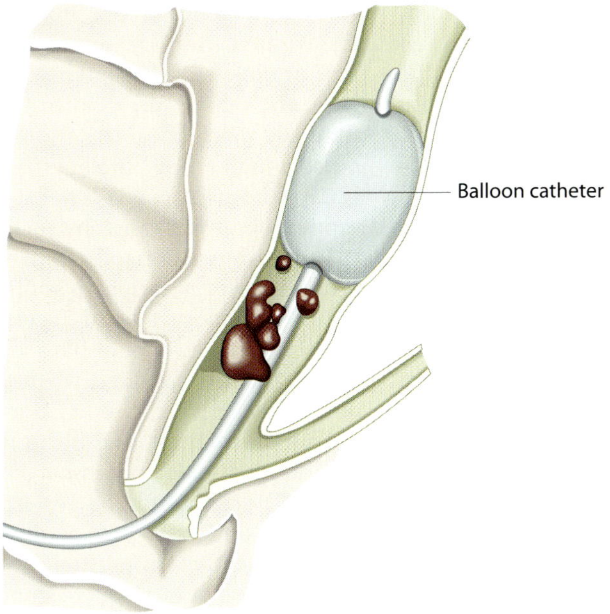


Figure 8B

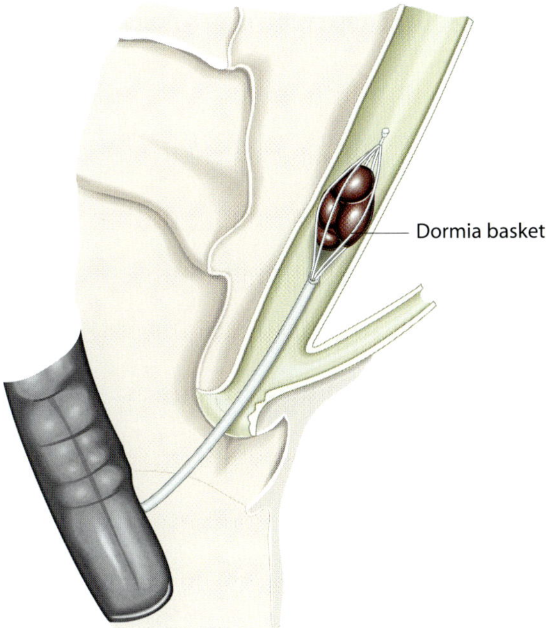

## Figure 8C, D: Stone Extraction

■ **Lithotripsy.** If stone extraction does not succeed, using the Dormia basket or the balloon catheter, then several methods of lithotripsy can be applied. In the case of mechanical lithotripsy, the outer plastic cover of the Dormia basket and the endoscope are removed and a firm metal coil is inserted over the in situ basket wire under radiological control just up to the stone. Once the Dormia basket has trapped the stone, the basket is then pulled strongly towards the metal coil using its central core shaft, until the concrement breaks into pieces. It is also possible to smash the stone using electrohydraulic waves or a laser beam under direct vision using a cholangioscope. Modern laser instruments possess a stone recognition system, which limits iatrogenic damage of the bile duct. Finally there is the possibility of extracorporal shock wave lithotripsy (ESWL). When using this method the stones are located either by sonography or by X-ray after instillation of contrast medium using a nasobiliary tube. High energy sound waves destroy the stones. The multiple small pieces of the stone are then removed using a conventional ERCP with a Dormia basket or balloon catheter (Fig. 8C and D).

■ **Pitfalls.** One should differentiate between complications of the ERCP, the papillotomy, and the stone extraction procedure itself. The most frequent complication after ERCP is iatrogenic acute pancreatitis, with an incidence of 5%. Prophylactic prevention of this complication by somatostatin, nitro preparations or diclofenac has not been successful in clinical trials, and only a very gentle method of cannulation can avoid mechanical irritation of the papilla. There is also a high risk of cholangitis as a consequence of ERCP if the endoscopist is not successful in complete removal of any existing obstruction to bile drainage.

The main risk of papillotomy is bleeding, followed by duodenal perforation. In addition, precut papillotomies predispose towards acute pancreatitis. As a consequence one should have all the equipment for bleeding control at hand when performing a papillotomy (sclerosing needle, double lumen needle, adrenaline solution, and fibrin glue). In the case of postinterventional abdominal pain or signs of infection, a CT scan should be performed immediately to recognize and treat any perforation, which occurs most frequently retroperitoneally.

In the case of incomplete stone extraction there is again a risk of cholangitis or acute pancreatitis due to impacted stone fragments. Furthermore there is always the possibility of a mismatch between the size of the stone and the orifice of the bile duct after papillotomy. Because of this there should always be a mechanical lithotripter available; however, in rare cases a stone caught in a Dormia basket can become impacted in the papilla and in these cases operative intervention can become necessary.

Figure 8C

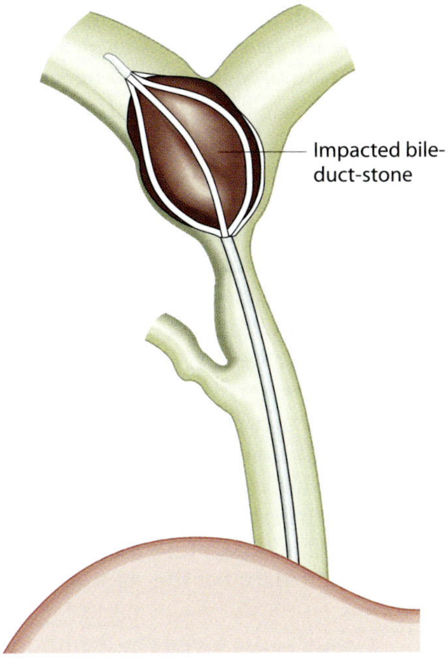


Figure 8D

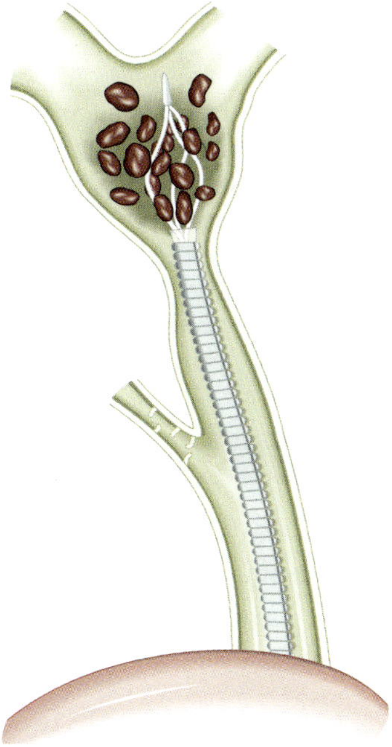

Stone fragmentation by pushing a metal tube against the stone in the dormia basket

## Figure 9: Stenoses

**Indications.** The indication to treat stenoses in the biliary or pancreatic duct depends on symptoms such as pain, jaundice, pancreatitis, or cholangitis. However, the optimal method of treatment will depend on the origin and nature of the stenosis, which should always be clarified before any intervention. When operative treatment of the stenosis is planned to be undertaken imminently, e.g. a Whipple resection in the case of a tumour of the pancreatic head, preoperative endoscopic drainage is only indicated in the case of complications, such as cholangitis.

**Special Conditions and Instruments.** A sideviewing therapeutic endoscope, contrast medium catheters, a variety of ERCP wires, precut and guidewire papillotomes, dilatation balloons, bougies, plastic endoprostheses with corresponding guidewires and pushers, and covered and non-covered metallic stents are the necessary items.

**Technique.** An initial endoscopy with the sideviewing endoscope is required, especially looking at the duodenum, to exclude duodenal infiltration of malignant tumours and to inspect the papilla and exclude neoplastic changes. Thereafter the bile duct is examined, in which excessive use of contrast medium should be avoided because of the risk of cholangitis. After this, passage of the stenosis using an ERCP wire is performed. This can be technically very demanding depending on the type, length, and size of stenosis. If the passage of the stenosis is not possible, one should change to a percutaneous transhepatic procedure or use a combination of such an approach with ERCP (rendezvous procedures). However, if one succeeds in crossing the stenosis with a guidewire, this wire is used to perform a sphincterotomy and eventually for bougienage or balloon dilatation of the stenosis. Finally a plastic endoprosthesis is inserted. The length of the endoprosthesis is related to the length of the stenosis and the distance from the papilla. The prosthesis should protrude beyond the papilla only for a short distance, whereas it should extend well beyond the proximal border of the stenosis. The treatment of biliary stenoses which involve both hepatic ducts can be extremely demanding and difficult, and in those cases where there is a lack of duct communication, a so-called double stenting procedure becomes necessary (Fig. 9).

Because of their relatively high cost, metal stents have not played a central role in the endoscopic insertion of prostheses into the biliary system to date. Furthermore they are contraindicated in the case of benign post-inflammatory or postoperative stenosis since they cannot be extracted endoscopically. However, in the case of locally inoperable tumours in the absence of metastases, the implantation of metal stents can be cost effective due to their longer patency. The insertion of metal stents is undertaken in a similar manner to that of plastic stents. When using covered stents, it is important not to allow the stent to cause an obstruction of uninvolved biliary ducts. Furthermore, the tendency for a stent to shrink should be taken into consideration to ensure a complete bridging of the stenosis.

**Pancreatic Stenoses.** Symptomatic pancreatic stenoses, especially those due to chronic pancreatitis, can also be treated effectively by means of insertion of a pancreatic endoprostheses. The only problem in many cases is the very high resistance of the pancreatic tissue when chronic calcifying pancreatitis is present. Technically the procedure is similar to the bile duct endoprostheses insertion as described above.

**Pitfalls.** A wrong choice of endoprostheses can lead to complications such as cholangitis due to inadequate drainage. In later stages occlusion can occur when using relatively narrow plastic endoprostheses. Therefore large calibre endoprosthesis (more than 10F in the bile duct) should be inserted and the patient should be followed closely. In the absence of cholangitis, exchange of endoprostheses can be performed on an outpatient basis in most cases.

### Figure 9

Bridging a hilar biliary tumor with two endprostheses (Klatskin tumor)

Figure 9

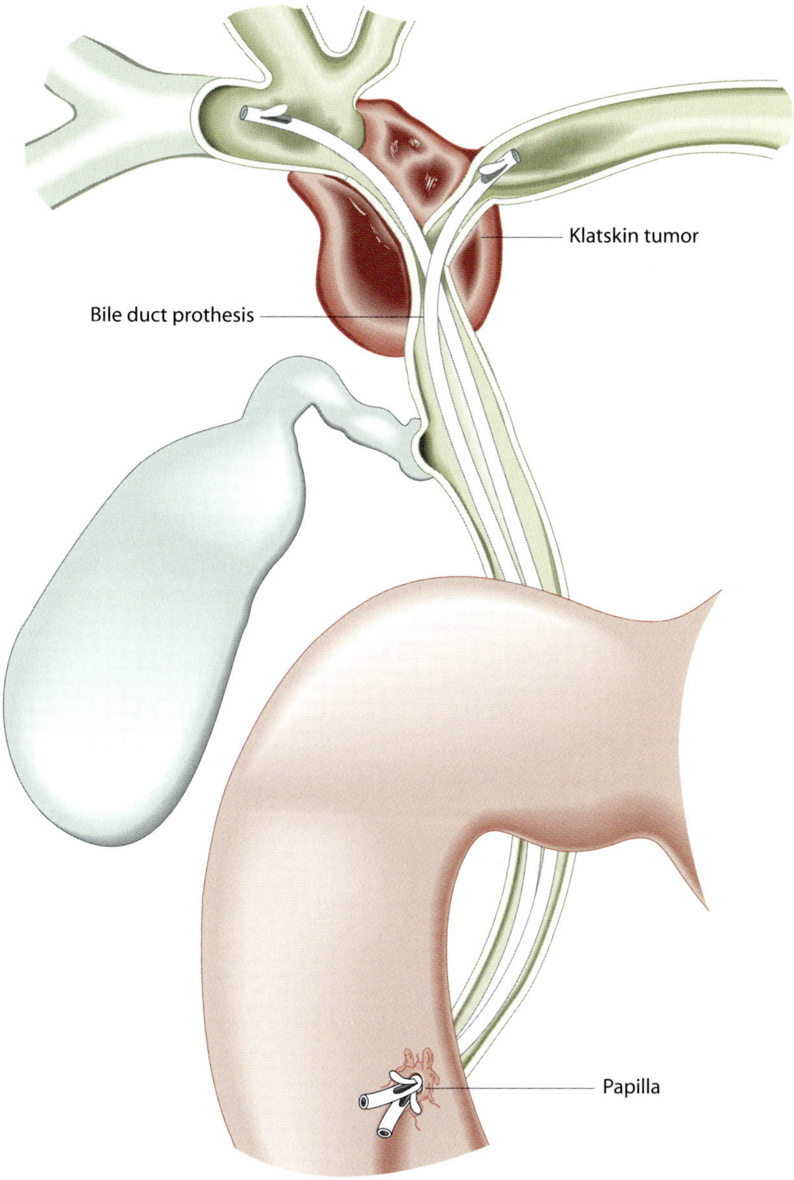

## SELECTED REFERENCES

Binmoeller KF, Schafer TW (2001) Endoscopic management of bile duct stones. J Clin Gastroenterol 32:106–118

Colombo-Benkmann M, Unruh V, Kocher T, Krieglstein C, Senninger N (2003) Modern treatment options for Zenker's diverticulum: indications and results. Zentralbl Chir 128:171–186

Dormann AJ, Huchzermeyer H (2002) Endoscopic techniques for enteral nutrition: standards and innovations. Dig Dis 20:145–153

Ferguson JW, Tripathi D, Hayes PC (2003) Review article: the management of acute variceal bleeding. Aliment Pharmacol Ther 18:253–262

Fogel EL, Sherman S, Park SH, McHenry L, Lehman GA (2003) Therapeutic biliary endoscopy. Endoscopy 35:156–163

Hartmann D, Jakobs R, Schilling D, Riemann JF (2003) Endoscopic and radiological interventional therapy of benign and malignant bile duct stenoses. Zentralbl Chir 128:936–943

Inoue H, Fukami N, Yoshida T, Kudo SE (2002) Endoscopic mucosal resection for esophageal and gastric cancers. J Gastroenterol Hepatol 17:382–388

Khulusi S, Morris T (2000) Endoscopic palliation of gastrointestinal malignancy. Eur J Gastroenterol Hepatol 12:397–402

Lerut T, Coosemans W, Decker G, De Leyn P, Nafteux P, van Raemdonck D (2002) Anastomotic complications after esophagectomy. Dig Surg 19:92–98

Lew RJ, Kochman ML (2002) A review of endoscopic methods of esophageal dilation. J Clin Gastroenterol 35:117–126

Luketic VA, Sanyal AJ (2000) Esophageal varices. I. Clinical presentation, medical therapy, and endoscopic therapy. Gastroenterol Clin North Am 29:337–385

Mergener K, Kozarek RA (2002) Stenting of the gastrointestinal tract. Dig Dis 20:173–181

Mulder CJ, Costamagna G, Sakai P (2001) Zenker's diverticulum: treatment using a flexible endoscope. Endoscopy 33:991–997

Ortner MA, Dorta G, Blum AL, Michetti P (2002) Endoscopic interventions for preneoplastic and neoplastic lesions: mucosectomy, argon plasma coagulation, and photodynamic therapy. Dig Dis 20:167–172

Siersema PD, Marcon N, Vakil N (2003) Metal stents for tumours of the distal esophagus and gastric cardia. Endoscopy 35:79–85

Vidyarthi G, Steinberg SE (2001) Endoscopic management of pancreatic pseudocysts. Surg Clin North Am 81:405–410

Vitale GC, Zavaleta CM (2003) Endoscopic retrograde cholangiopancreatography for surgeons. Semin Laparosc Surg 10:19–27